THE
AUGUSTAN
WORLD

harper ✤ torchbooks

EDITORS' NOTE: *A check-list of Harper Torchbooks, classified by subjects, is printed at the end of this volume.*

THE AUGUSTAN WORLD

Society, Thought, and
Letters in Eighteenth-Century England

By A. R. HUMPHREYS

> 'The Spirit of the Time' does not exist independently of the activities which manifest it. —
> GEOFFREY SCOTT, *The Architecture of Humanism*

HARPER TORCHBOOKS ♦ The Academy Library
HARPER & ROW, PUBLISHERS, NEW YORK AND EVANSTON

THE AUGUSTAN WORLD

Printed in the United States of America

This book was originally published in 1954 by Methuen & Co., Ltd., London, and is here reprinted by arrangement.

First HARPER TORCHBOOK edition published 1963 by
Harper & Row, Publishers, Incorporated,
New York and Evanston.

To
MY DEAR WIFE
IN ALL AFFECTION AND GRATITUDE

PREFACE

In the world of scholarship the eighteenth century has received abundant honour, but in that of the general reader a good many misconceptions still seem to survive. This book arose from my desire to explore outwards from literature into society and then return from society to literature again. Its intention was as much critical as social-historical, and if the critical aim is imperfectly realised that is my own shortcoming: to examine six major topics and still preserve a sense of critical relevance proved anything but easy, and success may well have eluded me. My hope at least is that Augustan literature may be more understandingly and percipiently read by those who sense how the writer might feel in his world.

Each chapter may be taken by itself yet has also its place in a pattern. Social life leads to the economic activities which supported it, and those to politics into which social life and economics so readily ran. Religion follows on the politics to which it was closely related, and is followed by philosophy to complete the framework of moral thought. Lastly the visual arts are included to reflect the taste of the age. Certain other subjects, such as education and linguistic conditions, had perforce to be left out, since they could have been accommodated only by considerable enlargement of the book or by serious abbreviation of the restricted space allowed to what is already here. In each chapter the last section tries more specifically than the others to show how literature was influenced. A certain amount of repetition proved unavoidable; the subjects of more than one chapter may affect literature similarly, and some writers are equally relevant to more than one subject. I hope, however, that passages which have echoes in the book may still be found essential to their own contexts.

Many colleagues at the University College of Leicester have given generously of their time and scholarship to help me in fields where they are much more at home than I: I thank the Principal, Mr C. H. Wilson, the former Principal Mr F. L. Attenborough, Dr A. S. Collins, Mr H. P. R. Finberg, Mr M. Hookham, Mr C. J. Horne, Dr W. G. Hoskins (now of Oxford University), Professor H. P. Moon, Mr J. C. Rees, Professor Jack Simmons and Professor T. G. Tutin for discussing larger or smaller parts of the book, while Miss Rhoda Bennett the librarian and her staff have been assiduous in the procuring of material. Further afield it is a pleasure to acknowledge my debts to the Reverend James Currie of Renton, Professor W. D. Niven of Glasgow University and the Reverend C. W. Dugmore of Manchester University for advice on chapter iv, on the subject of which I felt particularly vulnerable, and to Professor Basil Willey for critical comment on chapter v. Mr Wilson Steel and the staff at Glasgow University Library afforded me willing attention at a time inconvenient for themselves, and the editors of *The Cambridge Journal*, *The Modern Language Review*, *The Review of English Studies* and *The Journal of Ecclesiastical History* have allowed me to use some material first published in their pages. My thanks for permission to quote from Professor G. M. Trevelyan's *English Social History* are tendered to Messrs. Constable & Co., Ltd., and from Geoffrey Scott's *Architecture of Humanism* to Messrs. Longmans Green & Co., Ltd., and Charles Scribner's Sons, Ltd. Above all it is to my father, whose scrupulous detective power brought to light in an earlier draft scores of obscurities and errors, that my gratitude is due and acknowledged. For all the faults remaining I of course am responsible: I can only trust that they may not seriously distort this portrait of an age.

> *This let me hope, that when in public view*
> *I bring my pictures, men may deem them true.*

My wife, finally, has surrendered some thousands of hours of my company to the exigences of scholarship, and hers is the in-every-respect-deserved recompense of the dedication.

CONTENTS

		PAGE
I.	SOCIAL LIFE	
	i. The Spirit of Society	1
	ii. London	5
	iii. The Country	22
	iv. Society and Literature	41
II.	THE WORLD OF BUSINESS	
	i. National Expansion and National Pride	52
	ii. Change in the Country	59
	iii. Aspects of Industry	66
	iv. Communications	74
	v. Wider Horizons	77
	vi. The National Spirit	82
	vii. Business and Literature	90
III.	PUBLIC AFFAIRS	
	i. The Political Settlement and Locke	98
	ii. Political Parties	103
	iii. Men of Letters and some Major Events	109
	iv. Parliament	123
	v. Politics and Literature	127
IV.	RELIGIOUS LIFE	
	i. An Active Interest	138
	ii. Modes of Faith	142
	iii. Attack and Defence	149
	iv. 'An Inward Chearfulness'	163
	v. Religion and Literature	168
V.	PHILOSOPHY MORAL AND NATURAL	
	i. The New Temper	179
	ii. Locke and the Enlightenment	183

			PAGE
	iii.	Discourse of Reason	189
	iv.	Reason Deposed	194
	v.	The Culture of the Heart	197
	vi.	'The New Philosophy'	202
	vii.	Philosophy and Literature	210
VI.	THE VISUAL ARTS		
	i.	The Polite Imagination	217
	ii.	Order and Harmony	223
	iii.	The Main Stream	229
	iv.	Divergent Currents	240
	v.	The Arts and Literature	250
READING LISTS			261
INDEX			270

THE AUGUSTAN WORLD

I. SOCIAL LIFE

i. THE SPIRIT OF SOCIETY

In travelling thro' *England*, a Luxuriance of Objects presents itself to our View: Where-ever we come, and which way soever we look, we see something New, something Significant, something well worth the Traveller's Stay, and the Writer's Care.

DEFOE
A Tour Thro' the whole Island of Great Britain, preface

THE history of Augustan society has been written often and well, and this account, which is neither history nor sociology, does not attempt to rival the special knowledge of experts. Historians and sociologists have not neglected literature, yet there is still room for a sketch of social life specifically as it affected the writer, as it meant for him a world with certain social feelings and a certain range of material, in which on the whole he knew where he stood, and whose particular form and character, because of this knowledge, he could convey with peculiar clarity. This chapter will consider what kind of society surrounded the man of letters (the man of letters not as a special person but as a representative Englishman), and how it affected his writing.

The Augustan age is noted for its sense of man as a social being, divinely intended to collaborate in a great task. That task, which the age made particularly its own, was to live in widespread harmony, abjuring the hazards of war and fanaticism which had convulsed the seventeenth century. By instinct and intention men strove for a congenial society: they pondered on the principles of a civilised community and hoped to extend doctrines of 'sympathy', on both a Christian and a rational basis, as widely as possible. The social philosophy which is one of their main contributions to civil life is considered in the fifth chapter; here we may note in passing how prevalent were social aims in Locke, Shaftesbury, Addison,

Hutcheson, Hume and Adam Smith (to cite only the most prominent names), how confident the faith in which they were pursued, and how deep the satisfaction they afforded.

Practice, it is true, often halts behind precept. The tide of social sympathy which set through eighteenth-century thought did not imbue the whole nation with fraternity. There was much hardship and suffering, and much ignorant or selfish apathy about them, and if the clash of conflict was less violent than in the seventeenth or nineteenth centuries that is because the scheme of things was unrebelliously tolerated. Yet the age thought much about the ethical principles of society and did something to put its thought into practice. In 1791 a visiting German pastor, Friedrich August Wendeborn, published his *View of England*, and while he praised the intellectual theorising which had preceded the French Revolution on the continent he praised still more the practical energy which in England had progressed further towards social justice. The British combination of moral persuasion, practical energy and good fortune tended towards a social order of reasonable sense and human understanding, an order based on 'the grand principle of subordination', moderately conservative in class-feeling, but not so rigid that the energetic poor man might not rise far in almost any walk of life.

Its ideal was less equalitarian justice than social sympathy and religious duty, 'each man walking in Godly wise in his state of wealth or poverty', as William Law's *Serious Call to a Devout and Holy Life* (1728) puts it. This could dwindle into the idea that the poor should know their stations, and that privilege was divinely approved. Yet the belief that the social order was ordained of God was not hypocrisy; the eighteenth century inherited the age-old faith that God had appointed the structure of society and that, though the rich should ease the burdens of the poor, poverty itself, like pain and death, was part of the mystery of creation. This faith was convenient for the rich but not thereby hypocritical. It was certainly not designed to condemn the poor to perpetual subjection, for if God had ordained gradations of wealth he had ordained also the duty of labouring in one's vocation and of earning those rewards by which the industrious apprentice might finish as Lord Mayor of London.

To say that the Augustan age progressed in social sympathy, and that this progress encouraged the human interests of literature, is not to deny its limitations. Its social conscience was superficial; it put up with much injustice (partly from ignorance of how to remedy it), and it relieved only the barest fringe of misery. The crowds who sotted on gin (as Hogarth drew and Fielding described them) were not seeking merely the zest of a spree. The debtors who decayed in prison, the mobs who rioted when harvests failed, the wretches press-ganged to sea-life, which Johnson called a degree worse than gaol—these and their like could not congratulate themselves on their time. Poets, journalists and novelists drew grim pictures of suffering: Augustan excellences were erected on much misery and despair. Yet with all its evils the age strove to become less brutal, and gave to many the sense of strong humanity bearing good fruit in art, letters, philosophy and social life.

It presents the double face of stability and change. The stability is that of settled desires and tempered ambitions.

> *Grant me, You Gods! before I die*
> *An happy Mediocrity,*

wrote Henry Baker at the opening of his *Original Poems* (1725). The ideal is that of Pope's *Ode on Solitude* and Pomfret's *Choice*, both dated 1700 and thus well-timed evidence (though Cowley's essays had already voiced the same spirit). It is the mood of Horatian urbanity, meditative friendship and classical reading. *The Choice* is not merely an individual's whim; Johnson believed that nothing in English had been more read, and spoke of it as 'a system of life adapted to common notions, and equal to common expectations'. This 'system' includes a modest house, near town yet in the country, a garden, a cool stream, and a grove surveyed from a 'silent study' furnished with the classics and such moderns as are

> *Men of steady Sense,*
> *Esteem'd for Learning, and for Eloquence.*

A moderate estate supports it, providing hospitality to friends and charity to the poor, 'a little Vault' of wine to whet the wit, companions 'in Reas'ning Cool, Strong, Temperate and Just', an intelligent lady, 'Faithful to her Friend, and Good to all', and at last 'a silent and a peaceful Death'. Few 'common expectations' could really hope for such benefits, but Pomfret's alert and surprising poem, piquant, persuasive and conversational, expresses his century's dream. In similar vein Matthew Green wrote gay octosyllabics in *The Spleen* (1737) to 'Contentment, parent of Delight', and others as happy appeared anonymously in Dodsley's *Collection* (1755) entitled 'A Little Wish'. Like Pomfret and Green, the poet desires a small house, prospect, garden, grove, 'a little wine. For a guest that comes to dine', and an easy bucolic life. That settled comfort, that pleasure in meadows, books and people, is a staple of Augustan life, and men like Shenstone, Cowper and Gilbert White achieved it.

Yet equally staple is that other face, of change. Energy and enterprise, without engendering a revolution, gave life its breadth and force. Their achievements are postponed to the following chapter, yet any study of social life must recognise their existence. Moralists might deplore the 'luxury' which this enterprise was supposed to encourage, but their laments availed little against a chorus of joy. Every page of Defoe's *Tour Thro' Great Britain* (1724–7) shows how strong was the approval. In 1754 *The Gentleman's Magazine* (xxiv. 347) said that if those who toured England in the 1720s did so again 'they would find themselves in a land of enchantment', improved as much over that earlier time as over Borneo or Madagascar. In his *Journal* (31 March, 1781) John Wesley remarked, as did Josiah Wedgwood in 1783, on the remarkable advance of the Potteries since the 1750s. If one aspect of the century is stable, the other shows not only change but a vigorous philosophy of development. Only an age alive to social activity would have prompted that patriotic passage in James Thomson's *Summer* (1730: 653–67):

> *O Thou! by whose almighty* NOD *the scale*
> *Of empire rises, or alternate falls,*

> *Send forth the saving* VIRTUES *round the land,*
> *In bright patrol; white* PEACE, *and social* LOVE;
> *The tender-looking* CHARITY, *intent*
> *On gentle deeds, and shedding tears thro' smiles;*
> *Undaunted* TRUTH, *and* DIGNITY *of mind;*
> COURAGE *compos'd, and keen; sound* TEMPERANCE . . .
> *Rough* INDUSTRY; ACTIVITY *untir'd,*
> *With copious life inform'd, and all awake;*
> *While, in the radiant front, superior shines*
> *That first paternal Virtue,* PUBLIC ZEAL.

Only an age with a sense of the great nobleman's opportunities and a great poet to express that sense could have produced the conclusion of Pope's *Epistle to Burlington* (1731). In lines of complex opulence the Earl is encouraged to enrich the beauty and bounty of his estates, further the arts, and adorn 'happy Britain' with monuments and public works. The Elizabethan patriotic poets had sung of England's beauty, history and spirit, but the full praise of social life remained for the Augustans to express, in the private sphere of Pomfret and Green or the public of Defoe, Thomson and Pope.

The following pages treat London by itself, and then the rest of the country. This division reflects a real distinction, for though country towns had their local life London was always a special case: there one could be a complete citizen in the complex of metropolitan culture, and the countryman was, and felt, like a stranger in a strange land.

ii. LONDON

> All London increasing in architecture and inhabitants conveys no other idea but that of bustle and business.
>
> JOHN SHEBBEARE
> *Letters on the English Nation* (1756)

THE social phenomenon which aroused most interest was perhaps the growth and activity of the capital, the channel of that 'full tide of existence' which, said Johnson, flowed at Charing Cross.

'When we came upon Highgate Hill and had a view of London,' Boswell records, 'I was all life and joy' (*London Journal*, 19 November, 1762). Pastor Wendeborn's praise is that of an impartial visitor (*View of England*, 1791, i. 257):

> There is no place in the world, where a man may live more according to his own mind, or even his whim, than in London. For this reason, I believe that in no place are to be found a greater variety of original characters.... The friend of arts and science, the friend of religious liberty, the philosopher, the man who wishes to be secure against political and ecclesiastical tyrants, the man of business, the man of pleasure, can no where be better off than in this metropolis.

Such tributes prevail, on the whole, over objections to dirt, rowdyism and poverty, though by an odd chance Johnson, the capital's sturdiest admirer, gained his first fame with *London* (1738), modelled on Juvenal's diatribes against Rome, and asked (remarkable question from a Scot-baiter) whether anyone

> *would leave, unbrib'd,* Hibernia's *land,*
> *Or change the rocks of* Scotland *for the* Strand?

Johnson was either following Juvenal too closely or feeling the loneliness of a young provincial immigrant, or both. The general voice extolled London's merits. 'Happy *Augusta*!' sang Gay in *Trivia* (1716: iii. 145–50):

> *Happy* Augusta! *law-defended town!*
> *Here no dark lanthorns shade the villain's frown;*
> *No* Spanish *jealousies thy lanes infest,*
> *Nor* Roman *vengeance stabs th'unwary breast;*
> *Here tyranny ne'er lifts her purple hand,*
> *But liberty and justice guard the land.*

London had its perils, though not perhaps the more picturesque forms of Mediterranean ambush. Swift told Stella, on 8 March, 1712, about 'a race of Rakes calld the Mohacks that play the devil about this Town every Night', and Gay wrote *The Mohocks, a Tragi-Comical Farce* (1712) about them. *Trivia* describes the thugs infesting Lincoln's Inn, and Shenstone wrote to Richard Jago, on 30 May, 1744, of footpads bludgeoning their victims by day in Fleet Street and the Strand, and by night lurking in the Covent Garden piazzas to catch playgoers emerging from the theatres. There is rarely a week throughout the century when the journals fail to record at least one violent crime among the London news. But murders and riots were looked on as nuisances incidental to life in so stirring a city.

Most of all it was London's growth which attracted attention. Defoe, as usual, is to hand with evidence; he speaks of 'a particular and remarkable Crisis', namely the fact

> that the great and more eminent Increase of Buildings in, and about, the City of *London*, and the vast Extent of Ground taken in, and now become Streets, and Noble Squares of Houses, by which the Mass or Body of the whole is become so infinitely great, has been generally made in our Time, not only within our Memory, but even within a few Years.
>
> *Tour*, ed. G. D. H. Cole, i. 326

The capital had about 500,000 citizens in 1700, about 750,000 in 1750, and about 900,000 in 1800. This magnitude was the more remarkable in that its nearest competitors were so small—in 1700 Bristol and Norwich with about 30,000, in 1800 Manchester and Liverpool with about 80,000. Some concern darkened the general approval: London was called 'a great wen' long before Cobbett stamped his authority on the phrase. Defoe himself was perturbed; he admired bustle and success, but 'this great and monstrous thing' at times daunted him (*Tour*, i. 316):

> It is the Disaster of *London*, as to the Beauty of its Figure, that it is thus stretched out in Buildings, just at the Pleasure of every Builder, or Undertaker of Buildings, and as the Convenience of the People directs, whether for Trade or otherwise; and this has spread the Face of it in a most straggling, confus'd Manner, out of all Shape, uncompact and unequal, neither long or broad, round or square.

The complaint is still familiar and the process—the engulfing of neighbouring townships—familiar too. London had grown greatly since the Restoration and remorselessly encroached on its rural surroundings.

The nucleus was still the City itself within its gates and bars (removed in the 1760s), with perhaps 200,000 inhabitants. Eastwards spread the industrial area, a rapidly-extending proliferation of workshops, small houses and hovels, towards Shadwell and Limehouse, Whitechapel and Wapping, which Johnson advised Boswell to see as the centre of the seafaring world. Westwards advanced the march of civilisation with those squares—Bedford, Russell, Berkeley, Cavendish, Gordon, Hanover and the rest— whose names still sound with oligarchical distinction and whose dignity, wherever it precariously survives, is still a beacon of the civilised mind. From Greenwich to the West End the newly-fashionable Portland stone gave churches, public offices and private mansions their monumental character, varying the tide of red, yellow or grey brick. Here took place the crowded life of the streets, that world of Hogarthian comedy and tragedy, with its unruly populace, its sewage and offal in the roads, cobbles slippery with mud, iron-sheathed posts to guard jostling pedestrians from the wheels of carriages, shop-signs hiding the sky and creaking in the wind, and traitors' heads on Temple Bar. The London of Anne and George I is mirrored in Swift, Gay, the journalists, and Ned Ward, that garrulous, combative master of vernacular rhyming, whose *Hudibras Redivivus* (1705–7) is the essence of civic tumult:

> *Young Drunkards reeling, Bayliffs dogging,*
> *Old Strumpets plying, Mumpers progging,* [beggars scrounging]
> *Fat Dray-men squabling, Chair-men ambling,*
> *Oyster-Whores fighting, School-Boys scrambling,*
> *Street Porters running, Rascals batt'ling,*
> *Pick-pockets crowding, Coaches rattling,*
> *News bawling, Ballad-wenches singing,*
> *Guns roaring, and the Church-Bells ringing.*
>
> (Canto vii. 20–7)

Swift's pictures, in the *Journal to Stella*, the *Description of the*

Morning, and *A City Shower*, are as vigorous and comic; here he records the results of a downpour:

> *Now from all Parts the swelling Kennels flow,*
> *And bear their Trophies with them as they go;*
> *Filths of all Hues and Odours seem to tell*
> *What street they sail'd from, by their Sight and Smell . . .*
> *Sweepings from Butchers Stalls, Dung, Guts and Blood,*
> *Drown'd Puppies, stinking Sprats, all drench'd in Mud,*
> *Dead Cats and Turnip-tops, come tumbling down the Flood.*

(As late as 1782 C. P. Moritz, a visiting German, complained that 'guts and all the nastiness are thrown into the middle of the street, and cause an insupportable stench'.) Gay is as animated, though not so unsavoury. The third book of *Trivia* describes a traffic jam in the narrow part of the Strand by St. Clement Danes: colliers' carts from the Thames wharves (Seacoal Lane and Newcastle Street still survive near the Temple) block the road; the crowds gather; the long wagon-teams strain; harnesses snap; shafts break; bullocks for Smithfield bellow; drivers lash out, quarrel, and end fighting in the mud. Hogarth inevitably comes to mind. Through the reigns of George I and George II the same exuberant popular energy arises from Swift, Pope, Hogarth, Fielding and Smollett, from the ragged images of Grub-street poverty in *The Dunciad*, from the irresistible enthusiasm of Defoe's *Tour* and the realism of *Moll Flanders* and *Colonel Jack*, from the grim city scenery of Fielding's *Jonathan Wild* and *Amelia*, from Smollett's *Roderick Random*, *Peregrine Pickle* and the more genial *Humphry Clinker*, and from Hogarth's demotic melodramas.

By degrees the streets were widened, old houses demolished, creaking signs removed, illumination improved, cobbles and kennels changed for paving-stones and gutters, and Fleet-ditch's 'disemboguing streams' rolled their large tribute of dead dogs to Thames beneath a brick vault. Wendeborn compares London thus modernised with Paris, and finds it cleaner, safer, and 'infinitely better lighted'. Moritz describes with pleasure the paved and kerbed footways, and the lighting which even on ordinary nights looks like a festivity—a visiting princeling thought it to be an illumination in his honour. Sophie von la Roche, the intelligent wife of a German nobleman, visited England in 1786 and recorded the new order (*Sophie in London, 1786,* 1933, 86, 89).

How happy the pedestrian on these roads, which alongside the houses are paved with large, clean paving-stones some feet wide, where many thousands of neatly-clad people pursue their way.... Buildings... simple but lofty, always sensible.... The houses are mostly brick, and have no decoration other than big, well-kept windows, whose panes are framed in fine white-painted wood.

Pastor Moritz presents the panorama from Westminster Bridge in 1782 (*Travels in England,* ed. Matheson, 1924, 21):

The prospect from this bridge alone seems to afford one the epitome of a journey, or a voyage in miniature, as containing something of every thing that most usually occurs on a journey. It is a little assemblage of contrasts and contrarieties. In contrast to the round, modern and majestic Cathedral of St Paul's on your right, the venerable, old-fashioned, and hugely noble long Abbey of Westminster, with its enormous pointed roof, rises on the left. Down the Thames to the right you see Blackfriars Bridge, which does not yield much, if at all, in beauty to that of Westminster; on the left bank of the Thames are beautiful terraces, planted with trees, and those new tasteful buildings called the Adelphi. On the Thames itself are countless swarms of little boats passing and repassing, many with one mast and one sail, and many with none, in which people of all ranks are carried over.

Such, in its better aspects, was the London of Fanny Burney, and of Johnson's and Horace Walpole's later years.

Of all London's features it was the Thames, the channel of trade, which inspired the most eloquence. Defoe described it as

glorious by the Splendor of its Shores, gilded with noble Palaces, strong Fortifications, large Hospitals and publick Buildings; with the greatest Bridge, and the greatest City in the World, made famous by the Opulence of its Merchants, the Encrease and Extensiveness of its Commerce; by its invincible Navies and by the innumerable Fleets of Ships sailing upon it, to and from all Parts of the World.

Tour, i. 173–4

It was, said Thomson in *Liberty* (1736), the chief of rivers,

> *On whose each tide, glad with returning spoils,*
> *Flows in the mingled harvest of mankind.*

And Savage's *London and Bristol Delineated* (1744), before insulting Bristol (which had imprisoned him for debt), showered praises on London:

> *Wide, deep, unsullied Thames meandering glides,*
> *And bears thy wealth on mild, majestic tides;*
> *Thy ships, with gilded palaces that vie,*
> *In glittering pomp strike wondering China's eye;*
> *And thence returning bear, in splendid state,*
> *To Britain's merchants, India's eastern freight.*

London's Pool was a spectacle the average citizen saw more often than he does today. Docks were few, and ships many; Defoe reckoned that above 2,000 sea-going vessels might be on view at one time, and his exaggeration was probably not as lavish as usual —a modern estimate is that something like 1,400 ships might gather between Limehouse and the Tower. As Moritz bowled by postchaise from Dartford to London he saw 'a little forest of masts' whenever the Thames was in sight. The century's pride in sea-power and enterprise comes out in Burke's third *Letter on a Regicide Peace* (1797), which eulogises the wealth of London and the trade which congests the Thames, overloads wharves and roadways, and is limited only by the capacities of the distributive trades. The river was busy too with local traffic: Dryden's *Essay of Dramatick Poesie* (1668) is a discussion between friends who take a boat at London Bridge, thread their way through crowded shipping to Greenwich, and return to Somerset Stairs. A century later Moritz refers to 'countless swarms of little boats'; except for London Bridge, and until Westminster Bridge was finished in 1747, they were the only means of crossing the river.

Defoe's account of the City is confident and proud. He records the great offices of the Bank of England and the trading companies;

the Bank 'very convenient, very spacious' and prodigiously efficient; the East India and South Sea Companies planning new premises; the African Company 'a very handsome well-built and convenient house'; the Customs House intended to 'outshine all the customhouses in Europe', and the Royal Exchange 'the greatest and finest of the kind in the world'. The new churches rise clean and classical; so does the Monument, outdoing 'all the obelisks and pillars of the ancients'. There are 'many noble streets and beautiful houses' between the Strand and the river; there is Wren's Hospital at Chelsea—'the noblest building and the best foundations of its kind in the world'; Bethlehem Hospital, 'the most magnificent thing of its kind in the world' and a grievance to Louis XIV, it is said, by resembling one of his palaces; and Guy's Hospital, 'a most magnificent building, not yet quite finished'. There are developments in Soho and north of Piccadilly and in the Haymarket, which Defoe reckons 'more in bulk than the cities of Bristol, Exeter and York if they were all put together'.

The citizens could, if Anglicans, worship in the churches of Wren, Hawksmoor, Gibbs and the rest, and particularly in St. Paul's, rising serenely above the dark red tide of brick houses. If Dissenters, they chose among a hundred or so meeting-houses, filled in general with humbler but more zealous worshippers than the Anglican churches; Ward's *Hudibras Redivivus* is pungently satirical at their fervour. And the current of life which on Sunday set to and from places of worship and amusement flowed on weekdays into the shops and markets, with corn-chandlers at Bear Key and Queen Hithe, cattle-dealers at Smithfield, clothiers at Blackwell, and fish-mongers at Billingsgate, handsomely housed in tall formal ranges of buildings with open arcades below, and exercising, as Wendeborn remarked (*View of England*, i. 333), their

natural powers of speech, figures of oratory, well chosen epithets, strong expressions delivered with an audible voice in the vulgar English tongue.

In heraldic colours Gay depicts the kaleidoscopic pattern of the fish-market (*Trivia*, ii. 413–18):

> *When fishy stalls with double store are laid;*
> *The golden-belly'd carp, the broad-finn'd maid:* [young skate]
> *Red-speckled trouts, the salmon's silver joul,*
> *The joynted Lobster, and unscaly soale,*
> *And luscious 'scallops, to allure the tastes*
> *Of rigid zealots to delicious fasts.*

The daily comedy, caught so well in Gay's detail, meets one in all the literature of the time, intimate and familiar, moving among the affectionately-observed surroundings of a daily life controlled to the scale of man in his normal stature.

Man in his normal stature needs the country to supplement the town, and it was nowhere more than a mile away. Knyff's *Britannia Illustrata* (1708-20) shows Lambeth, Chelsea, Kensington Palace and Burlington House in Piccadilly, with wide fields around them and tree-grown hills rising to the horizon. Open fields came into Bloomsbury as far as the present British Museum site; the occupants of nearby Queen Square left its north end unbuilt so as not to interrupt their view of Highgate and Hampstead Hill. Swift, he tells Stella on 17 May, 1711, went to Vauxhall with Lady Kerry and Mrs. Pratt to hear the nightingales; two days later, at Chelsea, 'we are mowing already and making hay, and it smells so sweet as we walk through the flowry meads'. The parks were little less pleasant than the country; St. James the most accessible, Hyde Park with a deer-herd which Royalty hunted until 1768, and Kensington Gardens remodelled for Queen Caroline in the 1730s, when the Broad Walk, Round Pond and Serpentine were made. Kensington itself, on its gravel-beds, was for health and holidays; Swift tells Stella on 31 May, 1712, that he wants to lodge there for the air: Garth's *Dispensary* (1699) contrasts it with the dampness of Kent: Tickell's *Kensington Garden* (1722) unites nature and mankind there in a glimpse of vernal brilliance (lines 1-12):

> *Where Kensington high o'er the neighbouring lands*
> *'Midst greens and sweets, a regal fabric, stands,*
> *And sees each spring, luxuriant in her bowers,*
> *A snow of blossoms, and a wild of flowers,*

> *The dames of Britain oft in crowds repair,*
> *To gravel walks, and unpolluted air.*
> *Here, while the town in damps and darkness lies,*
> *They breathe in sunshine, and see azure skies:*
> *Each walk, with robes of various dyes bespread,*
> *Seems from afar a moving tulip bed,*
> *Where rich brocades and glossy damasks glow,*
> *And chints, the rival of the showery bow.*

Villages now urbanised were still rural—Tottenham, Islington, Sadlers Wells, Bethnal Green, Stepney and Newington: Moritz speaks of Paddington as in 'a rustic and pleasant situation'. Defoe praises Hackney ('remarkable for the retreat of wealthy citizens'), Tottenham ('there is not any thing more fine in their degree than most of the buildings this way') and Hampstead. Middlesex is 'a county made rich, pleasant and populous by the neighbourhood of London', with three thousand fine houses built in sixty years. Richmond evoked many a tribute: it figures in Defoe as George and Caroline's summer-resort when Prince and Princess of Wales, with fine houses for 'the first and second class gentry', with assembly rooms and mineral wells where company gathered for music and the waters. Sophie von la Roche saw 'hundreds of villas dotted about, shimmering between the fine verdure'; Richmond Park, where she disturbed the fallow deer among the tall bracken, brought *Ossian* to her mind. Moritz speaks of sunset there as a dream of paradise (*Travels in England*, 105–6):

> Instead of the incessant, distressing noise in London, I saw here at a distance sundry little family parties, walking arm in arm along the banks of the Thames. Every thing breathed a soft and pleasing calm, which warmed my heart, and filled it with some of the most pleasing sensations of which our nature is susceptible. Beneath, I trod on that fresh, even and soft verdure which is to be seen only in England: on one side of me lay a wood, than which nature cannot produce a finer; and on the other, Thames with its shelvy bank and charming lawns rising like an amphitheatre, along which, here and there, one espies a picturesque white house aspiring, in majestic simplicity, to pierce the dark foliage of the surrounding trees.

There was Epsom, also with music and wells, tree-grown so as to seem, says Defoe, 'a great wood full of houses scatter'd every where', busy in summer with merchants' families and with sportsmen racing, hunting and cricketing on Banstead Downs; there were spas at Islington, Hampstead and Sadlers Wells, which makes a placid rural appearance in Hogarth's *Evening* and which Sophie von la Roche describes agreeably (p. 132):

> This district is very lovely: large meadows alive with herds of excellent cows: lakes with trees in front of the house itself, numerous avenues with delightful tables and benches for visitors, under trees hung with tiny lamps. In the open temple, lower-class lasses, sailors and other young people were dancing.

Farther away were Dulwich and Sydenham, crowded in summer, and still further Tunbridge, of whose 'gaming, sharping, intriguing, as also fops, fools, beaus and the like' Defoe is firmly censorious.

One can hardly rejuvenate so venerable a theme as that of London's pleasure-gardens and coffee-houses, yet to avoid them would be to omit something indispensable not only to social life but to that kinship between literary men which comes from their recurrent dealings with the same material. Above all, Vauxhall and Ranelagh offered irresistible attractions. The former was livelier and less select: Fanny Burney's Evelina was frightened there by rowdies. It provided shady groves (the scenes of Evelina's alarm), *al fresco* concerts, and modish boxes in frivolously rococo Gothic and Moorish-Chinese. Not often was it indecorous; Wendeborn found it quiet and refreshing (*View of England*, i. 353):

> Even a philosopher may spend there agreeable hours at a small expence. He may hear good music and singing: he may refresh himself in the cool of the evening: he may make observations on men and manners, retire in good time, and rise the next morning without in the least repenting the pleasures of the last evening.

But popularity had the drawbacks Horace Walpole described to George Montagu on 11 May, 1769—the occasion was a *ridotto al fresco:*

Mr Conway and I set out from his house at eight o'clock—the tide and torrent of coaches was so prodigious, that it was half-an-hour after nine before we got half way from Westminster Bridge. We then alighted, and after scrambling under bellies of horses, through wheels, and over posts and rails, we reached the gardens, where were already many thousand persons.... We walked twice round and were rejoiced to come away, though with the same difficulties as at our entrance, for we found three strings of coaches all along the road, who did not move half a foot in half an hour. There is to be a rival mob in the same way at Ranelagh to-morrow; for the greater the folly and imposition, the greater is the crowd.

Ranelagh had its famous Rotunda, which Walpole told Horace Mann about on 26 May, 1742:

There is a vast amphitheatre, finely gilt, painted and illuminated, into which every body that loves eating, drinking, staring, or crowding is admitted for twelve-pence. The building and disposition of the garden cost sixteen thousand pounds. Twice a-week there are to be Ridottos at guinea-tickets, for which you are to have a supper and music.

Smaller than Vauxhall and better behaved (since, as Wendeborn observed, 'only tea and coffee are served'), it had its piquant moments. The Duchess of Northumberland notes in her diary for 21 July, 1761 (*Diaries of a Duchess*, 1926), that

a quarrel happened this Evening at Ranelagh, between Poll Davis & Kitty Fisher, two very pretty Women of the Town, (the first kept by Lord Coventry, the second by Mr. Chetwynd), in which the former not only boxed the others Ears, but also hit Ld. Coventry a Slap on the Face, for which she was turned out of Ranelagh & forbid to come there any more.

From 1771 there was also the Pantheon in Oxford Street, open in winter when Vauxhall and Ranelagh closed. Walpole, who called it 'the new winter-Ranelagh in Oxford Road' (to Mann, 26 April, 1771), said it rivalled the glory of Baalbec, which, more or less literally, it did, since its late-Roman style brought its young architect James Wyatt his precocious fame.

Another source of lively diversion was the theatres, limited in number by the 1737 Licensing Act to two, but by various means reaching an actual total of about six. Some were outside civic jurisdiction like that at Sadlers Wells where Sophie von la Roche saw farce, ballet, pantomime, acrobatics, operetta and a strong-man act, and noticed the spectators depositing hams, chops, pasties, bottles and glasses on the shelf behind each row of seats. More serious performances were not always more seriously received: according to Walpole the social year would have been incomplete without a theatrical riot. For their rowdy behaviour *The Guardian* castigated 'the most unmannerly Race of young Men that ever were seen' (2 April, 1713): in 1737 footmen, denied their customary free entry, attacked Drury Lane in force. Other riots occurred there in 1744 and 1755; in the latter year after five nights of increasing excitement (French dancers were performing at a time of hostility to France) on the sixth a free fight broke out resulting in heavy damages. No playwright or manager could discount the audience's temper; it could lead to triumph or to intolerant violence prompted at times by nothing more relevant than political enmity or a rival's jealousy reinforced by his friends. Even a friendly audience was high-spirited; Moritz saw Foote's *Nabob* at the Haymarket in 1782 and describes the house, with pit benches rising in an amphitheatre and prices graded from one shilling in the second gallery to five in the boxes. Rotten oranges (one hit his hat) flew about in a 'perpetual pelting from the gallery', the first and second galleries shouted and thumped sticks, and servants keeping boxes for their masters hid themselves from the showers of missiles. Yet except when an inaudible actress was barracked the play was received with enthusiasm.

Whether this degree of spirit, so natural to the age, was good for drama is debatable. On the one hand such Augustan plays as are still alive (all comedies, incidentally) are robustly phrased, and this (like the lively style of contemporary pamphleteering, and of Restoration drama) may be credited to an eager but unruly audience. On the other hand, that audience expected such unsubtle qualities as obvious humour, genteel sentiment and strong situation. Yet

Shakespeare and great acting could move it: when Garrick as Macbeth entered after Duncan's murder, Fielding observes, 'it is scarce an Hyperbole to say, I have seen the Hair of the Audience stand on end' (*Enquiry into the Late Increase of Robbers*, 1751), and his tribute in *Tom Jones* where Partridge denies Garrick's greatness as Hamlet because he acts so naturally is a stroke against village simplicity but not against town taste (Book XVI. v). The reputations of Cibber, Quin, Garrick, Barry, Foote, Mrs. Oldfield, Kitty Clive, Mrs. Siddons and others outshine those of most contemporary plays they acted in. 'The golden age of the English theatre', Lecky called the later eighteenth century, for its illustrious performers, for Goldsmith's and Sheridan's plays, and for its revival of Shakespeare (*History of England in the Eighteenth Century*, xxi). In a sense that is true—the sense of a strong, even flamboyant relationship between actor and audience, not indeed comparable with that of the Elizabethan stage yet still intimate and unsophisticated. Prologues and epilogues were still devices by which author, player and spectator shared each other's minds, a sign of the frank (if sometimes hostile) communion between the parties.

The best-known institution of Augustan social life, and the most difficult not to be tedious about, is the coffee-house. With the inn, the tavern and the club this created much of the mental world in which literature lived, and it contributed, as Swift said to Stella (*Journal*, 21 June, 1711), 'to advance conversation and friendship'. Augustan London had something like five hundred coffee-houses, differentiated often by social or professional distinctions but fertilising society's intermingling. They originated about the middle of the seventeenth century, and among the most famous were Garraway's in Change Alley, frequented by merchants, and the centre of South-Sea-Bubble speculation: Jonathan's and the Turk's Head, also in Change Alley (a later Turk's Head in Soho was the home of the Turk's Head Club which included Burke, Gibbon, Adam Smith, and the artists whose meetings gave rise to the Royal Academy): Lloyd's, which became the present shipping registry: Child's near St. Paul's, convenient for the clergy: the Chapter in Paternoster Row, for the near-by booksellers, the scene of that fortunate meet-

explained in his *Proposal for Making an Effectual Provision for the Poor* (1753),

the Sufferings of the Poor are indeed less observed than their Misdeeds; not from any Want of Compassion, but because they are less known,

and in the same year (8 February) Wesley's *Journal* recorded in tragic terms the conditions he found among the slums:

> Such scenes, who could see unmoved? There are none such to be found in a pagan country. If any of the Indians in Georgia were sick, those that were near him gave him whatever he wanted. Oh who will convert the English into honest Heathens! I found some in their cells underground, others in their garrets, half starved both with cold and hunger, added to weakness and pain. But I found not one of them unemployed who was able to crawl about the room. So wickedly, devilishly false is that common objection, 'They are poor only because they are idle.'

Public dispensaries founded in the second half of the century discovered how much medical help was needed for a larger, less comfortable circle than that of paying patients, and the more social conditions were examined the more concern was felt. London was not all large mansions, orderly terraces and West End squares. The fringes of the town, Fielding declared, would show 'such pictures of human Misery as must move the compassion of every Heart'. A symptom, rather than the root, of poverty was drunkenness, the traditional folly of the nation. Defoe denounced the tolerance which approved of 'an honest drunken Fellow' (*The Poor Man's Plea*) and trounced high and low (but mainly low) in *The True-Born Englishman:*

> *Good Drunken Company is their Delight,*
> *And what they get by Day, they spend by Night . . .*
> *In* English Ale *their dear Enjoyment lies,*
> *For which they'll starve themselves and Families . . .*
> *Slaves to the Liquor, Drudges to the Pots,*
> The Mob are Statesmen, and their Statesmen Sots.

That scorn, that colloquial wrath, that angry pun in 'dear Enjoyment', are signs of the impatience such folly provoked in the

ing in 1777 when it was decided to invite Dr. Johnson to write the lives of the English poets. Around the Strand moved authors and wits; Shenstone went to George's in the Strand, Cowper to Dick's in Fleet Street, Goldsmith to the Grecian in Devereux Court, famous for scholarship. Near Temple Bar were Will's (immortalised by Dryden's custom), Button's (where Addison held court) and the Bedford (the favourite of Hogarth, Fielding, Murphy, Colman and Foote). Fashion made for Pall Mall and St. James Street, to White's for the Tory élite, St. James's its Whig counterpart, and the Smyrna, the rendezvous of Swift, Prior, and the Kit-cat Club, which enrolled many of London's notables whom Kneller painted at that slightly-more-than-waist-length still known as kit-cat size. The ladies eventually counterpoised this male monopoly, though on a restricted scale, with salons where they could prove (as enlightened minds were ready to admit) that Nature shared her intellectual gifts fairly between the sexes. Under the encouragement of Mrs. Montagu, Mrs. Boscawen, Mrs. Vesey and others, society achieved an integration it had lacked—the collaboration of masculine and feminine tastes in cultural matters—and a necessary strand was woven into the fabric of London's life. Clubs of all sorts, professional, intellectual, artistic, political, musical, literary, eccentric, or merely companionable, were signs of a community conscious of similar tastes, and ready semi-formally to organise its growing sociability.

There is, however, another side of society to be considered. The eighteenth century was not mainly an age of the lighter social functions, of *Rape of the Lock* elegance, Sheridan's wit, or the graces of Arne's operettas. Such things sparkled on the surface of a deep, strong and often dark current of life, in which many were immersed in a struggle for survival. In the circumstances, historians have commented, the poor were remarkably law-abiding; Defoe at the time praised the wretched Thames lightermen for their honesty, and Wendeborn noted that Paris had far more murders than London. Yet violence was frequent, a symptom of conditions which for the submerged tenth must have been all but unendurable, and of which the general public was ignorant. As Fielding

> *She went, to plain-work and to purling brooks,*
> *Old-fashion'd halls, dull Aunts, and croaking rooks:*
> *She went from Op'ra, Park, Assembly, Play,*
> *To morning-walks, and pray'rs three hours a day.*

The vivacious Mrs. Sullen, in Farquhar's *Beaux' Stratagem*, is no less depressed by her country exile; so is Euphelia, in Johnson's *Rambler* (Nos. 42, 46); and Lady Teazle in *The School for Scandal* explains that her girlhood amusements were to play cards with the curate, read sermons to her aunt, and strum her father to sleep after a hunt. She accepted Sir Peter, she tells him, as the best, the only, way out.

Pope, Farquhar and Sheridan liked the country, and Johnson was not averse from it, yet in jesting at their heroines they strengthen the notion (strongly pressed by Restoration comedy—though not, incidentally, in Shadwell's *Bury Fair*) that outer darkness peopled by Sir Tunbelly Clumsys and Squire Sullens began at the Hyde Park turnpike. The idea is still current that apart from a few unusual poets the Augustans felt the country to be *terra incognita* and its remoter parts (as Defoe said of the Pennines and Lake hills) 'all barren and wild, of no use or advantage to man or beast'. Boswell's friend Sir Michael le Fleming, it is assumed, spoke for his age when invited to admire the scents of a May evening. 'This may be very well,' he replied coolly, 'but for my part I prefer the smell of a flambeau at the play-house.'

Yet England was not manned entirely by Sir Michaels; indeed, Sir Michael himself may sometimes have softened to natural beauty, since his seat was Rydal Hall, with Rydal Crag behind and, as William Gilpin's *Observations on the Mountains and Lakes of Cumberland* (1786) relates, a view to Windermere and a cascade visible from a summer-house. Johnson might agree with Boswell that Greenwich Park was not equal to Fleet Street; still, when he did so they had both enjoyed a sunshine sail down the Thames and been 'entertained with the immense number and variety of ships that were lying at anchor, and with the beautiful country on each side of the river'. Pope, reputed apostle of the town, was capable of *Windsor Forest* and of the 425th *Spectator*, praising the cool of evening after a sultry day, when the moon shining on his garden provided 'the pleasantest Hours I pass in the whole Four and twenty':

> The Reflection of it in the Water, the Fanning of the Wind rustling on the Leaves, the Singing of the Thrush and the Nightingale, and the Coolness of the Walks, all conspired to make me lay aside all displeasing Thoughts, and brought me into such a Tranquillity of Mind, as is I believe the next Happiness to that of hereafter.

Even a liking for wilder scenery, though rarer, was not uncommon: Pope himself could admire 'the shapeless rock, or hanging precipice', and Johnson was not blind to the grandeur of the Western Isles. What did the country mean to the Augustans?

To most it meant a place to live and work in, to improve and enjoy. Professor Trevelyan has described the feelings of those responsible for its management (*English Social History*, 1944, 308):

> The impression left by turning over many hundreds of letters to the better-to-do gentry of the reign of Anne is neither that of country scholar nor of country bumpkin. We read the actual thoughts of squires, anxious about their account books, their daughters' marriages, and their sons' debts and professions; attending to their own estates, and to the county business on the bench of magistrates, as well as to their hounds and horses; devoted to their gardens and their ponds a little more than to their books; living, as we should expect, a wholesome and useful life, half-public, half-private, wholly leisured, natural and dignified.

Into such an impression Sir Roger de Coverley fits as by natural right. The next chapter will describe the countryside's improvement, but here it may be noted that a desire to improve was widespread. The great landowners, the gentry, the tenant farmers, and many a merchant-turned-gentleman combined to evolve from the raw landscape England's greatest work of art. From many sources comes evidence (except when enclosures or rising prices impoverished the labourers) of a healthy bucolic England, with some mental and much physical vigour, and with that steadily-accepted relationship of classes which is typical of country society. *The*

Guardian (No. 6), for example, tells of Sir Harry Lizard, a sensible young man whose estates yield him £3,000 a year. His servants 'have a chearful, not a gay air', and they 'live in Plenty but not in wantonness'. The sons of 'gentlemen or lower people' have shared his education free and have become his friends; they have learnt to ride on his horses and they accompany him hunting. 'These and the like little joyful arts', *The Guardian* observes, 'gain him the Love of all who do not know his Worth, and the Esteem of all who do.' The portrait is held up as a model; not all the gentry were Sir Harrys. But human nature produces his like as often as that of Squire Sullen, and much Augustan writing about country life reflects a community of good sense and character. The merchant-proprietors reinforced those qualities: Adam Smith remarks that

> Merchants are commonly ambitious of becoming country gentlemen, and when they do are generally the best of all improvers. A merchant is accustomed to employ his money chiefly in profitable projects; whereas a mere country gentleman is accustomed to employ it chiefly in expense. The one often sees his money go from him and return to him again with a profit; the other, when once he parts with it, very seldom expects to see any more of it.
>
> *The Wealth of Nations*, ed. Cannan, i. 382

The land's attraction for such a man was not simply the chance of profit; other avenues—commerce or the Funds, for instance—might have brought more money. What he sought was that mixture of enterprise, interest, rural pleasure and social prestige which the successful cultivation of a country estate brings. The readiest purchasers of land were large merchants, judges, retired officers and civil servants, who were not merely investing in land but buying a hobby and social distinction. To quote Adam Smith again,

> The capital of the landlord which is fixed in the improvement of his land seems to be as well secured as the nature of human affairs can admit of. The beauty of the country besides, the pleasures of a country life, the tranquillity of mind which it promises, and, wherever the injustice of human laws does not disturb it, the independency which it really affords, have charms that more or less attract every body; and as to cultivate the

ground was the original destination of man, so in every stage of his existence he seems to retain a predilection for this primitive employment.

The Wealth of Nations, i. 357

If the new-rich rose in the world and bought land, the new-poor came down in it and sold; throughout the century many small squires farming their own acres yielded reluctantly to wealthier men. As Defoe's *Plan of the English Commerce* says, 'the rising Tradesman swells into the Gentry, and the declining Gentry sinks into Trade'. But the new money invested in land meant, on the practical side, a greatly improved and more productive cultivation, and, on the aesthetic, a fortuitous or deliberate landscape design which transformed the face of England with a lavish enrichment.

Defoe's *Tour* abounds with references to country estates improved by town wealth. The home counties in particular benefited; in one generation, he declares, fine houses and grounds have multiplied everywhere, particularly along the Thames, so that the scene from London to Richmond abounds in such 'rich habitations of gentlemen of quality' that (in his inevitable phrase) 'nothing in the world can imitate it' (*Tour*, i. 168):

the whole Country here shines with a lustre not to be describ'd; Take them in a remote view, the fine Seats shine among the Trees as Jewels shine in a rich Coronet; in a *near sight* they are meer Pictures and Paintings; *at a distance* they are all Nature, *near hand* all Art; But both in the extreamest Beauty.

Two astonished foreigners at Bushey Heath told him that 'England was not like other Country's, but it was all a planted Garden' (i. 388):

They had there on the right Hand, the Town of St. *Albans* in their View; and all the Spaces between, and further beyond it, look'd indeed like a Garden. The inclos'd Corn-Fields made one grand Parterre, the thick planted Hedge Rows, like a Wilderness or Labyrinth, divided in *Espaliers*; the Villages interspers'd look'd like so many several Noble Seats of Gentlemen at a Distance. In a Word, it was all Nature, and yet look'd all like Art.

He always kindles to beauty as a by-product of prosperity—in the West, to the Vale of Evesham with its fruit; to Shropshire and Ludlow, 'exceeding pleasant, fertile, populous and the soil rich'; to Cheshire with its pastures and fine cheese, 'the soil extraordinarily rich'; in the Midlands to the 'most beautiful' meadows of the Nene from Peterborough to Northampton, and the Ouse's luxuriant water-meadows at Huntingdon; in the East, to Suffolk and Norfolk with flourishing countrysides and rich dairying, and opening up from Newmarket 'a rich and pleasant vale westwards cover'd with cornfields, gentlemen's seats, villages, and at a distance, to crown all the rest, that antient and truly famous town and university of Cambridge'.

Any selection from Defoe's lavish detail is the merest sample of God's plenty. Yet not only in him, but in scores of other writers also, one finds, praised with inexhausted delight, that quality still most to be cherished in the country, not its romantic grandeur but the beauty of its ordinary face, that wealth of 'landscape plotted and pieced, Fold, fallow, and plough', in which the powers of Nature and man have so incomparably combined. Other foreigners than Defoe's two gentlemen remarked on it. There is, for instance, the Danish Pehr Kalm's *Accounts of his Visit to England in 1748* (translated by Joseph Lucas in 1892). Essex, he said, 'resembles one continuous pleasure-garden from the many living hedges that are everywhere'. Pastor Moritz declared that the green hills along the Thames outdid in beauty anything he had seen, and like Kalm particularly observed (p. 15)

> those living hedges which in England more than in any other country form the boundaries of the green cornfields and give to the whole of the distant country the appearance of a large and majestic garden.

As unqualified a eulogy as any in Defoe or foreign visitors occurs in Smollett's *Travels Through France and Italy* (1766: letter xxxvi):

> I see the country of England smiling with cultivation; the grounds exhibiting all the perfection of agriculture, parcelled out into beautiful

enclosures, corn fields, hay and pasture, woodland and common . . . I see her meadows well-stocked with black cattle, her downs covered with sheep; . . . I view her teams of horses and oxen, large and strong, fat and sleek: . . . I see her farm-houses the habitations of plenty, cleanliness and convenience: and her peasants well fed, well lodged, well cloathed, tall and stout, and hale and jolly.

This indeed sounds too good to be true. The country's improvement did not render everyone hale and jolly. A steady price-rise in the latter half of the century made landowners richer and labourers poorer, and Smollett's own *Continuation of the History of Great Britain* (1760-1) records riots against the high cost of corn. Thomas Mortimer's *Elements of Commerce, Politics and Finances* (1772) says that farm-workers are being driven to wholesale migration, that 'flinty-hearted or prodigal luxurious landlords have swept away the inhabitants', that the competition for land is inflating rents, that owners are often absentees, and that 'the proprietor of lands and his tenants come to have separate interests, and the former is regardless of the condition of the latter'. Similar witness comes from Nathaniel Kent's *Hints to Gentlemen of Landed Property* (1775), George Dyer's *Complaints of the Poor People of England* (1793), and David Davies's *Case of the Labourers in Husbandry* (1795). Cowper's *Task* (1785) speaks of the labourer as 'angry and sad, and his last crust consum'd', 'ill-clad and fed but sparely', in winter without light or fire (i. 246; iv. 379). William Gilpin the 'picturesque' traveller writes in *Observations on the River Wye* (1782) of extreme poverty around Tintern, and on returning from the Lakes, where he found countrymen of dignity and independence, he was shocked by the misery of those around the Peak (*Observations on the Mountains and Lakes of Cumberland*). In countrysides growing in productivity and beauty the poor often had much to endure, of a kind which Cowper's pictures in *The Task* and Crabbe's in *The Village* (1783) scarcely exaggerate. Stephen Duck the thresher-poet knew country life from his own experience, and 'The Thresher's Labour' in *Poems on Several Occasions* (1738) is no idyll:

> *Thus, as the Year's revolving Course goes round,*
> *No Respite from our Labour can be found:*
> *Like* SISYPHUS, *our Work is never done;*
> *Continually rolls back the restless Stone.*
> *New-growing Labours still succeed the past,*
> *And growing always new must always last.*

Crabbe noted the gulf that separated proprietors and labourers:

> *I grant indeed that fields and flocks have charms*
> *For him that grazes, or for him that farms;*
> *But when amid such pleasing scenes I trace*
> *The poor laborious natives of the place,*
> *And see the mid-day sun, with fervid ray,*
> *On their bare heads and dewy temples play;*
> *While some, with feebler heads and fainter hearts,*
> *Deplore their fortune, yet sustain their parts;*
> *Then shall I dare these real ills to hide*
> *In tinsel trappings of poetic pride?*
> The Village, i. 39-48

But farmers too could have their complaints, and this sample of country hardship may include an extract from Wesley's *Journal* (5 November, 1766):

In the little journeys which I have lately taken, I have thought much on the huge encomiums which have been for many ages bestowed on a *country life*. But after all what a flat contradiction is this to universal experience! See that little house, under the wood, by the river-side! There is rural life in perfection. How happy then is the farmer that lives there? He rises with or before the sun, calls his servants, looks to his swine and cows, then to his stables and barns. He sees to the ploughing and sowing his ground, in winter or in spring. In summer and autumn he hurries and sweats among his mowers and reapers. And where is his happiness in the mean time? Which of these employments do we envy? Our eyes and ears may convince us there is not a less happy body of men in all England than the country farmers. In general, their life is supremely dull, and it is usually unhappy too. For of all people in the kingdom they are most discontented, seldom satisfied either with God or man.

Cowper admitted that the pastoral golden age was a myth, yet he yearned for a lost simplicity free from 'speech profane and manners profligate', before the town had 'tinged the country' and tarnished its natural honesty (*The Task*, iv. 513). Already (in 1767) Arthur Young had lamented the easier travel which brought country folk to London and spread London worldliness in the country, and in 1782 John Byng noted in his high-spirited *Diary* that 'the country is only improv'd in vice and insolence by the establishment of turnpikes' (*Torrington Diaries*, 1934, i. 72).

Yet in general what caught the eye was prosperity; those like Kalm, Moritz, Smollett and John Shebbeare who knew agriculture abroad found it better in England. Writing *Letters on the English Nation* (1755) under the pseudonym of 'Batista Angeloni, a Jesuit resident in London', Shebbeare declared that

> plenty bursts forth to every view; a cleanliness unknown to the peasants of any nation is visible in every village. The country seems yet untainted; the smiling face of liberty shines amongst the inhabitants: and a wealth which no people ever boasted, of their rank, is to be found among the farmers of this isle.

This reference to the 'untainted' country recalls that it was supposedly the home of virtue, as the town of vice. Johnson said so in *London*, before his conversion. 'Though Men for the general good of the world are made to love populous cities,' *The Guardian* observed (No. 22), 'the country hath the greatest share in an uncorrupted heart'; pastoral poetry, it continued, is popular because it breathes innocence and tranquillity. Far from being inveterate townsmen Augustan poets paid almost nostalgic homage to rural life; many felt about the city what the Reverend James Ward said of Dublin ('Phoenix Park', in Concanen's *Miscellaneous Poems*, 1724):

> *I learn her Vice and Follies to despise,*
> *And love that Heav'n which in the Country lies.*

Gay's *Rural Sports* contrasts town vanities with the 'happy plains remote from war's alarms', where barns bulge with corn and the thresher's flail whirls in peace: Gray's *Elegy* puts side by side the madding crowd's ignoble strife and the villagers' tranquil tedium, repressed by penury and circumscribed by fate, but keeping the noiseless tenour of their way in paths remote equally from great honours and great crimes. And Goldsmith's *Deserted Village* immortally idealises the dream that there was (or had recently been) a rural paradise where health and plenty cheered the labouring swain, and simple men lived a life of decent work, leisure, and faith.

The truth no doubt lies somewhere in that middle area so well drawn in a much more recent study of country society, George Bourne's *Change in the Village* (1912). Bourne studies his country community in the ultimate stage of an immemorial country pattern now radically changed. His account, unsentimental but deeply understanding, includes hardship, prematurely broken health, crippling disease and accident, and all the difficulties natural to a community with primitive resources and few reserves of wealth, dependent on fickle weather and far-away markets. There is corroboration here for the pessimist. Yet there is much also to balance pessimism—neighbourliness, courage, resilience, and enough basic sense and humanity to justify not a pastoral idyll but a deep respect for the seasoned philosophy which feels life not in sentimental extremes but as a tempered matter of ill to be borne and enjoyment to be taken. It is the spirit of Hardy's countrymen. To this degree there was justification for the opinion that the poor were less degraded in proportion to their distance from London and that, as Shebbeare remarked, 'good order, sobriety and honesty' marked the village as against the 'anarchy, drunkenness and thievery' of the town (*Letters on the English Nation*, ii. 6). Despite his sense of rustic coarseness Cowper found Olney a congenial place for his home.

However the distribution of wealth and poverty, or virtue and vice, might be disputed, the Augustans took pleasure in the country, though generally in its more cultivated aspects. Addison returns frequently to it in *The Spectator*. 'A tree,' Pope told his friend Joseph Spence, 'is a nobler object than a prince in his coronation robes,' and he delighted in his Twickenham villa, as later did

Horace Walpole at Strawberry Hill; Swift yearned for country pleasures—'Oh that we were at Laracor this fine day! the willows begin to peep, and the quicks to bud'—'The Cherry trees by the River side my Heart is sett upon' (*Journal to Stella*, 19 March, 1711, and 26 March, 1712). Fielding liked country life; Goldsmith portrays the scenes of a rural pastorate in *The Vicar of Wakefield*, Richard Graves those of a gentleman's estate in *The Spiritual Quixote*, and Smollett those of the country tour in *Humphry Clinker*. There is pleasant rusticity in scores of poems and letters, novels, diaries and tours. The country was a place of cheerful visiting or occupation, where a man might stay sociably with friends or in his inn, or superintend his estate, designing and cherishing vistas, not always unawares of the introspective promptings of solitude, of self-communing pleasure and peace perhaps flavoured with mild melancholy, and indeed of philosophy and religion— spiritual excursions from which he returned to the reinforcement of a laden table. This last point is not negligible in Augustan country life; it features memorably in Parson Woodforde's *Diary* and it inspires some lines in William King's *Mully of Mountown* (1704) so vivacious and so richly appreciative in imagery as to deserve repetition:

> MOUNTOWN! *Thou sweet Retreat from* Dublin *Cares,*
> *Be famous for thy* Apples *and thy* Pears;
> *For* Turnips, Carrots, Lettice, Beans *and* Pease;
> *For* Peggy's *Butter, and for* Peggy's *Cheese.*
> *May clouds of* Pigeons *round about thee fly,*
> *But condescend sometimes to make a* Pye.
> *May fat* Geese *gaggle with melodious Voice,*
> *And ne'er want Gooseberries or Apple-sauce.*

It is an admirable thing in Augustan poets to do that kind of thing so naturally and well.

The country provided other pleasures than landscape, meditation and good living; literature, paintings and prints abound in the comedies of country sports. England, in John Nixon's lines prefacing Somervile's *Chace* (1735), was a

> *Distinguish'd land! by Heav'n indulg'd to breed*
> *The stout sagacious hound, and gen'rous steed.*

Fielding's 'A-hunting we will go', Paul Whitehead's *Hunting Song*—

> *With the Sports of the Field there's no pleasure can vye,*
> *While jocund we follow the Hounds in full cry,—*

Gay's *Rural Sports*, Somervile's *Chace* and *Field Sports*, figures like Squire Western in *Tom Jones* and Sir Harry Beagle in Colman's *Jealous Wife*, and scores of such things, are testimonies of rural diversion. Sir Roger de Coverley appears as a huntsman in *Spectators* 115 and 116, and Mr. Spectator achieves the vivacity of a sporting print:

> Our hare took a large field just under us, followed by the full cry, In View. I must confess the brightness of the weather, the cheerfulness of every thing around me, the chiding of the hounds, which was returned upon us in a double echo from two neighbouring hills, with the hallooing of the sportsmen, and the sounding of the horn, lifted my spirits into a most lively pleasure.

Sir Roger, however, eventually rescues the hare and honourably retires it to the safety of his orchard.

Along with the cudgelling, wrestling, dancing and football which Budgell describes in the 161st *Spectator*, and other sports and games, went the amusements which diversified the business of markets and fairs. Gay describes a ballad-singer with the traditional poems of the country—*The Babes in the Wood*, *Chevy Chase*, *Lillibulero*, *Robin Hood*—and singing too of 'Fairs and shows' ('Saturday', *The Shepherd's Week*, 1714, 73-90):

> *How pedlars' stalls with glittering toys are laid,*
> *The various fairings of the country maid.*
> *Long silken laces hang upon the twine,*
> *And rows of pins and amber bracelets shine:*
> *How the tight lass, knives combs and scissars spys,*
> *And looks on thimbles with desiring eyes.*

> *Of lott'ries next with tuneful note he told,*
> *When silver spoons are won, and rings of gold.*
> *The lads and lasses trudge the street along,*
> *And all the fair is crouded in his song.*
> *The mountebank now treads the stage and sells*
> *His pills, his balsams, and his ague-spells:*
> *Now o'er and o'er the nimble tumbler springs,*
> *And on the rope the ventrous maiden swings:*
> *Jack Pudding in his parti-colour'd jacket*
> *Tosses the glove, and jokes at ev'ry packet,*
> *Of Raree-shows he sung, and Punch's feats,*
> *Of pockets pick'd in crouds, and various cheats.*

The best quality of Gay's intently-delighted manner is there, that vitality by which his images have a peculiar brilliance and colour as of things seen in their essential bright reality. As for the fairs themselves, the same intent delight characterises Defoe's account of the great annual gatherings at Stourbridge near Cambridge, a vivid piece of history, of kaleidoscopic variety and detail, showing the nationwide ramifications of the wool trade, the vast market in hops, the heavy transport up the Ouse to the fairground, and the

> Goldsmiths, Toyshops, Brasiers, Turners, Milleners, Haberdashers, Hatters, Mercers, Drapers, Pewtrers, China-Warehouses, and in a word all Trades that can be named in *London*; with Coffee-Houses, Taverns, Brandy-Shops, and Eating-houses, innumerable, and all in Tents and Booths.
>
> *Tour,* i. 81

Later Sophie von la Roche visited Staines in fair-time and described the brightly-painted carts, the stalls with miscellaneous stocks—'gingerbread, and household goods very nicely worked, copper and iron goods'—and 'farmhands and maids very cleanly dressed, bunches of flowers in their hats, seeking employment'. Such details are not peculiar to the Augustans; they are part of country tradition. But they show that tradition in its natural health, and the pride of ordinary folk.

As for the countryside's buildings, they reflect a general well-being. The reigns of Anne and the Georges saw great numbers of new houses and farms, palatial for the nobleman, modestly dignified for the middle class, utilitarian for the labourer, the mellow seemliness of which pleases the eye as much as do the squares and crescents of town building. Moritz speaks well of Dartford, the first village he saw (p. 17),

where an uncommon neatness in the structure of the houses, which in general are built with red bricks and flat roofs [*i.e.* low-pitched roofs behind parapets] struck me with a pleasing surprise, especially when I compared them with the long rambling inconvenient and singularly mean cottages of our peasants.

Country builders adopted new styles, with sash windows, pediments and classical orders; country purveyors brought from London or had locally made the silver and china, the clocks, carpets and furniture, which went with the new taste. Proprietors rich enough to build or rebuild drew incomes from their estates but also enhanced the prosperity of their own localities; many places subsisted largely by supplying goods and services to the neighbouring nobility and gentry. The new houses, as signs of a new way of life, deserved the interest travellers took in them as symbols of social improvement.

Augustan literature consequently is increasingly attentive to local scenes—to natural beauties and to fine buildings and estates. Not all of this writing is a province of social life, yet the countryside it describes was a reflection of human living, was landscape cultivated and humanised, and surveyed as prospects and vistas. The Elizabethans had written poems of rural life and topography but the vogue of scene-description begins perhaps with Sir John Denham who, with *Cooper's Hill* (1642), became, as Johnson said in writing his *Life*, 'the author of that species of composition which may be denominated *local poetry*'. After Denham there was Pope with *Windsor Forest* (1713) and Garth with *Claremont* (1715) and a swarm of others so numerous that 'they left scarce a corner of the island not dignified either by rhyme or blank verse'. As landowners plumed themselves on finer houses and grounds, and as the countryside became more accessible and appreciated, the fashion spread.

Art provides a parallel; the late seventeenth and the eighteenth centuries saw a growing vogue for topographical drawings, and the late eighteenth and the nineteenth centuries an unprecedented flowering of landscape painting. The picturesque antiquity or the elegant modernity of great houses, their owners' taste and magnanimity, the formal or informal beauties of their gardens, and the prominent features of the scenery found themselves recommended in hundreds of poems, poems neither hard to write nor often distinguished when written but collectively arousing a pleasant sense of the country house and its landscapes. Dr. R. A. Aubin's *Topographical Poetry in XVIII-Century England* (New York, 1936) sympathetically explores this by-way of letters, and credits the poets in question with 'an admirable capacity for deriving satisfaction from the world about them, a divine willingness to be pleased'. They deserve this pleasant praise—poor poets, many of them, but friendly recorders of their country. And not always poor poets; Dyer's *Grongar Hill* (1726) is a good minor poem, affectionately pictorial, and tranquil as an early water-colour:

> *Grongar, in whose Mossie Cells,*
> *Sweetly-musing Quiet dwells;*
> *Grongar, in whose silent Shade,*
> *For the modest Muses made,*
> *So oft I have, the Even still,*
> *At the Fountain of a Rill,*
> *Sate upon a flow'ry Bed*
> *With my Hand beneath my Head;*
> *And stray'd my Eyes o'er Towy's Flood,*
> *Over Mead, and over Wood,*
> *From House to House, from Hill to Hill,*
> *'Till Contemplation had her fill.*

Amateur painter as well as a poet, Dyer had an appreciative eye.

Besides the pleasures of improvement, retirement, sport, good living, and landscape the country had its social life. Defoe found 'good conversation and good company' at Lichfield, Shrewsbury, Derby, York ('a man converses here with all the world as effectually as at London'), Exeter ('full of gentry and good company'),

Salisbury ('good manners and good company'), and Bury St Edmunds ('crouded with nobility and gentry... ladies mighty gay and agreeable... abundance of the finest ladies'). Shebbeare noted a general decent level of enlightenment, the common people showing 'a degree of knowledge not to be found among the peasants of any other nation'. Horace Walpole went to King's Lynn in 1761 to put himself before his electors, and wrote to his friend George Montagu on 31 March, first poking fun at an alderman who displayed his taste by buying faked Rubens and Carlo Marattos, and then continuing:

Yet to do the folks justice, they are sensible, and reasonable, and civilised; their very language is polished since I lived among them [*i.e.* during Sir Robert Walpole's later years at Houghton, 1741–4]. I attribute this to their more frequent intercourse with the world and the capital, by the help of good roads and postchaises, which, if they have abridged the King's dominions, have at least tamed his subjects.

In his youth, Wilberforce recalled, Hull was 'one of the gayest places out of London', with its theatre, balls, supper- and card-parties and other assemblies. Augustan provincial life has been little investigated, apart from a few places like Bath, Edinburgh, Oxford and Cambridge, but evidence abounds that the larger towns were organic centres and that country gentry unable to afford a London season could, as time went on, satisfactorily hibernate in their neighbouring metropolis.

Early in the century, it is true, the country's resources lagged far behind London's. Country folk, to a Londoner's eye, were fair game, uncouth addicts of grotesque dialects, ludicrous sports and sometimes dangerous superstitions. Among those not positively primitive there reigned, as Addison pleasantly observed in the 119th *Spectator*, a quaint punctilio of etiquette instead of the town's 'agreeable negligence'. Outworn fashions held their own: the 129th *Spectator* likens 'all who live at a certain distance from the town' to a gallery of family portraits, and in *She Stoops to Conquer* Goldsmith has fun with Mrs Hardcastle's antiquated modes. In the 298th *Tatler* Swift contrasts the country's embarrassing hospitality with the restraint of good town breeding. Manners were roughest where roads were worst; William Hutton's *History of Birmingham* (1781) relates how civilised the Birmingham townsmen seemed on his first visit in 1741 and how, in contrast, those of Market Bosworth set their dogs on him:

> Human figures not their own are seldom seen in those inhospitable regions: Surrounded with impassable roads, no intercourse with man to humanise the mind, no commerce to smooth their rugged manners, they continue the boors of nature.

But better roads brought the 'sophistication' deplored by Arthur Young and John Byng, and welcomed by Horace Walpole and James Lackington. The latter was a prosperous London bookseller, and his *Memoirs* (1791) note that instead of the witch- and ghost-stories which were once the farmer's staple fiction the novels of Richardson, Fielding and Smollett now circulate in the country as well as in town. Finally an indignant conservative, T. J. Mathias, whose religion was the settled order and whose prophet was Burke, protested that the countryman was too advanced: 'our peasantry', he complained in *The Pursuits of Literature* (1797: Part iv, 'Advertisement'), 'now read *The Rights of Man* on mountains and moors and by the wayside'. Satire had a new butt, a rustic society which was catching up with the times.

There were of course interests other than the political. Thomas Holcroft's novel *Hugh Trevor* (1794) tells how the hero's uncle and his friends from neighbouring hamlets would meet to sing the songs of Purcell, Croft, Boyce, Greene and Handel to the accompaniment of flute, violin and bassoon. The scene recalls *Under the Greenwood Tree*, and much in Augustan country life leads straight into the novels of Hardy. Travelling actors, precursors of the immortal Crummles, made irregular but stimulating visits, as from time to time Woodforde describes them in his *Diary*; and all in all the resources of country towns are well displayed in *Letters concerning the Present State of England* (1772). Of rustic 'inferior tradesmen and shopkeepers' the anonymous author says (p. 230):

THE COUNTRY

Their tables are served as well as rich merchants were a hundred years ago; their houses good and ornamented; what formerly was a downfall gable end, covered with thatch, is now brick and tile; and a sashed front, with white pales before it: and the furniture strangely improved from the last age: in dress, see the sons and daughters tricked out in all the little ornaments which make a country church gay, grogram changed for silk and thousands of ribbons where pack-thread once sufficed. See the amusements of these people: they resort to their theatres, and are busy in visits and tea-drinking and cards: as much ceremony is found in the assembly of a country grocer's wife as in that of a countess.

To the pessimist, primitive virtue was being eroded by a fatal tide of luxury; to the optimist, it was acquiring comfort and civility.

Country society, then, was in general either quite rustic or else congregated into small towns intimately allied with the activities and outlook of farming. Hardy's Wessex and its centre Casterbridge-Dorchester still represent the eighteenth century. Such a life moved to a different rhythm from that of the city, to that steady seasonal cycle which is the countryman's expectation. It called for the traditional skill and the sober philosophy of the country. From a social standpoint this steady basic continuity, of which something more will be said in the next chapter, provided most men with a stabilising sense of sameness and recurrence, as their lives were regulated by the natural succession of the seasons.

It is easy to romanticise country life. An anonymous satirist in *The St. James's Magazine* (1762: i. 8) foresaw an outburst of Nature-poetry in which

> *Trim poets from the City desk*
> *Deep vers'd in rural picturesque . . .*
> *Shall thro' the seasons monthly sing*
> *Sweet Winter, Autumn, Summer, Spring.*

Johnson's young Templar Dick Shifter, having read the right authors, expects 'homely quiet and blameless simplicity' as soon as he leaves London (*The Idler*, No. 71); in consequence he is scratched by briars, soaked by rain, fleeced by the rustics, and threatened by an irate farmer. Such are the rewards of sentimentality. But though the townsman, like Shifter, sometimes ignores country realities, the basic conditions of country life (given reasonable circumstances) develop self-reliance, cautious judgment, manifold skill, and a phlegmatic balance in varying fortune. These are not romantic qualities, and on the border line of poverty they may disappear in apathy or brutality; it is again relevant to refer to Crabbe's poems, and to Bourne's *Change in the Village* for its account of the countryman's outlook. But the men who can make a tolerable living from the land tend to be sturdy in character as well as physique, resourceful but not rash, practical in temper and settled in opinion, seasoned by experience of the past, busy in the present, and looking towards an inscrutable but not unfriendly future.

In the eighteenth century the combination of increasingly skilled farming, steadily developing estates, and gradually spreading enlightenment helped to produce a sound and sensible, if sometimes too John Bullish, society. And it fostered the sensible appreciation of country beauty and country pleasure, realistic rather than mystical. Mr. Spectator enjoys Sir Roger's country estate; *The Guardian* (No. 125, by Tickell) recalls springtime at a country house, and the prospect of a ruined castle and a horizon of hills; Thomson has a good eye for hay-making (*Summer*, 352 ff.), sheep-shearing (ibid., 379 ff.), and the hunting feast (*Autumn*, 502 ff.). Somervile pictures the beagle (*The Chace*, i. 236), the fox-hound (i. 284—rather indebted to Shakespeare), the gathered harvest (ii. 51), the excited pack (ii. 94) and the hunt (iii. 64). Dyer (*The Fleece*) goes patiently through the whole process of sheep-farming. These things and many others in poems, letters, journals and novels show a characteristic liking for country life. *Satis beatus ruris honoribus* was the motto which Bolingbroke, after his fall from power, affixed to his farm at Dawley near Uxbridge. Pope wrote thence to Swift on 28 June, 1728, that Bolingbroke was reading one of Swift's letters 'between two haycocks', superintending his harvesters, and casting his eyes to the sky 'not in admiration of what you say but for fear of a shower'. It epitomises the century that the urban sophisticate should have come to terms with the country.

It is appropriate to such an age that one of its best books is one in which the true country-lover's intelligent eye, careful observation, honest interest in real things, and devoted comprehension of natural phenomena are everywhere evident. That book is Gilbert White's *Natural History of Selborne* (1789). Most of it concerns Selborne's flora and fauna but the first nine letters present the parish in a wider perspective, its geography, its soils, its inhabitants and anecdotes of its life. These letters form as pleasant and direct a picture as one could wish of the firm traditional pattern of country life. Gilbert White can make things stand before the mind's eye in their native truth, and enter into the affections in their very Englishness, and these letters are a good miniature picture of rural life in his time. This brief survey may end, however, with a reference not to White but again to Bolingbroke, to a letter of his to Swift (Elwin and Courthope, *Works of Pope*, vii. 113). Bolingbroke did not live up to them, for he returned to politics, but they well express his century's recognition of country stability:

> I am in my farm, and here I shoot strong and tenacious roots: I have caught hold of the earth, to use a gardener's phrase, and neither my enemies nor my friends will find it an easy matter to transplant me again.

iv. SOCIETY AND LITERATURE

> Humane Nature I always thought the most useful Object of humane Reason, and to make the consideration of it pleasant and entertaining I always thought the best Employment of humane Wit.
>
> POPE
> *The Spectator*, No. 408

THE Augustan sense of society, a society complex and varied but marked with unmistakable character, is one of its best sources of strength. To analyse this sense fully would be an exacting exercise in social psychology but a few plain aspects present themselves quite readily. Books, it is true, are not merely social products; they are written by men and women and are 'social' or 'individual' in degrees varying with the writer's nature. But literature was then strongly permeated by the corporate spirit of the age which affected subject-matter and style by conventions both deliberate and instinctive.

Literature has always dealt with social life. Is there then anything particular about its Augustan interests? Three points perhaps call for attention: first, that writers take as their main material man in society, not man as an individual soul faced with fateful metaphysical problems, or as a seeker for personal experience, an asserter of self; second, that man and society are shown in normal size and proportion, in normal concerns and aspirations, not as exceptional: and third, that the aspects of life treated in literature tend towards a family resemblance.

The first two of these characteristics mark the convergence of a general drift of opinion and social change. Stress was always being laid on man as a social rather than an individual person; in politics and religion dissension and separatism had been proved by experience to be disastrous, and the current set towards tolerance and co-operation. Man's religious duty came to seem not the beseeching of grace from a minatory God but the expression towards man of help and sympathy. Though economic policy was hard-headed, economic philosophy laid stress on collaboration and interdependence. Moreover, it is one of the main virtues of Augustan culture that it was all, practically speaking, within the comprehension of the normal intelligent person. This is no doubt a weakness when any real degree of expertness is desirable. But it meant that almost any subject was available for general discussion, and that a major part of one's social responsibilities was to be aware of and informed about current interests. Augustan society made knowledge readily available, and kept it still within the capacities of good normal intelligence. So letter-writing and conversation were among the arts of the age, signs of its social integration and of common interests widely shared. Its dominant literary forms were the essay, the novel, and satirical, moral or discursive poetry, forms which certainly can deal with the eccentric or unusual yet which as the Augustans used them are notable for their normality, without the vivacity and sensationalism of Elizabethan drama, the ingenuity of

Metaphysical poetry, the fancifulness of Caroline prose, or the subjective variety of the Romantics and Victorians.

The third characteristic concerns the familiar homogeneous impression writers give of their society. In the case of Augustan London, for instance, what impresses is not its magnitude but what seems, curiously enough, its small-town intimacy. To write so varied and vigorous a poem about modern London as Gay's *Trivia* and still preserve *Trivia*'s sense of a close-knit social world would be almost impossible. Social activity has increased, but it is that of megalopolis, of commercial, industrial or pleasure-seeking superhumanity. Lamb, Dickens and Thackeray could still convey the sense of community; modern writers like Virginia Woolf in *Mrs. Dalloway* can capture it but for familiar districts only. The intimacy that is strong in Gay, and fifty years later in Boswell and Johnson, has gone.

The industrial east, admittedly, was *terra incognita* to most writers, but then came the City with its well-understood activity and citizen-character, then the region of the law from the Temple to Gray's Inn, then the coffee-house-tavern-theatre area north of the Strand, then the fashionable district of St. James and Piccadilly, and Westminster with Parliament and the Abbey. The arts and society kept to the City and the regions west of it, and recurrently dealing with this familiar ground they create a sense of pattern and community of interest. *Trivia*, and Pope's satires, and Fielding's *Amelia*, and Johnson's *Life of Savage*, and Boswell's *Life of Johnson*, and dozens of other works, are portraits of a city on a human scale, with a complex sense of corporate activity but a significant prominence of personality. So, in miniature, is Swift's *Description of the Morning*, with its motley company of bawling itinerants who connect the Augustan scene with the brawling London of Jonson—mop-twirling housemaids, street-sweepers, bailiffs, duns, turnkeys, lagging satchel-swinging schoolboys, and prisoners slinking back to gaol after a night's freedom stealing for fees. This pattern of life re-appears in writer after writer until it is a stereotype ineffaceably impressing a familiar scene, a constant element in the experience of the generic Londoner.

Perpetually one seems to be part of a large but very real family. London provided an audience coherent enough to give writers an understood body of communal experience, expressed in the sharing of scandal, gossip, and allusion in a freely-comprehending way. This is clear in Steele and Addison, Pope and Swift, Defoe and Fielding, Johnson and Boswell, and particularly in Horace Walpole, in whose letters time and again one feels the social world of literate London bound together in a close linkage of experience. He relates for instance how the fourth Earl of Sandwich was nicknamed 'Jemmy Twitcher'. The Earl (for whom the portable snack was invented, since he would not stop gaming long enough to dine) had been a fellow-reveller with John Wilkes but in an unexpected burst of virtue supported the prosecution of Wilkes for an obscene poem, *An Essay on Woman*. The town took this for hypocrisy, and as *The Beggar's Opera* was being performed at Covent Garden the audience burst into applause at Macheath's line about a treacherous colleague—'That Jemmy Twitcher should 'peach me I own surprises me'—and applied the name to Sandwich, 'almost to occasion the disuse of his title' (*Memoirs of the Reign of George III*, 1894, i. 249). Such theatrical episodes are not uncommon; a sensational one is recorded of Drury Lane in 1820, when George IV had failed to get his marriage to Queen Caroline annulled, and the audience cheered the line in which Emilia castigates Othello— 'What should such a fool do with so good a wife?' This communal cohesion is still strong, especially among pantomime, music-hall, and repertory-theatre audiences, and the wireless has enormously extended its range. The Augustan sense, however, is not that of nationwide demotic culture but of a circle of initiates (mostly in London), large enough not to be a coterie yet not so large as to lose definition in an amorphous mass—in other words, a community of 'common readers' (Johnson's court of appeal) or common spectators, knowledgeable in the affairs of 'the Town', recognising nicknames and pseudonyms, initials and asterisks, as clues to notabilities, seizing allusions to character, morals, opinions, physiognomy, family history and public office, and even (showing its perspicacity) interpreting innocent comments as insinuations. The sense of community did not indeed unite the sea-dogs of Wapping and the exquisites of St. James's, but it made the citizens at least of the western half of town parts of a composite coherent picture. The writer could aim at an 'average man' of upper- rather than lower-middle-class level, supposedly a compound of mature knowledge, good sense, and judgment disciplined by worldly experience and (ideally) by classical and modern reading.

Literature, then, could be free with allusions within this considerable circle, free to refer itself to a definable and generally-held body of knowledge. It could also take its bearings among a number of accepted types, images, themes and conventions. Repeatedly one comes across the coquette, the prude, the harridan, the Gallican dandy, the sober citizen, the penniless hack, the bombastic bookseller, the young blood, the street wench, the corrupt politician, the honest merchant, the profligate, and so on. The list does not imply that the characterisations of Augustan literature were excessively limited, but at times the character-vogue of the seventeenth century seems merely to have taken on a larger flight; certain persons become familiar and recur in a series of family likenesses.

The same may be said of scenes and images. The garret-and-Grub-Street pattern is stable; so is the city-uproar of Ned Ward, Swift, Gay, Hogarth and others; so are the ingredients of the gossiping self-interested world which composes 'the Town'. Another pattern, that of social glitter, was set going perhaps by Restoration comedy and Congreve, certainly by Pope. He starts with the brilliance of *The Rape of the Lock* (first version 1712). He repeats the effects in a vision of Aurelia's heart (*The Guardian*, No. 106), full of 'Fans, Silks, Ribbonds, Laces, and many other Gewgaws which lay so thick together that the whole Heart was nothing else but a Toy-shop', a gay clutter of coaches-and-six, cards, church-going, play-house, the court, and pet animals. Gay then tries the same thing, more clumsily, in *The Fan* (1714: i. 111), and Lady Mary Wortley Montagu in *Town Eclogues* (1716), and so the pattern passes down the century, the social imagery, the light tone, the fans, laces, play-houses and play-things. Writers tread a familiar ground in these topics and attitudes. For a last illustration of social pattern, of accepted habits within a self-aware society, here is Horace Walpole writing on 29 December, 1763, to the Earl of Hertford, about the year's social round. Apart from its brilliance, many a pen between 1680 and 1830 might have written it, but the purpose in quoting it is to show the stability not so much of a literary mode as of the social scene accepted as pattern, life presenting itself in thoroughly-understood shape:

Posterity, who will know nothing of our intervals, will conclude that this age was a succession of events. I could tell them that we know as well when an event, as when Easter, will happen. Do but recollect these last ten years. The beginning of October, one is certain that everybody will be at Newmarket, and the Duke of Cumberland will lose, and Shafto [a well-known racing M.P.] win, two or three thousand pounds. After that, while people are preparing to come to town for the winter, the Ministry is suddenly changed, and all the world comes to learn how it happened, a fortnight sooner than they intended; and fully persuaded that the new arrangement cannot last a month. The Parliament opens; everybody is bribed; and the new establishment is perceived to be composed of adamant. November passes, with two or three self-murders and a new play. Christmas arrives; everybody goes out of town; and a riot happens in one of the theatres. The Parliament meets again; taxes are warmly opposed; and some citizen makes his fortune by a subscription. The opposition languishes; balls and assemblies begin; some master and miss begin to get together, are talked of, and give occasion to forty more matches being invented; an unexpected debate starts up at the end of the session, that makes more noise than anything that was designed to make a noise, and subsides again in a new peerage or two. Ranelagh opens, and Vauxhall; one produces scandal, and t'other a drunken quarrel. People separate, some to Tunbridge, and some to all the horse races in England; and so the year comes again to October.

The passage is long, but to shorten it would destroy its integral rhythm. As it is, it contains, beautifully suspended in its calendar of the year's circle, not only an individual but a generic flair for basic social reliability—'social' here in the narrow fashionable sense, but also widely applicable to Augustan life in no matter what circles.

Since social life was felt as a kind of pattern, men and women could be rendered in literature as beings with a fairly restricted range of attitudes and emotions, and with characters which might be extravagant and eccentric but were not particularly subtle or analytical. That is not to say that actual persons were thought of as stereotyped; the Briton prided himself on his individuality, and was as likely to be a nonconformist in behaviour as in faith. But the writer dealt much less in the analysis of individuals than in the portrayal of characters recognisable (even if eccentric) for their representative truth: that was in line with current critical doctrine. He worked moreover with generally-accepted frameworks both intellectually (in religion, philosophy and criticism) and socially (in the plotting of human relationships): he knew where he stood. To insist too much on uniformity would be misleading and would strengthen the common delusion that the Augustans lacked variety. But more than in any other period there were family resemblances between one writer and another, and agreement as to how literature was to treat its subjects and what in its various kinds it was for. A sign of this is the acceptance of literary forms—couplet, ode, blank verse, periodical essay, satirical poem, and so on—to be handled in much the same fashion (though with varying quality in the performance) by whoever practised them. Literature, like society, was a more orderly spectacle than at any other time; a certain general shape of behaviour, a certain general order stressing not the individual so much as the communal form, prompted art and literature to model themselves to comparatively set moulds. The degree to which critics repeated similar judgments, and poets reproduced each other's successes, seems surprising until one appreciates the strength of this sense of community, and the sense too that experience had evolved the 'right' forms, and the 'right' treatment of accepted subjects. Literature reflected a society fairly stable in structure and expectations.

Characterisation, then, is exercised largely in formulas, sharply outlined with something like the vitality of caricature, and filled with well-understood features. What the novelist, dramatist, essayist or poet does with these type-portraits—the prude, learned lady, pedantic doctor or lawyer, brutal squire or pedagogue, errant but lively hero—is to draw them with such graphic phrase, to animate them with such distinctive action, that they are as real as one could desire, though the reality is less psychologically skilful than in more modern writing. Augustan literary characters can be great figures, but their power comes from the fact that they are not subtly-understood individuals but representatives of a type, with a kind of collective force. Robinson Crusoe is any sensible castaway, psychologically simple but grasped firmly enough in his simplicity to represent not merely himself but his nation (John Bull, we recall, is himself an Augustan character, the typical Englishman of Arbuthnot's *Law is a Bottomless Pit*) and its spirit of practical adventure coloured by religious earnestness. Moll Flanders is any shrewd adventuress, very much a person yet with a composite and representative quality. Trulliber is any pig-breeding Hodge of a farmer-parson; Jonathan Wild any cowardly master-crook; Sir Charles Grandison and Lord Orville the type-figures of wealthy gentlemen; Sir Anthony Absolute, Sir Lucius O'Trigger, Tom Jones and Charles Surface, Lady Teazle, Lady Booby, and Mrs. Malaprop are, respectively, the typical peppery parent, fiery Irishman, good-hearted rake, country-girl-turned-lady-of-fashion, imperious mistress, and deranger of epitaphs. They are representative members of their species, though much better than average: they are their species raised to its best.

Original conceptions took second place to accepted practice. With reservations (for there are Swift, Richardson and Sterne to remember) it is generally true that the Augustan scene is crowded with figures whose quirks have a familiar air: Hogarth's subjects, for instance, however grotesque, render what a weary debauchee, a sleeping congregation, or a crowd of cock-fighters representatively is. Such portraits do not lack life, but it is life in an understood frame, not in the more complex relationships of the nineteenth and twentieth centuries. Much of it is in the old manner of comedy, hearty, popular, insular and traditional. Even some of the exceptions may be less exceptional than they seem: *Gulliver's Travels*, for instance, though highly original in its effects, recognises even by ironic dissection the accepted patterns of government, morals and conventions—it recalls the accepted order even in riddling it; and

Pamela, novel in its introspection, yet applies that introspection to the accepted types of squire and village maiden.

Much Augustan writing, then, gives us portraits and actions in an accepted mode, just as do most of its portrait paintings and conversation pictures. For that reason the greatest novelist, Fielding, is less an individual artist than the voice of his time. As Spenser's all-inclusive composition reflects the omnivorous Elizabethan mind, so Fielding's broad knowledge and firmly-made characters (even when, as with Adams, Western, Pounce and others, their basis may be in particular persons) reflect his age's firm comprehension of life, and result in the assured 'placing' of his picture's components. The journalists, too, like Steele and Addison, rectify the foibles of their time not by a revolutionary conception of man and society but strictly in terms of the acknowledged ideals of the age. The same assurance shows itself in Pope's authoritative ordering of social and literary values, Goldsmith's and Sheridan's comedy of manners (with everything settled in the name of mellow good sense), and the whole tone and content—different from Pope, Goldsmith and Sheridan as they are—of Johnson's literary and moral philosophy. Even Swift's destructiveness is, with a few exceptions, the outcome of a wish to disentangle from bigotry and hypocrisy a healthily-conservative state of society.

If much in the age suggests a society stratified by rank, yet the better minds penetrate through rank to the humanity beneath. Swift, Defoe, Pope, Gay, Hogarth, Fielding and Johnson, for instance, observe society high and low conforming to the same morals. Roxana, Defoe's 'Fortunate Mistress', plays her cards to keep a precarious station in the affections of men, just as the great Harley, Godolphin, and Walpole play theirs in the game of statecraft. Moll Flanders struggles for life with the only commodity she has—sex—just as the politicians struggle for power with their only (and no more moral) commodity, patronage. Defoe, the tribune of the people, is a great leveller because he shows the rough-and-tumble of existence all men are involved in. Coleridge recognised this: Defoe's excellence, he said, 'is to make me forget my specific class, character and circumstances and to raise me, while I read him, into the universal man' (*Lectures of 1818*, in *Literary Remains*, 1836, i. 189). Swift, though a Tory, gives no credit to rank as such—a Lord Wharton is a disgrace to his species, and *Gulliver's Travels* levels all mankind. In Gay's *Beggar's Opera*, Peachum, Lockit and Macheath equate the mercenary treachery of their underworld with that of Walpole and 'statesmen': Fielding's *Jonathan Wild* deliberately parallels the 'great man' dispensing rewards and punishments in the underworld of the gaol, and the Prime Minister doing the same thing at Cabinet level. This difference of planes and identity of motives is congenial material for satire. Writing on *The Beggar's Opera* in *Some Versions of Pastoral* (1935) Professor Empson suggests that a stratified society needs works of art which break down the stratification and show men as really the same. Augustan stratification was not rigid, yet to have writers and artists (like Hogarth) promoting a sense of unity across the class-structure was healthy. It is as though society were a cone standing on its base, with social ranks marked by lines scored round it at different heights. Viewed from the side it shows each rank as higher or lower, narrower or wider, than the others, but viewed from above or beneath it shows only concentric rings, less or more extensive but all seemingly on the same level. Gay and Swift, Hogarth and Fielding, do something like that—they enable the reader to see each level as essentially the same thing, centred on the same point. The purpose is of course ironic, and not serious objective sociology. But insofar as society is healthy or corrupt, moved by honour or deceit, it is so at each level, and one looks at the cone again from the side with a renewed sense that although each class has a different altitude in society all classes are part of a unity. In an unsatiric way Johnson's poems, essays and *Rasselas* do the same thing, and Gray's *Elegy* too: Miltons vocal and glorious, or mute and inglorious, Cromwells guilty or guiltless of their country's blood, are the same kind of man.

Augustan writing, then, is soberly humanistic, dealing with men in society (their resorts, enterprises, occupations and opinions) and in relation to their moral and social duties. Poets, as Professor Sutherland has said in *A Preface to Eighteenth-Century Poetry*

(1948), wrote poems rather than poetry, the finite social object rather than the indefinite personal emotion, pieces often justified mainly by their good craftsmanship, like the furnishings of a Georgian house. Both their styles and their subjects were largely matters of common acceptance. The scenes of town life—news, theatres, the streets, visiting, gaming, politics, 'singing, laughing, ogling and all that'—and of the country—its pleasures, activities, the beauty of its views, and its benefit to mind and body—these topics, abundantly treated in poems, essays, novels and letters (it is the first great age of letter-writing) reflect society still under control, still run by man as a normal-scale being, not as multi-millionaire, industrial tycoon, totalitarian despot or efficient bureaucrat, and still (despite surface flurries) giving no cause for fundamental alarm. It was, we have concluded, in some ways limited in the experience it undertook to express in the arts; but its sense of being sure of itself, of knowing how men should address each other, on what subjects and in what styles, gave a striking certainty to the expression of what it wrote, to the portraits it drew of men and women, to the actions it put them through, and to its idea of the world they lived in. The houses they built, the furnishings they made, the paintings they produced, the philosophy they evolved, the connoisseurship they propounded in taste and morals, the enthusiasm they felt in an expanding national life, and the literature they created—these things suggest that Augustan society with all its imperfections was a sterling collective achievement of the British people.

II. THE WORLD OF BUSINESS

i. NATIONAL EXPANSION AND NATIONAL PRIDE

The present and future grandeur, fame, riches and happiness of Great Britain depend so entirely on the ingenuity, industry and commercial spirits of its inhabitants, and on the wisdom of its legislature, that no study seems more important than that which tends to convey proper ideas of those most essential subjects, Commerce, Politics and Finances.

THOMAS MORTIMER
Elements of Commerce (1772)

To relate literature to economic life is to enter a jungle of controversy. In one view, a writer's sole concern with his economic world is that he shall not starve; in another, he is its product nearly as much as a cloth is that of a loom. Discreet rather than valiant, the present chapter limits itself to the fact that many Augustan writers were interested in economic affairs; around them they saw business affecting their world for good or ill (good, they concluded, on the whole), and helping to create a philosophy typical of the age. These pages will try to describe that business and that philosophy.

The prevalent mood may first be sampled at random. In the 21st *Spectator* Addison congratulates his countrymen on the activity of their trade, which makes all men useful; the professions are liable to overcrowding but trade increases with the increasing numbers of participants, and merchant ships open up markets wherever they sail. *The Guardian* (No. 76) sees in trade a force of unity because it enriches both businessmen and their rivals the landed gentry. Unity was a frequent theme; commerce clearly fostered interdependence. It was part of Heaven's plan, Pope declared in the *Essay on Man*, that the individual should need his fellows' help, so that 'one man's weakness grows the strength of all', and this providential disposition was true of commercial as well as of social life. In *Liberty*, a very Whiggish poem on the prosperous effects of constitutional government, Thomson pronounced it Britain's mission

> *Instead of treasure robb'd by ruffian War,*
> *Round social Earth to circle fair exchange,*
> *And bind the nations in a golden chain.*
> (iv. 436-8)

The Fleece (1757), Dyer's Georgic on the wool trade, observes how the globe

> *Is now of commerce made the scene immense,*
> *Which daring ships frequent, associated*
> *Like doves or swallows, in th' aetherial flood,*
> *Or like the eagle, solitary seen.*
> (iv. 168-71)

And Mallet's *Amyntor and Theodora* (1747) proclaims it Heaven's wish

> *With ev'ry wind to waft large commerce on,*
> *Join pole to pole, consociate sever'd worlds,*
> *And link in bonds of intercourse and love*
> *Earth's universal family.*
> (i. 165-8)

The Augustans were sure that such comprehensive ministration to human needs must strengthen human brotherhood; commerce, Adam Smith said in one of their philosophical classics, brings both individuals and nations into co-operation and harmony. Gain indeed entered into this ministration but not so coarsely as to tarnish the brightness of co-operation; a man seeking his own profit, Adam Smith believed, is led insensibly to promote the welfare of others, by a providence as wise in economic as in physical science.

Satisfaction, then, on the whole prevails; the idea of prosperity kindles the imagination. Thomson's *Castle of Indolence* (1748) is only the most engaging of many tributes to enterprise. The villain of this romance is the wizard Indolence (an appealing character, it must be admitted), luxuriating in his 'pleasing Land of Drowsy-hed' until routed by the paragon 'Sir Industry', a strenuous apostle of hard work who galvanises Britain 'to freedom apt and persevering pains' (II. xx):

> *Then Towns he quicken'd by mechanic Arts,*
> *And bade the fervent City glow with Toil;*
> *Bade social Commerce raise renowned Marts,*
> *Join Land to Land, and marry Soil to Soil;*
> *Unite the Poles, and without bloody Spoil*
> *Bring home of either* Ind *the gorgeous Stores;*
> *Or, should Despotic Rage the World embroil,*
> *Bade Tyrants tremble on remotest Shores,*
> *While o'er th'encircling Deep* BRITANNIA'S *Thunder roars.*

Britain having become a paradise of cheerful labour, Sir Industry retires to a country life. But Indolence once more spreads his enchantments, and the hero is compelled to final exertions which banish the magician and rescue his victims. It is an improving moral in the true spirit of militant busy-ness. Defoe, who might have been born to the role of Sir Industry himself, is not less zealous; trade and civilisation he considers almost synonymous, and he contrasts the uncommercial backward Turks with the commercial progressive Venetians. 'The commerce of England', he observes, 'is an immense and almost incredible thing'; trade awakens every corner of the land (*A Plan of the English Commerce*, 1927, 65):

> the Villages stand thick, the Market Towns not only more in Number but larger and fuller of Inhabitants; and in short, the whole Country full of little End-ships or Hamlets and scattered Houses, that it looks all like a planted Colony, every where full of People, and the People every where full of Business.

His *Essay on Projects* (1697) abounds in commercial proposals, and the Augustans' practical interests were furthered during the eighteenth century by encyclopedias of the arts and sciences, and columns of useful suggestions in journals like *The Gentleman's Magazine*.

This chapter will deal mostly with change and progress, but a counterpoise may well be proffered at the outset. Change and progress catch the eye, yet they are not the whole of Augustan economics, and while patriotic enthusiasts naturally celebrated the nation's expansion the great majority of men found the rhythms and occupations of their lives continuing with little change. For nine out of ten, especially in small towns and unenclosed country districts, things went on as before, calling for traditional skill and method but seldom requiring a new outlook. For these men the substance of life was established and traditional practice, the familiar modes of farming or trade, the accepted custom and occupation. Since observers generally noticed the new rather than the old, this chapter stresses the emergent rather than the persistent features of life, and compresses into a few pages the gradual changes of a century. But the background to many a diary, novel, and poem is the sense of unhurried ways, the old life persisting behind the newly-enclosed fields, rising factories, larger merchantmen, busier ports, smoother roads and reticulating canals. Much of Augustan writing took its steady unexcited pace from the predominance of tradition.

That being said, what strikes the attention is innovation. Interest was widespread in the fostering of enterprise. After the 1688 revolution it was Parliament rather than King and Court which tried to control economic life, until Adam Smith made *laisser-faire* the fashion. Most M.P.s were concerned for their own prospects and those of friends and constituents, and since, under the later Stuarts and Queen Anne, most of them though themselves gentry sat for boroughs the interests of country and town were not unbalanced. One of the things best known about Sir Robert Walpole is that he directed his policies to prosperous trade; at the beginning of his long ministry the King's Speech of 19 October, 1721, sounded the key-note (*Collection of Parliamentary Debates*, vii. 1740):

> In this situation of affairs, we should be extremely wanting to our selves, if we neglected to improve the favourable opportunity which this general tranquillity gives us, of extending our commerce upon which the riches and grandeur of this nation chiefly depend. It is very obvious, that nothing would more conduce to the obtaining so public a good, than to

make the exportation of our own manufactures, and the importation of the commodities used in the manufacturing of them, as practicable and easy as may be; by this means, the balance of trade may be preserved in our favour, our navigation increased, and greater numbers of our poor employed.

The Whigs traced Britain's prosperity ultimately to 1688, when toleration replaced bigotry, and proximately to Walpole; Savage's *Epistle* to him celebrates Britain's happiness under his liberal rule:

> *Abroad the merchant, while the tempests rave,*
> *Advent'rous sails, nor fears the wind and wave;*
> *At home untir'd we find th'auspicious hand* [*i.e.* of Liberty]
> *With flocks and herds and harvests bless the land* . . .
> *Thus stately cities, statelier navies rise,*
> *And spread our grandeur under distant skies.*
>
> (187–98)

Such satisfaction was increasingly widespread.

The London merchants, by lending the Treasury £200,000, had enabled William of Orange to meet his immediate expenses against James II, and their influence over the monarchy was strengthened when in 1694 the Bank of England was founded, for the Bank could place its resources behind a constitutional king and withdraw them from an absolute one. It was a major instrument of policy, encouraging trade by extending credit to those who could profit by it, and it was also an instrument of Whiggism, suiting the Whigs' constitutional politics and disturbing the Tories' tenderness for royal supremacy. The Whigs' fondness for it is reflected in the third *Spectator* (by Addison). Mr. Spectator looks into 'the great hall where the Bank is kept' and falls into a daydream, in which 'a beautiful virgin seated on a throne of gold' appears in a room hung with Acts of Parliament (guarantees of constitutional government) and particularly with Magna Carta and the Acts of Uniformity, of Toleration and of Settlement. The lady—Public Credit—periodically swoons and revives, and the entry of certain 'most hideous phantoms' afflicts her with dangerous collapse. These are the old

Whig bogies (in antithetical pairs) of Tyranny and Anarchy, Bigotry and Atheism, Republicanism and Absolute Monarchy. Happily a sextet of 'very amiable phantoms' is at hand to restore her, namely Liberty and Monarchy, Moderation and Religion, and the Elector of Hanover (this was in 1711, before George's accession) with 'the Genius of Great Britain'—a sight so agreeable that Mr. Spectator awakes from his reverie in a transport of joy.

The founding of the Bank was only the most significant of many Parliamentary activities in business. As had always been the case laws were propounded for all kinds of operations—to pay bounties on corn exports, to prevent the importation of Indian textiles, to promote timber and naval supplies from North America instead of the Baltic, to develop Greenland whaling, to subsidise the building of large ships, and so on. Treaties contained commercial clauses, as a natural result of wars fought largely for commercial reasons. The Methuen Treaty (1703) diverted Augustan wine-drinkers from burgundy to port, by admitting Portuguese wines at a lower duty than the French, in exchange for larger Portuguese purchases of British cloth. Shippers envious of the Spanish American slave trade helped to involve England in the War of the Spanish Succession (1701–13), and the famous 'Asiento' clause in the Treaty of Utrecht (1713) gave Britain the monopoly of carrying slaves to South America. Spain's later transfer of the Asiento to a French company contributed to Britain's entering the War of the Austrian Succession from 1742, and rivalry with the French was acute in eastern and western hemispheres. In this perpetual concern for commercial advantage or colonial expansion there was a great deal to agitate Parliament, newsmongers, military men, traders, and even poets, with an agreeable ferment. It was a living spectacle of unruly growth, and writers treated it not as a 'literary' theme but as an urgent concern to be influenced one way or another.

The case of the South Sea Bubble is symptomatic. The South Sea Company's shares rose nearly ninefold in three months (April to July, 1720) and then fell even more rapidly. Defoe comments on the Bubble's calamitous effects on county families obliged to sell their estates (*Tour*, i. 90, 159, 169). But City investors suffered no less, except, as Gay put it (*Fables*, xxxv), for certain

> *Proud rogues, who shar'd the* South-Sea *prey,*
> *And sprung like mushrooms in a day.*

Swift let fly a satirical ballad, *The Bubble* (1721), which, like the public, equated the directors with 'a savage race by shipwrecks fed', malevolently waiting on 'Garraway's cliffs' (the business was done at Garraway's coffee-house) to strip the bodies of their victims:

> *Ye wise Philosophers explain*
>   *What Magick makes our Money rise*
> *When dropt into the Southern Main,*
>   *Or do these Juglers cheat our Eyes?*
>
> *Put in Your Money fairly told;*
>   *Presto be gone—'Tis here ag'en,*
> *Ladyes and Gentlemen, behold,*
>   *Here's ev'ry Piece as big as ten . . .*
>
> *As Fishes on each other prey*
>   *The great ones swall'wing up the small*
> *So fares it in the* Southern *Sea*
>   *But* Whale Directors *eat up all.*

Revenge was inevitable, though in his *Autobiography* Gibbon, whose grandfather as a director was fined more than nine-tenths of his fortune by an irate Parliament, temperately suggests that it went too far. But what inflated the Bubble was more important than the Bubble itself; circles hitherto immune were taking an interest in business and suffering from economic growing pains. To quote Swift again (*The Run upon the Bankers*, 1720):

> *Money, the Life-blood of the Nation,*
>   *Corrupts and stagnates in the Veins,*
> *Unless a proper Circulation*
>   *Its Motion and its Heat maintains.*

Joint-stock financing enabled inexperienced investors to speculate; ignorance, fluctuation, greed for profit, and anger at losses were consequently too frequent. But money was circulating and maintaining its motion and heat. The Bubble with its smaller and crazier constellated bubbles was more than mere deception, intentional or not; it was a sign that business was becoming a popular pursuit.

It is now time, after these samples of public interest, to outline the development of economic life. The eighteenth century's changes were far less violent than those of the nineteenth, yet they were striking enough. They affected agriculture and industry, and trade at home and abroad. Farming must first be considered—'the parent of all other arts' as Thomas Mortimer calls it—and then its pushful rivals industry and commerce.

ii. CHANGE IN THE COUNTRY

Rich is thy Soil, and merciful thy clime;
Thy Streams unfailing in the Summer's Drought,
Unmatch'd thy Guardian-oaks; thy Valleys float
With golden Waves; and on thy Mountains Flocks
Bleat numberless; while, roving round their Sides,
Bellow the blackening Herds in lusty Droves.

JAMES THOMSON
Summer (1730), 538–43

THE changes of eighteenth-century farming centre upon 'the enclosures', the regrouping of the traditional strips of land distributed over a whole parish into the fields and farms of today, a development which largely transformed the face of England and was recognised from the beginning (which goes back to the later Middle Ages) as a most notable instance of social change. The old system had held from time immemorial throughout the arable districts of England—that is, through much of the east, south and midlands, the west and north being mostly pasture. By it, each parish, instead of being divided into compact areas centring on a number of farms, was partitioned into great fields (usually two, three or four), in each of which the villager occupied certain narrow strips scattered here and there. Though the strips were occupied by different men, by natural practice most of those in one field grew the same crop at the same time; under the three-field system, which is the easiest to describe, one field in turn lay fallow, one grew mainly a spring corn such as barley, and one mainly a winter corn such as wheat. Beyond the cultivation there lay whatever rough grazing there might be in the vicinity, and the villagers had communal rights upon it. The system obtained through much of Europe from the Middle Ages onwards, and though in Tudor England wealthy landowners turned much arable into pasture (thus bringing strip-cultivation to an end), and though more enclosure took place under the Stuarts, the old pattern still predominated in 1700 over the Midlands particularly, and even in 1800 was by no means extinct.

Generally speaking it gave every man a chance. Some chances were better than others, and some villagers became richer than others. But since everyone by and large did the same thing at the same time, working similar strips distributed over the same fields, the chance for variation was small. So too was the chance for improvement; no one man could do much to better his methods or suit his own tastes. The change from one system to the other meant that the traditional way of life on which an understood (though very conservative) pattern of country society had grown up was transformed by a revolution, and an agriculture of communal habit gave place to one of individual enterprise. The 'revolution' was spread over three centuries, and its violence thereby mitigated, but though change was not in the eighteenth century a novelty the pace of change greatly accelerated, and enclosure instead of being a voluntary agreement was often imposed from above by the larger landowners, with effects amounting to a social upheaval.

Two important classes of men disliked the old system. One was that of the traditional landed proprietors who, since land was the most obvious form of concentrated wealth, bore most of the country's taxation and therefore hoped to increase their revenues. The other was that of rich men, mostly in business, who invested money in land rather than in stocks or industry. Retiring from 'social commerce' like 'Sir Industry' they bought estates. Weary of the vicissitudes of trade, Sir Andrew Freeport takes leave of town and acquires 'a fine spread of improvable lands' which he proposes to drain, plough and plant (*The Spectator*, No. 549). In short, he says,

as I have my share in the surface of this island, I am resolved to make it as beautiful a spot as any in her majesty's dominions; at least there is not an inch of it which shall not be cultivated to the best advantage, and do its utmost for its owner.

Not unlike him is Mr. Charwell in *The Guardian* (No. 9), a London merchant who founds a flourishing estate in an undeveloped countryside, in a spirit which Defoe would have applauded. Robinson Crusoe too, after returning from his island,

bought a little Farm in the County of *Bedford*, and resolv'd to remove myself thither. I had a little convenient House upon it, and the Land about it I found was capable of great Improvement, and that it was in many Ways suited to my Inclination, which delighted in Cultivating, Managing, Planting and Improving of Land.
Farther Adventures of Robinson Crusoe (1927), ii. 116

To the great landowner, 'improvement' was a personal pleasure and national duty, a gratifying responsibility embodied in Pope's lines:

> *Who then shall grace, or who improve the Soil?*
> *Who plants like Bathurst, or who builds like Boyle.*
> *'Tis Use alone that sanctifies Expence,*
> *And Splendour borrows all her rays from Sense.*
>
> *His Father's Acres who enjoys in peace,*
> *Or makes his Neighbours glad, if he encrease,*
> *Whose chearful Tenants bless their yearly toil,*
> *Yet to their Lord owe more than to the soil;*
> *Whose ample Lawns are not asham'd to feed*
> *The milky heifer and deserving steed;*
> *Whose rising Forests, not for pride or show,*
> *But future Buildings, future Navies grow:*
> *Let his plantations stretch from down to down,*
> *First shade a Country, and then raise a Town.*
> *Epistle to Burlington*, 177-90

Yet these ambitions could be fulfilled only by abolishing the old system. A petition to enclose land was normally presented to Parliament, signed by the owners of three-quarters or more of the territory (who might in fact be a small minority or even—though rarely—one person). The petition usually became an Act of Parliament and commissioners were appointed to redistribute the land in compact lots corresponding to the value of the strips each owner surrendered. In general, it seems, the commissioners really tried to ensure a just exchange, yet the smaller men were inevitably squeezed out, either at once or within a few years. They found themselves with very small farms indeed, which they had to hedge, drain and equip, while the commons which had provided free grazing were also enclosed for cultivation. This was the death-blow to the independent 'bold peasantry, their country's pride', who on small farms unsupported by common pastures could not make a living as they had done, on the whole, under the old system. They were far more vulnerable than bigger men: bad weather, crop-failures, and falling prices were misfortunes which could be absorbed by the resources of a large but not of a small estate. The middling owners—small gentry, richer yeomen, larger tenant farmers—survived because the land was more productive. But the smallholder and even more the cottager who needed the commons for subsistence lost irremediably, sank to the status of a labourer, or drifted into the new factory towns.

The balance of good and ill in the process of enclosure is still a matter of argument and was so more urgently then. In some districts productivity multiplied and employment abounded; in East Anglia, for instance, much common was put under plough, and labour was in demand. In others, arable yielded to pasture, and labour was less needed; this was generally so in the Midlands, where great areas were grassed and many small farms absorbed into larger ones needing fewer hands. Arthur Young's *Inquiry into the Maintenance and Propriety of applying Wastes to the Better Support of the Poor* (1801) spoke bitterly for the deprived labourer:

Go to an ale-house kitchen of an old inclosed country, and there you will see the origin of poverty and poor-rates. For whom are they to be sober? For whom are they to save? (Such are their questions). For the parish? If I am diligent, shall I have leave to build a cottage? If I am sober, shall I have land for a cow? If I am frugal, shall I have half an acre for potatoes? You offer no motives; you have nothing but a parish officer and a work-house!—Bring me another pot!

Goldsmith's *Traveller* (1764) and *The Deserted Village* (1770) are the best-known reflections of enclosure's harsher side. The former castigates that greed for power or money which 'breaks the social tie' (397-404):

> *Have we not seen, round Britain's peopled shore,*
> *Her useful sons exchang'd for useless ore?*
> *Seen all her triumphs but destruction haste,*
> *Like flaring tapers brightening as they waste?*
> *Seen Opulence, her grandeur to maintain,*
> *Lead stern Depopulation in her train,*
> *And over fields where scatter'd hamlets rose*
> *In barren solitary pomp repose?*

The Deserted Village, in words as familiar as proverbs, presents a landscape which 'blooms a garden and a grave', where 'one only master grasps the whole domain'. Whether Goldsmith's protest had a general or only a limited validity was in dispute; his prefatory letter to Sir Joshua Reynolds anticipated the criticism that depopulation was merely a figment of his mind, by avouching that his picture was drawn from recent observation. Indeed, it would be true of many parts of the enclosed Midlands, though his reverie of a ruined paradise was certainly idealisation. Whatever the poem's precise value as 'truth', it expresses a haunting regret, oversentimental as Crabbe was to complain, but sentimental with such sincere affection that it recommends itself more truly than any verdict of accurate sociology.

Despite some unhappy consequences, enclosures and reclamations, both by redistribution of open fields and cultivation of waste lands, were desirable; much of the country had hitherto been largely useless. It is after all better to farm well than badly, to improve herds and crops than to persevere with poor strains, to reclaim wastes than to persist in the apathy of custom. Some improvers, like Jethro Tull (1674-1741), Lord Townshend (1674-1738), Robert Bakewell (1725-95) and Coke of Holkham (1754-1842) are famous. But as with the inventors whose machines revolutionised industry their successes grew out of obscure work by many predecessors and contemporaries, and while modern research confirms them in their pre-eminence it recalls too the widely collaborative nature of the movement. Impressive as might be the spectacle of a few lonely innovators, that of general experiment is still more so, even though for each improver there were scores of traditionalists, yielding only reluctantly to the logic of events. The greatest publiciser of the new movement was perhaps Coke of Holkham; he indefatigably held meetings and demonstrations to convince the sceptical, and assembled his annual 'Sheep-shearings' like agricultural congresses to draw visitors from all over Britain and from abroad. Good farming was his passion, quite apart from its profitableness, though indeed good farming far from minimising profit multiplied the rental of his Norfolk estates tenfold, increased Holkham's population from two hundred to a thousand, and rendered superfluous its previously full poor-house. Less remarkably elsewhere but steadily the countryside developed towards fertility and its present orderly landscaping of trim farms and hedged fields. Wet lands were drained, so that, as Dyer somewhat preposterously observes (*The Fleece*, ii. 162-3):

> *Moors, bogs and weeping fens may learn to smile,*
> *And leave in dykes their soon-forgotten tears.*

Sandy soils and poor pastures enriched, root crops introduced for food and for a cleaner ground, and livestock improved—these were processes in which Nature provided the raw material, man the art. The pace of progress, slow from the Middle Ages, quickened rapidly in an age which applied to agriculture the experimental methods of science and the ambition of individual enterprise. In the upshot the country fed more people better than before (the population of England and Wales rose from five-and-a-half millions to nine between 1700 and 1800) and avoided starvation in the Napoleonic Wars.

CHANGE IN THE COUNTRY

This activity stimulated the writing of descriptive tours. Defoe's and Arthur Young's are the most famous, to be followed in the next century by Cobbett's *Rural Rides*, but they are only the most eminent of many. Some, like those of William Gilpin, who was in search of 'picturesque' beauty, rather deprecated cultivation, preferring an ungroomed countryside and (like the Dutch painters) finding in its roughness a source of pleasure. But more numerous were those who approved; the Augustans naturally took pleasure in signs of activity and success. The supreme approver is Defoe, and though he wrote when agricultural development was not fully under way his account has a full measure of the right spirit. The 'vast quantity' of sheep in Kent and on the Downs; the Cotswolds 'so eminent for the best of sheep and finest wool in England'; the Midlands also notable for flocks, and Yorkshire and Lincolnshire too, with sea-transport to the manufacturing towns of Norfolk and Suffolk; the black Welsh cattle sent yearly to English markets; 'innumerable droves' in Lincolnshire, destined for London; fine herds along the East Anglian river-pastures and in Norfolk; wheat crops on the newly-fertilised Downs and on the rich lands of Gloucestershire, Warwickshire and Essex; corn-markets at Bedford and St. Albans; barley in the Eastern counties with markets and maltsters at Royston and Ware; fruit-growing in Kent and the West; cloth-weaving evolved from the wool-trade in Yorkshire, East Anglia, Shropshire and Devon; towns like Brentford, Ingatestone, and Chelmsford 'maintained by the excessive multitude of carriers and passengers who are continually passing this way to London, with droves of cattle, provision and manufactures'—all these are the themes of his travels through the Eastern and Home counties, the South Downs and Wessex, the Midlands and the North and West, his notebooks garnering comment. The light of modern statistics may shine rather coldly on his figures, but as with Goldsmith on depopulation Defoe is to be valued for his sentiments as much as his 'facts'. If his zeal paints too coloured a picture, the course of the century was to bring nearer the prosperity he praised.

iii. ASPECTS OF INDUSTRY

> The New Buildings erected, the Old Buildings taken down; New Discoveries in Metals, Mines, Minerals; new Undertakings in Trade; Inventions, Engines, Manufactures, in a Nation pushing and improving as we are: These Things open new Scenes every Day, and make England especially shew a new and differing Face in many Places, on every Occasion of surveying it.
>
> DEFOE
Tour, ii. 535

To do justice to eighteenth-century industry in less than a large volume is manifestly impossible, and the present aim is much humbler. It is, by a somewhat arbitrary glance at four industries—wool, iron, coal and pottery—to sense the national spirit which was active throughout the larger field of general industrial life, and to feel in miniature the confidence of that spirit.

The woollen industry makes a natural transition from farming to manufacture. Defoe travels through Wessex into Devon and notes the flannel-work of Salisbury—'the people gay and rich, and have a flourishing trade': he finds serge at Honiton, and Devon so busy with manufactures, so full of 'great towns and those towns so full of people' that he fancies there can be no equal county in England. The ships in his novels, incidentally, are never without their cargoes when outward-bound of serges, druggets and bays, to pay for the inward-bound freights of sugar, spices, silks and other luxuries. The industry slowly migrated during the century from south to north, but predominantly it remained as Defoe described it, mainly in the West country, East Anglia and the Pennine valleys. In the West, wool towns clustered along the Stroud valley and along the base of Dartmoor and the Cotswolds, where streams ran down to provide power. In East Anglia the industry centred on Norwich, where the big clothiers had their houses, and in the North it followed the rapid Pennine streams.

The main literary monument to this is Dyer's long work *The Fleece* (1757). Johnson disliked it, partly on the neo-classic grounds of 'the meanness naturally adhering, and the irreverence habitually annexed, to trade and manufacture', and quoted a quip to the effect that the aged author would be 'buried in woollen'. Yet *The Fleece* is a reasonably entertaining work and Wordsworth found a word of praise for it. Dyer shares Defoe's zeal for trade: he sees rivers crowded with barges, roads with carts, packhorses plodding, buildings rising, and fleets sailing all the seas. He ambles along under some of the heaviest poetic diction ever shouldered by an English poet, yet he remains alert to the country scene, often vivid in portraying it, and alive to natural interest. To describe a ram's forehead as

> *fenc'd*
> *With horns Ammonian, circulating twice*
> *Around each open ear, like those fair scrolls*
> *That grace the columns of th'Ionic dome*
> (i. 210–13)

may verge on the ludicrous, yet the lines convey not only a precise effect but an appropriate and almost heroic satisfaction. It is not at all ludicrous to write of

> *The ram short-limb'd, whose form compact describes*
> *One level line along his spacious back;*
> *Of full and ruddy eye, large ears, stretch'd head,*
> *Nostrils dilated, breast and shoulders broad,*
> *And spacious haunches, and a lofty dock.*
> (i. 220–4)

That is an admirable picture of a fine animal, done with the Augustan instinct for real things. Even when Dyer describes simple operations in learned language, the elaboration in itself adds something of baroque richness to a theme which gave him pleasure, and an ornamental opulence to a topic as plump as a fertile field. Here is Dyer not learned but clear and clean, observing a sunlit countryside:

> *See the sun gleams! the living pastures rise,*
> *After the nurture of the fallen shower*

> *How beautiful! how blue th'ethereal vault,*
> *How verdurous the lawns, how clear the brooks;*
> *Such noble warlike steeds, such herds of kine,*
> *So sleek, so vast; such spacious flocks of sheep,*
> *Like flakes of gold illumining the green,*
> *What other paradise adorn but thine*
> *Britannia? happy, if thy sons would know*
> *Their happiness.*
>
> (i. 163-72)

The Latin words—'nurture, ethereal, verdurous, spacious, illumining'—and the Virgilian reminiscence at the end, are enrichments, not encumbrances. Together with the details of colour, light and fostering life they create a splendid abundance and beauty.

Wool not only in its natural state but through all the processes of manufacture is his subject: 'houses of labour, seats of kind constraint' are to be built 'for those who now delight in fruitless sports'. Even now, the idle are informed,

> *Even now the sons of trade,*
> *Where'er their cultivated hamlets smile,*
> *Erect the mansion; here soft fleeces shine;*
> *The card awaits you, and the comb, and wheel.*
>
> (iii. 250-3)

Inside the mill he glows with a bland content:

> *By gentle steps*
> *Uprais'd, from room to room we slowly walk,*
> *And view with wonder and with silent joy*
> *The sprightly scene, where many a busy hand,*
> *Where spools, cards, wheels, and looms, with motion quick,*
> *And ever-murmuring sound, the unwonted sense*
> *Wrap in surprise. To see them all employed,*
> *All blithe, it gives the spreading heart delight.*
>
> (iii. 263-70)

Finally the cloth is despatched by wagon, packhorse and barge:

*Wide around
Hillock and valley, farm and village, smile;
And ruddy roofs and chimney-tops appear
Of busy Leeds, up-wafting to the clouds
The incense of thanks-giving: all is joy:
And trade and business guide the living scene,
Roll the full cars, adown the winding Aire
Load the slow-sailing barges, pile the pack
On the long tinkling train of slow-pac'd steeds.*
(iii. 306–14)

Dyer often provokes a smile, and the superior wisdom of hindsight can see that 'ruddy roofs up-wafting to the clouds The incense of thanks-giving' was soon to be a misleading impression of Leeds. Yet a certain magnanimity and pleasure in national prosperity make the grandiloquence not entirely absurd, and only a bold man would nowadays undertake to write a poem as long as *The Fleece*, grandiloquently or not, which would carry over two centuries an industrial panorama as agreeably as Dyer's does.

As for iron and coal, both industries were ancient but neither in 1700 was more than primitive. In the development of iron the moving spirit was a certain Abraham Darby, who set up a foundry in 1699 and in 1708 took over an old forge and furnace at Coalbrookdale on the Severn, a name henceforth to be historic. Smelting with coke instead of charcoal he ran the liquified ore into finer moulds and produced better cast iron. Members of the Darby dynasty spread the process to Wrexham in 1726 and expanded the industry in Coalbrookdale: in 1760 the Carron works, which have been outstanding ever since, were opened on the Carron River in Stirlingshire: by 1770 foundries had spread through Shropshire, Staffordshire, south Yorkshire and Clydesdale. The way was prepared for the technological revolution which the alliance of iron and steam-power made possible. Manufacturing towns began to take on a forbidding appearance: Defoe had noted Yorkshire as abounding in manufactures, and Sheffield as being 'very populous and large, the streets narrow, and the houses dark and black, occasioned by the continual smoke of the forges' (*Tour*, ii.

569). Dyer put the same thing in a Rembrandtesque chiaroscuro, describing

> the sounding caves
> Of high Brigantium [i.e. Sheffield], where, by ruddy flames,
> Vulcan's strong sons, with nervous arm, around
> The steady anvil and the glaring mass
> Clatter their heavy hammers down by turns,
> Flattening the steel.
>
> The Fleece, i. 556–61

Horace Walpole travelled through Leeds and Sheffield in 1756 and 1760 respectively, finding the former 'a dingy large town' and the latter 'one of the foulest towns in England'. His distaste and Dyer's pleasure are contemporaneous: art is a corner of nature seen through a temperament. Heavy industry was producing its by-product of squalor, and Blake was soon to contrast England's green and pleasant land with the dark satanic mills spreading upon it. Uvedale Price, an enthusiast for picturesque beauty, forthrightly denounced the desecration of the landscape; a century and a half has not made his protest obsolete (*Essays on the Picturesque*, 1810, i. 198):

> When I consider the striking natural beauties of such a river as that at Matlock, and the effect of the seven-story buildings that have been raised there, and on other beautiful streams, for cotton manufactures, I am inclined to think that nothing can equal them for the purpose of disbeautifying an enchanting piece of scenery; and that economy had produced what the greatest ingenuity, if a prize were given for ugliness, could not surpass.

Yet as will be suggested later (cf. pp. 83–4), the dramatic novelty and the visible benefits of the new technology gave a sense of confidence which eclipsed its disadvantages. As Matthew Boulton said when he took visitors round his Soho factory, 'I sell here what all men desire—power'.

Power depends on fuel, and coal entered into that collaboration with iron which has since seemed like one of the laws of nature. At the beginning of the century it was used to fire pumping-engines in the coal-mines themselves, later as coke for iron-smelting, and later again for every kind of operation. Two million tons of it were raised in 1700, five million in 1750, and over ten million in 1800.

Its poet, less eminent than Dyer, is the Reverend Thomas Yalden, friend of Addison despite extreme High-Toryism, Fellow of Magdalen, and incumbent of two Hertfordshire parishes. He gets a perfunctory notice in Johnson's *Lives of the Poets* and an interesting one in F. D. Klingender's *Art and the Industrial Revolution* (1947). In 1710 he wrote a poem *To Sir Humphry Mackworth on the Mines*. Mackworth, also a Tory, was under fire from the Whigs for allegedly defrauding investors in a mining company, and the poem was a demonstration in his favour. Yalden claims to be the first British bard to invite the Muse not to soar but to descend, and it must be admitted that she duly obliges. The result is an enthusiastic puff for the industry: we hear how Wales bulges into mountains because of her inward riches, how

> *all beneath deep as the centre shines*
> *With native wealth, and more than India's mines;*

how Dovey's waters shall outshine the wealth of Tagus; how the Welsh miner (an 'ancient Briton') is 'resolv'd to conquer tho' he combats death', and how

> *Night's gloomy realms his pointed steel invades,*
> *The courts of Pluto and infernal shades.*

Finally there is an outburst of patriotic jubilation meant no doubt to divert the House of Commons from the question of Mackworth's finances:

> *How are thy realms, triumphant Britain, blest;*
> *Enrich'd with more than all the distant West:*
> *Thy sons no more, betray'd with hopes of gain,*
> *Shall tempt the dangers of a foreign main,*
> *Traffic no more abroad for foreign spoil,*
> *Supplied with richer from their native soil*

(a forecast remarkably impercipient). Spain's trade will dwindle, Britain's swell, and prosperity lies waiting in the rocks.

It was not the poem but the fall of the Whigs in 1710 which saved Mackworth. But Yalden's verses, though they did not promote an extensive poetry of coal-mining, reflect the prevalent gratification at Britain's good fortune, gratification partly at man's skill, his subjugation of Nature's manifold and dangerous resources, his technological imagination and the heroic ingenuity of his inventiveness, but partly also of the kind that rings through Defoe, that Britain was outpacing her rivals and that prosperity might bring universal peace. These sentiments inspired Burke also: his *Observations on a Late Publication entitled 'The Present State of the Nation'* (1769) celebrates the prosperity of Yorkshire wool, the 'infinite variety of admirable manufactures' of Manchester, the busy-ness of Glasgow and Paisley, the Carron ironworks and the rising output of Sheffield, Birmingham and Wolverhampton.

The making of pottery, finally, is peculiarly significant since it unites the useful and the fine arts, and its leading figure represents the best qualities of his time. English pottery had been little more than a peasant art of crudely-painted earthenware, unsophisticatedly pleasant to the eye but lumpish in form and clumsy in use. Some improvements had recently come from Germany; John Philip Elers's red Staffordshire stoneware of about 1700 is a worthy anticipation of Wedgwood's work in its admirable texture and its formal shapes finely designed with classical discipline and grace. But it is Wedgwood himself (1730–95) who gave the industry greatness and whose accomplishment typifies the leadership not only in industry but also in good taste to which the ethical and aesthetic traditions of the century could prompt the practical humanist. Self-educated but widely read, he corresponded with writers and archaeologists (especially with Sir William Hamilton the ambassador at Naples) and undertook to revive the styles of classical antiquity. His art was not confined to luxury, for his Queens ware (named after Queen Charlotte) is ordinary Staffordshire cream pottery sufficiently improved to satisfy the rich and sufficiently cheap to serve the poor: one of his best qualities was the broad humanity which took the whole of his intellectual and social world for its province. Yet after all it is not his popular ware that best shows his genius but the superb taste which produced—or caused his designers to produce—the basaltes and jasper, the former with its severe but noble dull black, perhaps brightened with a coloured medallion, austere or graceful in line, statuesque or sculpturesque in form; the latter with its white decoration of impeccable classical motifs—plumes, garlands and figures at times almost microscopically minute yet perfect in grace and poise of line—shown against an immaculately smooth coloured ground. They are masterworks of technical brilliance directed by a taste at once refined, exacting and confident. Wedgwood was not the only maker of good pottery: from about 1750 the works at Bow, Chelsea and Derby turned out gay and graceful wares lively in line and brilliantly fresh in colour—applied art of a sparkling vivacity. But it was Wedgwood alone who produced an art not only of charm but of greatness. He was a firm but reasonable employer, politically advanced (he approved the American and French Revolutions) and a strong supporter of the Society for the Abolition of Slavery, for which he devised a medallion with a chained Negro and the legend 'Am I not a man and a brother?' Under the stimulus of his energy and imagination the pottery industry flourished and Staffordshire exported its products to Europe, the East and West Indies, and North America, with the results he indicates in an *Address to the Young Inhabitants of the Pottery* (1783):

I would request you to ask your parents for a description of the country we inhabit when they first knew it; and they will tell you, that the inhabitants bore all the marks of poverty to a much greater degree than they do now. Their houses were miserable huts; the lands poorly cultivated, and yielded little of value for the food of man or beast, and these disadvantages, with roads almost impassable, might be said to have cut off our part of the country from the rest of the world, besides rendering it not very comfortable to ourselves. Compare this picture, which I know to be a true one, with the present state of the same country. The workmen earning near double their former wages,—their houses mostly new and comfortable, and the lands, roads, and every other circumstance bearing evident marks of the most pleasing and rapid improvements. . . . Industry has been the parent of this happy change.

In that confident assertion one hears the voice of practical Augustanism finding that experimental science and co-ordinated skill could point man to an entirely new level of accomplishment. In the combined sense of personal achievement, national benefit and heightened civilisation the enterprising army of innovators found their faith.

iv. COMMUNICATIONS

> Every thing wears the Face of Dispatch; every Article of our Produce becomes more valuable; and the Hinge upon which all these Movements turn is the Reformation which has been made in our publick Roads.
>
> HENRY HOMER
> *Enquiry into the Means of Preserving and Improving the Public Roads of this Kingdom* (1767)

As Wedgwood says, the 'happy change' depended partly on 'pleasing and rapid improvements' in transport. While commerce largely relied on infrequent fairs (even if as protracted and popular as the Stourbridge Fair at Cambridge), while carriage was by pack-horse or wagon on bad tracks, the novelties of thought and practice could not far extend their stimulus. Eighteenth-century roads were not perhaps on the whole as bad as travellers alleged; had they been so, no-one other than a pedestrian would ever have journeyed anywhere save at the peril of his life. An anthology of complaints is not hard to compile; the bad is more readily blamed than the good is praised. Road-conditions varied with the weather and the means of transport; a dry day or season made things tolerable, and a horse could go easily where a coach would stick. But in general, travel was wearisome and unpredictable, and the spread of goods and ideas was hindered. Bad roads run through Defoe like a refrain—'dirty roads, scarce passable', 'the deepest, the dirtiest country', 'deep, stiff, full of sloughs', 'deep stiff clay'. When Arthur Young toured the North of England he found the roads even worse than elsewhere because of the strain industry was putting on them, and words failed him for that between Wigan and Liverpool—'I know not, in the whole range of language, terms sufficiently expressive to describe this infernal road'. The most striking evidence, perhaps, is that bad communications prevented the Hanoverian army for a long time from coming to grips with the Jacobites in 1745.

The alarm caused by that military hazard brought to a head the desire for better communications, and acts for the maintenance of highways passed through Parliament in rapidly-increasing numbers —over four hundred and fifty between 1760 and 1774. Road-making came to be considered, as Defoe said it should, 'more an honour and ornament to the country' than almost any other undertaking. Between the 1750s and 1780s the time taken between London and such towns as Birmingham, Bath, Manchester and Newcastle was curtailed by a half or even three-quarters, and by 1800 the mail-coach had entered on that brief glory which the railways were to extinguish. When Pastor Moritz landed at Dartford in 1782 he took a postchaise for London along 'incomparable' roads, 'so firm and solid', and enjoyed the experience:

> These carriages are very neat and lightly built, so that you hardly perceive their motion as they roll along these firm smooth roads. The horses are generally good, and the postilions particularly smart and active, and always ride on a full trot.
>
> *Travels in England*, 19

A lively sense of what this transformation meant can be gathered from the Reverend Henry Homer's *Enquiry*, quoted at the head of this section. Homer was rector of Birdingbury in Warwickshire and chaplain to Lord Leigh, the commissioner for two Warwickshire turnpikes. He describes the drawbacks of bad roads, the difficulty of distributing abundance or relieving scarcity, and 'the slow Progress which was formerly made in the Improvement of Agriculture', and then contrasts with it the transformation by which 'our very Carriages now travel with almost winged Expedition':

> There never was a more astonishing Revolution accomplished in the internal System of any Country, than has been within the Compass of a few Years in that of *England*. The Carriage of Grain, Coals, Merchandise,

&c. is in general conducted with little more than half the Number of Horses with which it formerly was. Journies of Business are performed with more than double Expedition. Improvements in Agriculture keep pace with those of Trade.

If roads made transport fast, canals made it cheap. The seventeenth century had started the process; the Aire and Calder rivers in Yorkshire, for instance, had been deepened at the instance of the clothiers of Leeds, Halifax and Wakefield, and joined by a canal with locks. From 1701 onwards the Trent and Derwent were dredged for the benefit of Nottingham and Derby, and from 1720 the Mersey. But the coal which was among the main commodities to be carried did not always lie conveniently for river carriage, and the story of how, instead of coal's being brought to the water, James Brindley between 1759 and 1761 brought water to the coal, for the Duke of Bridgewater's mines, is among the familiar pages of history. His success gave canal-digging an enormous impetus: the great London firm of Childs lent the Duke money to link his canal with the Mersey; noblemen eager for profitable investment joined in; Lord Anson and the Marquis of Stafford engaged Brindley to design the Grand Junction Canal between Mersey and Trent, and Wedgwood, whose heavy raw material and fragile manufactures alike needed water-carriage, became their treasurer and in 1766 cut the first sod of the system which opened up the Midlands and reached the Severn. Three thousand miles of canals were dug in the next thirty years.

The total consequences of better transport are incalculable. They include great material and great cultural benefits. That the quality of taste, among those capable of it, was higher in 1780 than in 1680 would be hard to prove beyond cavil, but that its dissemination, in an appreciation of good building, good furnishing, good painting and good writing was far more extensive admits of no question at all. In the cultural circumstances of the eighteenth (though not of the nineteenth) century, better communications made for an improvement in taste, not as an elegant superficiality but as an intelligent code of living. 'Good roads and postchaises', as Horace Walpole observed, were the agents of civilisation.

V. WIDER HORIZONS

The commercial spirit of the age hath also penetrated beyond the confines of Great Britain, and explored the whole continent of Europe; nor does it stop there, for the West Indies and the American world are intimately acquainted with the Birmingham merchant; and nothing but the exclusive command of the East-India Company over the Asiatic trade prevents our riders [*i.e.* agents] from treading upon the heels of each other, in the streets of Calcutta.

WILLIAM HUTTON
History of Birmingham (1781), 70

BEFORE the literary influence of economic life is assessed, there is one more facet, that of overseas trade, to be considered. It formed only a minute fraction of the nation's economy, yet by its exotic variety and its dependence on remote countries it worked potently on the imagination. Strictly speaking, economic and imaginative profits were inversely proportionate to each other; the interesting continents of Africa and Asia, and the island-strewn spaces of the Pacific, were powerful mental stimuli but comparatively small items in the financial balance-sheet; Europe and the American colonies, on the other hand, the main channels of overseas trade, were relatively familiar and unexciting. It was the distant rather than the nearer markets, the sources of romantic luxuries rather than of practical necessities, which broadened the mind's horizons.

The first development of these distant territories had been undertaken by bodies like the Levant and East India Companies, established in the sixteenth and seventeenth centuries. Long trading voyages were of course nothing new, but the competition for trade and trading-posts became increasingly intense. The Sir Andrew Freeports were prompt to secure free ports and other facilities for themselves, and often equally prompt to exclude others from them. The great explorations of Dampier (between 1675 and 1711), Anson (1740–4), Byron (1764–6), Wallis (1766–8) and Cook (1768–71, 1772–5, and 1776–9) were the most striking sign of this interest in remote countries, an interest bearing fruit in theories of

Noble Savages (encouraged by Wallis's discovery of Tahiti in 1767 and a more momentous visit there by the French Bougainville in 1768), Virtuous Orientals, and primitive or exotic societies in general, like the Madagascans in whose folkways Defoe shows an interest in *Captain Singleton*. Commerce brought into view new possibilities of life. The East in particular was a source of interest, the storehouse of strange and ancient civilisations. Through the great trading companies not only was Europe, like Pope's Belinda, decked with glittering spoil—

> *This casket India's glowing gems unlocks,*
> *And all Arabia breathes from yonder box—*

but ethical and aesthetic novelties accompanied material luxuries with effects on taste to be described later (cf. pp. 96–7). Tickell's lines *On the Prospects of Peace* (1713) bring into view these new panoramas (238–45):

> *Fearless our merchant now pursues his gain,*
> *And roams securely o'er the boundless main;*
> *Now o'er his head the polar Bear he spies,*
> *And freezing spangles of the Lapland skies;*
> *Now swells his canvas to the sultry line,*
> *With glitt'ring spoils where Indian grottos shine,*
> *Where fumes of incense glad the southern seas,*
> *And wafted citron scents the balmy breeze.*

The full sense of this physical and mental expatiation is caught in Addison's Royal-Exchange *Spectator* (No. 69), that prose-poem to the glory of commerce. His vanity as an Englishman is gratified, Mr. Spectator declares, to see so many foreign merchants busy in London—Japanese, Indians, Russians, Armenians, Jews, Dutch, Danes, Swedes, Frenchmen and Egyptians. His heart 'overflows with pleasure at the sight of a prosperous and happy multitude'. Felicitously he evokes the interchanges of trade—Portuguese oranges and China tea sweetened with West Indian sugar; Philippine spices flavouring the 'concoctions' of Europe; muffs converging for the ladies' pleasure from the frozen north and fans from the burning south, gold rising from the mines of Peru and diamonds from those of India. Luxuries of remote provenance systematically assemble to gratify the taste of Britain:

> Our rooms are filled with pyramids of China, and adorned with the workmanship of Japan. Our morning's draught comes to us from the remotest corners of the earth. We repair our bodies by the drugs of America, and repose ourselves under Indian canopies. My friend Sir Andrew calls the vineyards of France our gardens; the Spice-Islands our hot-beds; the Persians our silk-weavers, and the Chinese our potters.

Defoe's novels show a striking familiarity (however he acquired it) with the trade-routes and commodities of the Atlantic, Pacific, and Indian Oceans. Crusoe finally returns to England having crossed Asia by camel-caravan with a load of silk, tea, calicoes and spices. Captain Singleton takes a cargo of cloth to the East Indies, spends his time as a pirate in the Indian Ocean watching the passage of East Indiamen, Spanish treasure-ships and Chinese junks, and at last returns through Persia disguised as a Persian or Armenian merchant (a ruse in which—Defoe not being one to waste a good idea—Captain Avery imitates him). And Dyer's *Fleece*, having dispatched British woollens abroad, greets as briskly as Defoe the arrival of

> *cotton's transparent webs,*
> *Aloes, and cassia, salutiferous drugs,*
> *Alum and lacque, and clouded tortoise-shell,*
> *And brilliant diamonds.*
> The Fleece, iv. 339–42

It accords with the spirit of the age that in Thomson's *Liberty* the Genius of the Sea should welcome Britons to his empire (iv. 410–18):

> *All my dread walks to Britons open lie,*
> *Those that refulgent, or with rosy morn*
> *Or yellow evening, flame; those that, profuse,*
> *Drunk by equator suns, severely shine;*

> Or those that, to the poles approaching, rise
> In billows rolling into *Alps* of ice.
> E'en, yet untouch'd by daring keel, be theirs
> The vast *Pacific;* that on other worlds,
> Their future conquests, rolls resounding tides.

That, over thirty years before Cook's first expedition, was a shrewder prophecy than Yalden's delusion that Britain would 'traffic no more abroad for foreign spoil'.

These developments were widely welcomed, but did not go entirely unprotested. There was the old bogy of 'luxury', which pessimists suspected of softening the national fibre. There was the enormous problem of India; consciences were increasingly uneasy about East-India-Company exploitation. Samuel Foote wrote *The Nabob* (1772) to castigate the corrupt grandee, the novelist Robert Bage asserted that in the Company's service 'not to grow rich is beyond the power of human virtue' (*Mount Henneth*, 1781, p. 184), Wendeborn spoke of immense riches gained from victimisation, and Warren Hastings was impeached for corruption in the century's greatest trial, in which Burke pursued his long campaign against the Company with the vehemence of monomania. And finally there was the slave-trade, profitable, established, justified by economic arguments that Negro labour was indispensable to the West Indian and American plantations, and even by humanitarian arguments that slaves lived better there than in their native Africa.

The average Englishman thought little about such evils, of which he was more or less ignorant. But a trickle of protest which started with seventeenth-century Quakers, which was nobly expressed in Aphra Behn's *Oroonoko* (1688), and which led Defoe to portray the moderate humanitarianism of the Quaker surgeon Walters (in *Captain Singleton*) and the passionate humanitarianism of *Colonel Jack*, grew in volume. Pope's *Essay on Man* imagines the Indian's dream of heaven (i. 107–8),

> Where slaves once more their native land behold,
> No fiends torment, no Christians thirst for gold.

Richard Savage, with that rough force which made him an awkward houseguest for his hosts but a strong-minded friend for Johnson, prophesied retribution against the trade (*Of Public Spirit in Regard to Public Works*), and finally Granville Sharp, Wedgwood, Thomas Clarkson, Wilberforce and others organised the movement for abolition. Most strikingly, Cowper turned from quiet meditations to write bitingly against slavery, particularly in a group of poems in 1788—*The Negro's Complaint, The Morning Dream, Pity for Poor Africans*, and *Sweet Meat has Sour Sauce*. The first of these, set to music and popularly sung as a street-ballad, was printed with a reproduction of Wedgwood's anti-slavery medallion; the last, to the tune of 'Which nobody can deny', is a notably grim ditty purporting to be sung by a slaver retiring from business and selling his stock of implements:

> 'Tis a curious assortment of dainty regales,
> To tickle the negroes with when the ship sails,
> Fine chains for the neck, and a cat with nine tails,
>   Which nobody can deny, deny,
>   Which nobody can deny.
>
> Here's padlocks and bolts, and screws for the thumbs,
> That squeeze them so lovingly till the blood comes,
> They sweeten the temper like comfits or plums,
>   Which nobody can deny.
>
> When a negro his head from his victuals withdraws,
> And clenches his teeth and thrusts out his paws,
> Here's a notable engine to open his jaws,
>   Which nobody can deny.

Some did deny it, but untruthfully and unavailingly, and to the relief of enlightened men the trade came to an end in 1807.

vi. THE NATIONAL SPIRIT

He that will diligently labour, in whatever occupation, will deserve the sustenance which he obtains, and the protection which he enjoys; and may lie down every night with the pleasing consciousness of having contributed something to the happiness of life.

JOHNSON
The Adventurer No. 67

An adequate answer to the question how such varied and sometimes novel activity affected the Augustans' outlook would assess a wide scope of opinion: thousands gained, thousands lost, and the gains and losses were of many degrees and kinds. It should always be remembered that the lives of most men kept to the placid continuity of the old rhythms, and their outlooks to the familiar horizons: this stable persistence is one of the fundamental things about Augustan life. But some conclusions are possible also about the changes which the eighteenth century was bringing about.

Crossing the stability there was, first, a widespread sense of national expansion, felt with pleasure and even exuberance. Richard Savage's poem *Of Public Spirit in Regard to Public Works* (1737) is symptomatic. As a poem it is as unappetising as its title, but it is addressed to the Prince of Wales and recommends itself to the highest quarters. Its interest lies less in its verses than its prospectus, which proposes as fit topics for poetry the subjects

> Of reservoirs and their use; of draining fens, and building bridges; cutting canals, repairing harbours and stopping inundations, making rivers navigable, building lighthouses; of agriculture, gardening, and planting for the noblest uses; of commerce; of public roads; of public buildings, viz., squares, streets, mansions, palaces, courts of justice, senate houses, theatres, hospitals, churches, colleges; the variety of worthies produced by the latter. Of colonies. The slave-trade censured, &c.

—all to be accomplished by 'Public Spirit, Liberty and Peace'. The poem is far from good but its intentions are impeccable, and its zeal for public improvements is a sign of ambitious citizenship. The spirit of enterprise spread through society; men of foresight vied with each other in advancing new ideas, and in 1754 the Society for the Encouragement of Arts, Manufactures and Commerce was founded to unite those interested in practical progress as for a century the Royal Society had been uniting the 'natural philosophers'. Dr. Johnson was a member and admitted that he tried to speak at several of its weekly meetings but never knew what to say —a confession which if nothing else did would qualify the Society for commemoration. After the Adam brothers erected the Adelphi Buildings in 1771, its meeting-place was the great hall there, where James Barry painted an allegorical frieze showing man's struggles with nature, and the philanthropist receiving his reward at the gates of Heaven.

Other signs of interest are to be found in art. Blake and Uvedale Price might condemn the desecration of nature, yet it was not always clear that industry would turn out ugly. Indeed, a new factory in a country valley, housing an ingenious and productive machine, might well be aesthetically interesting. Gilpin exploring the Wye for picturesque beauty was not dismayed by the signs of industry; he liked the bustle around the coal-wharves at Lidbrook; the smoke burst from the chimneys along the river with 'double grandeur' and forges and charcoal-pits 'happily adorned' the hills of Neath (*Observations on the River Wye*, 1782, pp. 25, 72). Some admirable plates in Mr. Klingender's *Art and the Industrial Revolution* illustrate the imaginative stimulus of early industry. There is, for instance, an anonymous painting of the 1790s showing a Midland coal-mine, with an almost idyllic feeling of primitive innocence about it. There is an 1805 aquatint, after Philip James de Loutherbourg, revealing the Coalbrookdale iron-works in a light fully justifying Gilpin's sense of the picturesque in nascent industrialism. In a darkly-wooded valley a cluster of broad chimneys rises above the gable-end of the works like a Gothic Revival vision of mediaeval towers: from them orange and purple smoke drifts to form a cloud impending over the shadowed waters of the Upper Forge pool and contrasting with a yellow-white glare from the forges, which spectacularly fills the centre of the picture. John Sell Cotman's water-colour of this Bedlam furnace in Coalbrookdale (reproduced in Arthur Raistrick's *Dynasty of Iron-Founders* [1952]) is a similar, though far finer, piece of romantic impressionism. Arthur Young too mentioned this scene, with its natural situation setting off the 'horridly sublime' works of industry, and other observers sensed the melodramatic aesthetics of the new age, particularly the painter Joseph Wright of Derby, whom science and industry deeply impressed.

The prestige of the practical life brought into the limelight a new kind of person, shown at its best by Wedgwood and by Matthew Boulton. The latter, whose Soho works near Birmingham rivalled in fame Wedgwood's at Etruria, was an honourable and generous man, who set high standards in the quality and design of his products, bold like Wedgwood in progressive causes, paternal towards his workers, and distinguished by a magnanimous bearing which earned him the title of 'princely Boulton'. His friends (who included Wedgwood) were as distinguished as Wedgwood's own, and he gathered them together in the Lunar Club, which met on full-moon-lit nights at his house for intellectual discussion and included in its membership Erasmus Darwin, Joseph Priestley, Wedgwood himself, R. L. Edgeworth the father of Maria, and James Watt (whose collaboration with Boulton is famous).

Wedgwood and Boulton, it is true, were exceptions, even rare ones, rather than the rule. They typify their time, nonetheless, in their eminence as gentlemen and businessmen, for the age was well aware that the two roles were not incongruous. Addison had already displayed Sir Andrew Freeport: Steele apologising for neglecting 'the industrious part of mankind' (*Spectator*, No. 552) paid tribute to his friend Peter Motteux, translator of Rabelais, man-of-letters-turned-man-of-business. 'An English Merchant', commented Johnson, 'is a new species of Gentleman'. While Walpole was ruling England, Voltaire observed, his younger brother was running a warehouse in Aleppo. The prejudice which had allowed the fashionables of Restoration comedy to lord it over the citizenry declined. There were of course exceptions; with his feudal principles Boswell disliked the idea that titles of nobility might be conferred on men like Henry Thrale, friend of Johnson, eminent brewer, and a cultured man. But whether or not titles were to be given merchants were claiming distinction. Thorowgood, in Lillo's famous melodrama *The London Merchant: or, the History of George Barnwell* (1731), asserts that 'as the name of Merchant never degrades the Gentleman, so by no means does it exclude him'. Steele's aptly-named Mr. Sealand in *The Conscious Lovers* (1722) holds his own against Sir John Bevil the squire:

we merchants are a species of gentry that have grown into the world this last century, and are as honourable and almost as useful as you landed folks that have always thought yourselves so much above us.

At a time when the Royal Academy had recently been instituted, Thomas Mortimer's *Elements of Commerce* (1772) spoke up for the applied rather than the fine arts on the grounds that their practitioners, the most useful members of society, should receive as much honour as any others. They did not indeed lack recognition; a French visitor in 1788 remarked that the great industrialists 'command such credit and respect that in the eyes of everyone they are on a level with the greatest in the land'. On the whole, those who directed Britain's economy received their meed of praise, and that economy was a general source of pride.

The pride, indeed, was not unblemished. Mortimer commented on strikes and riots among miners, weavers and other labourers, and advised Parliament to amend their grievances since excessive toil could not earn them a living. Defoe spoke of the Peak lead-miners as 'subterranean wretches', and noticed the grime of industrial towns. In the last decades of the century a strain of crusading humanitarianism entered into many a novel and poem, a contribution to the long and bitter struggle to vindicate the rights of labour and, more widely, of human beings as such. Godwin's *Fleetwood* (1805), for instance, contains a searing account of child-labour in the Lyons silk-mills which is relevant also to England. Protests against political and social injustice are scattered about the work of Robert Bage and Thomas Holcroft and many a pamphleteer. Not every diligent labourer enjoyed 'the pleasing consciousness of having contributed something to the happiness of life'.

Yet not all these evils were obvious at first, and even when obvious they were not always new. The poor had suffered throughout history. What was new was the greater abundance of goods, and the worldwide interchange that abundance promoted. The virtues that led to business success came in for special emphasis: even 'dull and phlegmatic tempers', Budgell points out in *The Spectator* (No. 283), can prosper by methodical work, whereas 'the greatest parts and most lively imaginations' may fail by lack of it. This to be sure was no new discovery: the prehistoric trader must have come to the same conclusion. Yet a work like Benjamin Franklin's *Autobiography*, that perfect exemplar of the practical life, belongs in a special sense to its time; its progressive politics, shrewd business intelligence, and rational science and religion, express this phase of Anglo-Saxon civilisation. Such qualities, Professor Tawney argues in *Religion and the Rise of Capitalism* (1926), are peculiarly the offspring of Puritanism, both inside and outside the Church of England. Trade and business, in this view, are prosecuted as the religious duty of being diligent in one's vocation, and the Puritan spirit, in energetic self-justification and in zeal for the works of this world, inspires an earnestness which achieves success. Idleness is ungodly; hard work is the path of Christian morals; Hogarth's Idle and Industrious Apprentices point out the alternatives.

The assertion of special kinship between Puritanism and the business mind has been criticised as too narrow, since not Puritanism alone but all forms of Christianity came to approve the practical virtues. It may need adjustment, then, but mainly by extension of scope. All the churches were having to reckon with the hard-working and hard-headed man who laboured stoutly for his own (and perhaps others') good and was not disposed to abnegation. It is true that Dissenters were often more prominent in business and industry than Anglicans or Roman Catholics: many early ironmasters were Nonconformists (often Quakers), with Biblical names —three Abraham Darbys, Benjamin Huntsman, Isaac Hawkins, Shadrach Fox, Aaron and Jonathan Walker, and so on; Quakers were eminent in milling, brewing and banking; and all branches of Dissent provided inventors (Newcomen a Baptist, Watt a Presbyterian, Roebuck an Independent, Wedgwood a Unitarian). Excluded from Oxford, Cambridge and the professions, they took to other occupations, and having at their dissenting academies or Scottish universities often received an excellent education, especially in science and mathematics, they rose in the world. Many Scots engineers were well-qualified sons of the manse and graduates of Glasgow and Edinburgh (universities far more progressive than Oxford and Cambridge, whose neglect of modern studies was often criticised): many clear-sighted men, in and out of business, like Defoe, John Howard, Boulton, Priestley, John Dalton, Godwin, and Malthus were schooled in dissenting academies. Dissenters then, though not alone in cultivating the practical virtues, had a special impulse to justify themselves.

At its best this philosophy of life could evolve an admirable code of which men like Boulton were an embodiment. It interpreted religious values differently from the century before: man tended to be, as Professor Tawney observes, not primarily a spiritual being prudently acknowledging economics to keep alive, but an economic being prudently acknowledging religion as an insurance for his soul. But if virtues and values were more secular, they were not absent. In the 174th *Spectator* Sir Andrew Freeport refutes Sir Roger de Coverley's contention that trade is illiberal; he pleads the trader's extensive knowledge, intelligent foresight and social worth. William Hutton's *History of Birmingham* makes a similar, confident, claim:

> That property which arises from honest industry is an honour to its owner; the repose of his age; the reward of a life of attention; but, great as the advantage seems, yet being of a private nature it is one of the least in the mercantile walk. For the intercourse occasioned by traffic gives a man a view of the world and of himself; removes the narrow limits that confine his judgment; expands the mind; opens his understanding; removes his prejudices; and polishes his manners. Civility and humanity are ever the companions of trade; the man of business is the man of liberal sentiment; a barbarous and commercial people is a contradiction.
>
> (1781 : 61-2)

The young merchant, Thomas Mortimer advises, is to aim not only at private profit but at public service also, to keep constantly in his mind's eye 'the honours of magistracy and the important charge of a British legislator', to abide by 'the soundest principles of religion and morality, and a sacred veneration for truth', and to take as his aim

> a firm attachment to the true principles of honour, a religious adherence to his word, clearness and integrity in his contracts, prudent generosity in his dealings with the industrious poor, with a becoming dignity and moral rectitude in his manners.
>
> *Elements of Commerce*, 215

Anyone uneasy about economic results might find comfort in the semi-religious sanction Adam Smith gave to business by detecting the hand of Providence in the working of economic laws. All in all the businessman could consider himself a public benefactor, strong in moral worth and active in promoting civilisation and the good life.

Much of this feeling is conveyed in *The Wealth of Nations* (1776). Without ever supposing that man is merely an economic animal—his own *Theory of Moral Sentiments* is a plea for social sympathy—Adam Smith urges, with careful lucidity, that wealth increases best when each man seeks his own good unhampered by external control. The economic bases of his argument have not stood the test of time, nor have his deductions, but his work reflects one of his century's preoccupations, how to see man's self- and social-love as harmoniously related. He rejects the current mercantilist practice which regulated trade from the centre, and he argues that Providence best knows how to produce the good of the whole. A natural order which so admirably regulates the courses of the stars and the life-cycles of insects must surely extend its wise guidance to other spheres; in the case of economics it must turn the great natural force of individual enterprise to a richer result than any human contrivance can do. All this is part of that humility which, along with a modest pride in their own powers, the Augustans felt before Nature. The individual, says Adam Smith,

> generally indeed neither intends to promote the public interest nor knows how much he is promoting it. By preferring the support of domestic to

that of foreign industry he intends only his own security; and by directing that industry in such a manner as its produce may be of the greatest value, he intends only his own gain, and he is in this as in many other cases led by an invisible hand to promote an end which was no part of his intention. Nor is it always the worse for society that it was no part of it. By pursuing his own interest he frequently promotes that of society more effectually than when he really intends to promote it. I have never known much good done by those who affected to trade for the public good.

The Wealth of Nations, ed. Cannan, i. 421

By government interference trade becomes a part of politics and therefore a source of rancour, whereas in itself it is 'a bond of union and friendship'; it should therefore be freed from 'the unreasonableness of restraints'.

Adam Smith's doctrine is stimulating, whatever its dangers. It breathes the free air of the open world, even if two centuries of experience have shown reasons for revising it. As significant as the doctrine is the humanity of style and tone. Economics is here not the dismal science Carlyle was to call it; the most noteworthy thing about Adam Smith, at least to a non-economist, is the pervading sense that the operations he discusses are not an abstract set of processes dehumanised by a technical vocabulary but normal human activities, the natural cycle of daily occupations. His illustrations are pictures of countryside, village and town life, of trafficking and seafaring and cultivating. Everything has human reality and is on a human scale. Without ignoring the fact that thousands of the labouring poor fared very badly in the eighteenth century, and still worse as *laisser-faire* grew in prestige, we may still feel that small-scale free enterprise looks more compatible with human nature (even if experience qualifies the notion) than do combines, cartels, unions, Boards, Authorities and Mass Observations. Necessary as modern organisation is, it dwarfs the individual; dangerous in its consequences as *The Wealth of Nations* was, it breathes the air of humanity. The tragedies to which a philosophy of uncontrolled enterprise led cannot be denied, nor indeed can the impossibility of leaving economic practice to itself; this apparently 'human' faith became the cover for hideous inhumanity, and the laws of nature turned out, in science and economics alike, to be not beneficent but morally neutral. But the point here is not whether or not the Augustans were mistaken but how they thought and felt, and there is no doubt that as they surveyed Britain's expanding economy they believed that industry was justifying itself and that man, provided he were steady and foresighted, was master of his fate. The result was the confidence Akenside expressed in his *Ode to the Country Gentlemen of England* (1758), at the thought of the nation's prosperity:

> *Thou art rich, thy streams and fertile vales*
> *Add Industry's wise gifts to Nature's store;*
> *And ev'ry port is crouded with thy sails,*
> *And ev'ry wave throws treasure on thy shore.*

It was a confidence widely shared.

vii. BUSINESS AND LITERATURE

> While courts are disturbed with intestine competitions, and ambassadours are negotiating in foreign countries, the smith still plies his anvil, and the husbandman drives his plow forward; the necessaries of life are required and obtained, and the successive business of the seasons continues to make its wonted revolutions.
>
> JOHNSON
> *Rasselas*, ch. xxviii

THE literary consequences of this complex activity must now be deduced. Clearly the attention focusses on aspects of life different from the focal points of previous ages; it seeks for instance less the heroic passions of Elizabethan drama or the ideal ethics of Elizabethan poetry than the practical virtues embodied in Defoe or Franklin, less the soul in its religious experience than the social man in his daily environment. It brings out more and more the features of the tradesman or merchant, in essays, verse and drama. The advice Crusoe's father gives him is characteristic—it is to settle steadily in the middle way of life, safe from the luxury of the rich and the penury of the poor. In actual fact many great fortunes were made and the gap between rich and poor widened; but literature dwelt rather on the moderately well-to-do, on those who, like Steele's friend Motteux, showed 'that modest desire of gain which is peculiar to those who understand better things than riches' (*The Spectator*, No. 552).

Literature then speaks for the gradually more vocal middle class, and its normal range is between the level where the struggle for survival is veiled only slightly if at all, and that of almost aristocratic power and dignity. Whatever its level it deals mainly with the real world of men and manners, and these dealings may be urbane, as they are in Addison, Horace Walpole or Gibbon, manly and forthright, as they are in Fielding, Adam Smith or Burke, or uninhibitedly combative, as they are in Defoe or Smollett, where self-preservation is the urge. Whereas Elizabethan romance, and the traditions of drama up to Restoration tragedy stress the heroic passions, typical Augustan work is the record of normal life. The difference is not exactly due to greater realism in middle-class taste than in aristocratic, yet a middle-class public, even though it often wishes to escape from its own codes, naturally wants to recognise its own sort of truth in what it reads.

Not only were the middle classes conscious of their importance, but they were increasingly the author's main support. The nature of the book-buying public was the more important as patronage gradually yielded before the establishment of a popular market. Writers, particularly novelists, show an increased interest in the question of earning a living. Defoe's characters are face-to-face at every stage with this problem; after each 'husband' Moll Flanders counts her gains and losses, covers half a page with arithmetic, and explains how she invested the balance, if any. It is true that the literature of social realism has always dealt with this side of life, from Langland's *Piers Plowman* through the Elizabethan pamphleteers and the plays of Jonson and Massinger. But with the Augustans poverty and struggle can form the main substance of major novels and—for example in Johnson's *London* and *Life of Savage*—of poems and biography.

How far was this an outcome of economic conditions? To some

extent at least it reflected the existence of a literate poor class, unprotected from economic strain, though such a class had long existed and was no novelty. The decline of patronage which had provided, if not security, at least a cushion against penury threw writers directly on to an unpredictable public market, and the fact that they were often struggling dipped their work into social reality as it had done that of the Elizabethan pamphleteers.

The economics of Augustan authorship have been a good deal studied, and certain melodramatic notions of tyrannical booksellers (the counterpart of modern publishers) browbeating reluctant hacks have been modified. Those notions have some basis in fact, it is true; hacks existed, and booksellers might well seem to them more like slave-drivers than allies. John Shebbeare referred to 'that harpy, a book-seller', and declared it a national scandal that authors 'should be constantly haunted by that fiend, necessity'. *The Dunciad* is a famous genre-picture of Grub-street misery, and Fielding's *Author's Farce* presents Bookweight the unscrupulous publisher, and Scarecrow, Dash, Quibble and Blotpage his exploited dependants.

Yet the truth is more complex and creditable. Until the reading public became large enough to support a crowd of authors, patronage was almost indispensable for anyone wishing to maintain himself by his pen. It had been given for political advantage or from disinterested love of the arts: the former motive was prominent during the party strife preceding the rise of Walpole, and blazed up again in the late 1730s when the Opposition enlisted the help of Thomson, Glover, Mallet and Paul Whitehead; the latter motive had a reign of glory extending into the first decades of the century when the influential Montagu, Somers, Harley, St. John and Burlington helped philosophers, writers and artists like Locke, Addison, Newton, Congreve, George Vertue and William Kent. It was a valuable system which established friendship between men of high place and men of great gifts in letters and the arts. This was the relationship of Harley to Swift, the Queensberry family to Gay, and Burlington to Kent and other architects. That alliance between letters and the aristocracy so prominent under the Restoration was continued; each party gave lustre to the other.

The more writers abounded, however, the less patronage sufficed; the public market therefore became crucially important. Early in the century political pamphlets and the best periodicals could sell in thousands, though not yet on such a scale as to make their authors independent. About 1720 there were signs of a good market for other kinds of work; *Robinson Crusoe* (1719) sold three editions in four months and made more than £1,000 for its publisher; *Gulliver's Travels* (1726) was exhausted a week after publication; the sale of Gay's *Polly* (1729), stimulated by its banning from the stage, exceeded ten thousand copies and Thomson's *Sophonisba* (1730) had four editions in a year. The best instance is Pope's success with his Homer: the *Iliad* (1715–20) brought him (according to different accounts) between £4,000 and well over £5,000, and the *Odyssey* (1725-6) nearly £4,000 more. Pope achieved the independence he so prized, and though at that date this was a unique triumph it remains a landmark in the progress of authorship.

Yet the ordinary writer's lot might be tragically different. Booksellers found for him whatever work the market would support, but they were primarily concerned with profits and could not fairly be blamed (though satirists in fact blamed them unceasingly) if too many writers chased too few readers. They did in fact encourage authors when they could and often showed a personal interest in those who provided their commodity: Johnson spoke well of them, and Robert Anderson in his *Life of Smollett* (1796) said that there were no more generous men in business. Grub Street's sufferings were the fault less of booksellers than of general economics.

They grew less severe as, with the passing years, the body of readers expanded. The number of schools increased; journals like *The Gentleman's Magazine* (from 1731), *The Monthly Review* (from 1749) and Smollett's *Critical Review* (from 1756) provided a useful publicity. In 1740 the first circulating library was opened in London, to be followed by others there and in the provinces so much in vogue as to provoke satire—Sheridan's jest at the 'evergreen tree of diabolical knowledge' in *The Rivals* (1775) is famous. Sunday schools were founded from the late 1760s onwards; Methodism, and radical pamphlets, stimulated a desire to read; and better roads made reading matter available. Not all these factors operated at the level of 'polite' literature, but they helped to make authorship possible as a profession. Fielding's *Tom Jones* (1749) and *Amelia* (1751) brought him £700 and £1,000; Macpherson's *Works of Ossian* (1762–3) £1,200; Robert Henry's *History of England* (1771–85) £3,300; Hume's *History* £3,400 between 1754 and 1762; and Robertson's *Charles V* (1769) £4,500. By 1800 the transition from authorship dependent on a patron to authorship supported by the public was far advanced.

This revolution made the writer's position more dangerous and more exhilarating—more dangerous in that he risked failure and ruin, more exhilarating in that the prizes of success, both material and psychological, could be enormous. The assurance by which the early Augustans appealed to a known taste and audience gave way to the dynamism by which purveyors of 'sensibility' like Richardson and Sterne or of Gothick mystery like Horace Walpole and Mrs Radcliffe could spread their intoxications, and popular enthusiasm could later sweep Scott or Byron to the pinnacle of fame. The process was inevitable and it brought benefits to compensate for the loss of Augustan concentration, as the open ocean has advantages over the sheltered river. Changes in the reading public are among the main reasons why the literature of 1850 differs so profoundly from that of 1750.

Yet literature did not sail at once into the maelstrom of romantic emotion. The man with only his pen for keeping hunger at bay had to consider the public taste, and the public taste was particularly interested in normal social life, of a kind with which the writer's own preoccupations made him familiar. Swift, Defoe, Fielding and Smollett for instance are men whom an incessant concern with the circumstances of life, at the level where survival means struggle and even callousness (as well, often, as generosity), stamps with a mark of hard-headed practicality, keeping their phrases direct, their comment trenchant, and their substance near to the muscular effort that life requires. That Augustan literature so often keeps close to fact is a sign not so much perhaps of economic influence directly as of the exigences of the time which moulded both literature and economic life. The mass of detail surrounding Crusoe's colony, and the calculations of Moll Flanders, Roxana, Colonel Jack, Captain Singleton and Captain Avery are signs of the times. So too is Defoe's imagery—moidores, Bills of Exchange, pieces of eight, woollen goods, '*Indian* stuffs of sundry Sorts, Silk, Muslins and fine Chints . . . Bales of very fine *China* silks . . . Packs of Bales of Spices, particularly Cloves and Nutmegs' (*Captain Singleton*), hogsheads of sugar, bags of cotton-wool, barrels of indigo, bundles of ivory and casks of rum (*Colonel Jack*). Such things, together with the abundant material details of Dyer's *Fleece*, Grainger's *Sugar-Cane*, Addison's Royal-Exchange *Spectator*, or Belinda's dressing-table in *The Rape of the Lock*, are the overflow into literature of the extraverted interests of the men of commerce.

The mark of such literature is that of minds moving familiarly in the world of real things. Defoe for example treats the realism of seafaring with brisk interest, Smollett with angry satire in *Roderick Random* (1748), and William Falconer with mixed vividness and tedium in *The Shipwreck* (1762), a poem inexcusably lengthy but now and then casting aside its classical pretence for the technical details of seamanship and convincing glimpses of the eastern Mediterranean. Defoe's work in particular belongs to its time, and most of all *Robinson Crusoe*, which in a sense examines the essential bases of life. The book is indeed a study (an incidental rather than a deliberate exercise in sociology) of what life would be like without the economic structure which normally supports it. Crusoe has the implements of simple technology (a few tools) but he is deprived of that division of labour which makes life relatively easy. To get a plank he must work a whole tree into shape; to store grain he must find clay and make pots; to bake bread he must plant, harvest, mill, bolt and finally cook the grain, in an oven he has himself made. Much of the book's interest is in the stratagems of a man outside the framework of social organisation and in that primitive condition in which life is a laborious though adventurous thing. It is a parable of the lesson the age was making explicit, man's practical need of his fellows.

Yet not all economic influence was severely practical; there was also an extension of imaginative life. In particular the art of the East was elegant, strange, and the product of subtle aesthetics. The same qualities affected letters; Europe translated Eastern tales, wrote Eastern imitations, studied Eastern (and especially Chinese) morality, and sought novelties of imaginative strangeness and fanciful colour which its own civilisation tended to deny it. Even Pope once thought, he told Joseph Spence, of trying a Persian fable; it 'would have been a very wild thing'. Galland's French version (1704–17) had introduced *The Arabian Nights* to the West, to be followed by (allegedly) Persian, Turkish, Chinese, Mogul, Tartarian and Peruvian tales (all these had appeared in England by 1760), which opened the way for Oriental stories in the periodicals, in Collins's *Persian Eclogues*, Johnson's *Rasselas*, Goldsmith's *Citizen of the World*, and Beckford's *Vathek*, and for the eventual spectacular efflorescence of Byron's Eastern tales and the Prince Regent's astonishing Pavilion at Brighton.

The contents of the mind, as well as of the house, became more colourful. As the preface to *Mogul Tales* (1736) observes,

the late humour of reading Oriental romances ... has extended our Notions, and made the Customs of the East much more familiar to us than they were before.

It would be pleasant to go into all the consequences; there were satirical consequences in the appearance of Eastern travellers to criticise the European scene, like Montesquieu's Usbek and Rica or Goldsmith's Lien Chi Altangi; there were imaginative consequences leading to Vathek in his fantastic palace with sky-piercing towers, crowds of strange faces, and hideous apparition with the magic sabres. But we must let the quaint procession pass—'dusk faces with white silken turbans wreath'd'—the Tartar sages, Chinese anchorites, Persian notables, Arabian philosophers, Indian kings, Babylonian wiseacres and princes of Abyssinia, commenting on the world with engaging obliquity of eye, in prose often flowery and bedizened, mildly sententious, and full of invocations to remote and improbable deities. If the commercial mind fostered in general a sober temper it also fed the imagination with unexpected nourishment, enriching and reinforcing the curious reports of explorers and missionaries.

A century's concern with the bases of its existence, the labour which keeps it alive, is clearly complex. Strains of practical realism on one hand, of exotic fantasy on the other; pride in national wealth or denunciation of the 'contracted spirit' of trade; zeal for progress or fear of it; human effort conserving tradition, or courting new enterprises—all these make a kaleidoscopic pattern. Of them all, perhaps three factors particularly influence letters: the first is the writer's changing public; the second is the accumulation of economic power, in the hands of men concerned for social stability provided that they were the beneficiaries of it; and the third is the normal human scale of economic operations. The first produced no spectacularly sudden results, but Pope's success of heroic classicism with his Homer, Richardson's of sentimental psychology with *Pamela* and *Clarissa*, and Macpherson's of heady romanticism with *Ossian* are signs of the totally different waters in which literature was in future to float or sink. The second establishes in literary psychology an assumption of basic stability, of developments based on traditional foundations and taking place not by convulsion but by intelligent steady foresight, in a sensible strong society ratified by practical reason, fortified (its ethos being set by the upper class) by the example of classical antiquity yet not subservient to authority, and ready to act in self-confident independence. And the third brings it about that economic forces do not seem to have struck the Augustans as hostile or superhuman. They might in fact be so, as might the forces of nature, and their victims might suffer bitterly. But the poor were too inarticulate to set the dominant tone, and that tone was one which believed both nature and business to be guided by Providence, and which, since it felt both to be reasonable, was cowed by neither. The Augustan thought the world made for him, and he bustled in it.

III. PUBLIC AFFAIRS

i. THE POLITICAL SETTLEMENT AND LOCKE

I feel myself a member of a regulated society, and I would maintain an established order.

T. J. MATHIAS
The Pursuits of Literature (1797) pt. iii
'Advertisement'

ON James II's first birthday as King, Edmund Waller presented him with verses entitled *A Presage of the Ruin of the Turkish Empire* (1685), celebrating his manifold virtues and his 'aspect propitious to mankind'. Three years later the eulogised monarch was in flight to France taking his infant son to be brought up in the Church of Rome. He had discarded Parliament because it would not allow him a standing army or repeal the Test Act excluding non-Anglicans from office; he had illegally insinuated Roman Catholics into official positions; he had threatened Church and Universities with royal but arbitrary authority; and he had packed the bench of judges. The country had quickly united: Whigs and Tories, sinking their differences for the moment, joined in a brief but fortunate alliance, and the results were the expulsion of James, the accession of William and Mary, and the meeting of the Convention Parliament (1689), which set the shape of political development throughout the next century.

This is not the place to go into the events leading to 1688, or indeed at much length into later political history. The purpose rather is to sense the political instincts of Hanoverian England and suggest how these directed writers into certain kinds of expression. But since of all historical events it is the 'Glorious Revolution' which most engrossed the Augustans, that must be the point of departure.

In *The English Revolution 1688–1689,* Professor Trevelyan has suggested a new baptism for this historic affair: it should rather, he remarks, be called 'The Sensible Revolution'. Not that it lacked glory; it was bloodless, it was not vindictive, and it made major change unnecessary until 1832. But such glory is the glory of good sense; it shows a true understanding of the Englishman as a political animal. The Revolution conserved instead of destroying—or if it destroyed it destroyed only infringements of law and order. In spite of satire on their fickle politics the English have never hungered for innovation, and they combined on this occasion rather against innovations they disliked than for the sake of change. When in his *Appeal from the New to the Old Whigs* (1791) Burke defended his support of the English revolution and his attack on the French, the distinction he made was that the former was and the latter was not a revolution of preservation. 1688, like the restoration of 1660, had reaffirmed the traditions of England as 'a scheme of government fundamentally and inviolably fixed in king, lords and commons'. Through James's folly, revolution had become 'the only means left for the recovery of that *ancient* constitution formed by the original contract of the British state'.

The results were fundamental. The Whig theory of 'contract' between people and ruler triumphed over the Tory theory of Divine Right; Parliament became the unquestioned supreme power; judges were emancipated from the King's will; the 1689 Toleration Act ended religious persecution as far as was then possible (though retaining the civil disabilities of non-Anglicans); and the crown was confirmed in a Protestant succession. The system seemed to guarantee the subject's rights and to ensure that nothing should be done contrary to the publicly-debated laws of the land and the safety of the Protestant faith. This, in internal affairs, is what the Augustans meant by freedom, and Locke, the great philosopher of Whig politics, expressed it in his *Second Treatise of Civil Government* (1690) in terms which have become almost Holy Writ throughout the Western world (ch. IX, sec. 131):

> Whoever has the legislative or supreme power of any commonwealth is bound to govern by established standing laws, promulgated and known to the people, and not by extemporary decrees, by indifferent [impartial]

and upright judges who are to decide controversies by those laws; and to employ the force of the community at home only in the execution of such laws, or abroad to prevent or redress foreign injuries and secure the community from inroads and invasions. And all this to be directed to no other end but the peace, safety and public good of the people.

Praise of Parliamentary government and a limited monarchy is thereafter a constant theme. Apart from Non-Juror and Jacobite extremists the Augustans felt that their political world was grounded in the natural order of things and that, as Thomson said in *Liberty* (iv. 813–16) of Simon de Montfort's Parliament,

> *Then was the full, the perfect Plan disclos'd*
> *Of* BRITAIN's *matchless* Constitution, *mixt*
> *Of mutual checking and supporting Pow'rs,*
> KING, LORDS, *and* COMMONS.

If it was a sensible revolution, its great vindicator was a sensible philosopher. Locke is not merely the propagandist of a particular event—his thought is too deeply-considered for that. But he is essentially the philosopher of sensible men, whose ideas his readers can easily share. His arguments were foreshadowed by centuries of philosophical tradition, yet they seem the inevitable processes of a fresh mind assessing the data of human nature itself. From the present point of view his most important works are four *Letters Concerning Toleration* (1689, 1690, 1692 and 1706) and two *Treatises of Civil Government* (1690), all long-pondered and stamped with authority. In its barest epitome Locke's thought is concerned with three questions:—is human nature sociable? why does man enter into political society? how can society satisfy man's needs? On the answers Locke gave depended much of the eighteenth century's social confidence.

Human nature, Locke asserts, is sociable and reasonable; men are not, as Hobbes had alleged, so combative that only by submission to an absolute ruler (one man or body of men) can they be safe from each other. Instead, even before political organisation, they can live peaceably together and their reason prompts them to do this by sociable collaboration. It tells them moreover that each man is equal to his fellows (since none has a superior right to exert authority), that he should be secure in his life, health and property, and that as a sociable being he should protect not only his own interests but those also of others, and 'preserve the rest of mankind'.

For certain reasons men exchange this unorganised sociability for organised society. They need, in particular, a recognised authority to administer justice, whenever natural reason is insufficiently persuasive. They enter a political society to ensure a settled existence, impartial judgment, collective security, and agreed laws. An arbitrary sovereign is clearly worse for this purpose than the pre-political 'state of nature' since it neither provides impartial judgment nor allows its subjects to defend themselves. The basic purpose of political societies is nullified if men yield complete power to an autocrat or autocratic body: the people therefore must retain the right of judging whether their rulers are serving their interests and of changing them, by force if need be, if they are not. To those who argue that this means little more than anarchy Locke replies that men revolt only after long provocation, and that the responsibility for revolution is that of the governors themselves, whose misdemeanours are the real 'rebellion' by reducing society to war ('rebellare').

'The great and chief end therefore of men's uniting into commonwealths', Locke writes, 'is the preservation of their property.' The statement is perhaps misleading; 'property' is not only material wealth but also life and safety. Moreover Locke is not openly saying that a man should acquire and preserve unlimited wealth for himself: property in material goods amounts only to such gifts of nature as he can use for his own needs and improve by his own or his servant's work—the timber he can fell, the house he can build, or the fields he can till. In a developed community, with division of labour and so on, this naturally becomes more intricate: later theorists urged more clearly than Locke had done that a man's own labour (which earns him his right to possess wealth) can be indefinitely extended by that of his servants, and that by the device of money he can own far more wealth than he can in fact use.

Locke's theory therefore becomes a defence of plutocracy. Yet in his own mind 'property' (which society defends) is not unlimited accumulation regardless of personal effort; man's right to possession derives from his own labour.

Locke's theories, it has been said, are faulty. He thinks of political activities as far more deliberate and rational than they really are, and underestimates those emotions which are so powerful a component in Burke's thought, and so abundantly evident in later history. Moreover he vindicates the people's rights against absolutism but strongly preserves the rights of 'property' (in our sense) and the governing class. And lastly, he gives the state little constructive function, little chance to plan the national life for the general good. Burke in the eighteenth century and socialism in the nineteenth were needed to bring some of these things into the forefront of thought. But Locke's reasonable arguments that the subject is the source of political power, that the laws should protect his interests and that society is a rational, humane thing were the perfect corollary to 1688 and blew like a refreshing wind at home and abroad.

Here then was sanity and reason, almost the voice of Nature herself; here, as *The Spectator* said, was England's 'national glory' in politics. Defoe, tribune of the people, strong for toleration and civil liberties, adopted Locke's theses for his main political tract *The Original Power of the Collective Body of the People of England* (1701). That vigorous Whig Bishop Hoadly, though basing his *Original and Institution of Civil Government* (1710) on Hooker (whom a Tory opponent, he says, called 'the Father of the *Whigs* and Latitudinarians'), yet chose from his source just those arguments which have the most whiggish and Lockeian flavour. Pope, who took much, in general and in detail, from Locke, declared that 'Nature knew no right divine in men' (*Essay on Man*, iii. 236), and versified man's search for political security (iii. 275–82):

> *How shall he keep what, sleeping or awake,*
> *A weaker may surprise, a stronger take?*
> *His safety must his liberty restrain;*
> *All join to guard what each desires to gain.*

Forc'd into virtue thus by self-defence
Ev'n Kings learn'd justice and benevolence:
Self-love forsook the path it first pursu'd,
And found the private in the public good.

Bolingbroke was a lifelong Tory but in the main he followed the Whig oracle: *The Idea of a Patriot King* (1738) propounds that men are by nature sociable and unite to preserve their liberties, that this is best done by limited monarchy deriving authority from the people, that the Patriot King shall recognise power to be a trust for the good of those who give it, and that 'the constitution will be reverenced by him as the law of God and man'. Men of all parties combined to echo Locke, from doughty Churchmen like Warburton (who calls him 'the honour of this age and the instructor of the future') to radical dissenters like Richard Price and Joseph Priestley. The measure of his influence is reflected in the fact that whereas in 1683 the University of Oxford denounced rejection of Divine Right as 'false, seditious and impious', and in 1686 Cambridge declared kings accountable only to God, such doctrines survived after 1700 only among the Jacobites, to lead to the valiant futilities of 1715 and 1745.

ii. POLITICAL PARTIES

The general division of the *British* Nation is into Whigs and Tories, there being very few, if any, who Stand Neuters in the Dispute, without ranging themselves under one of these Denominations.

ADDISON
The Freeholder, No. 34

Locke's thought provided an agreed foundation but not a uniform superstructure. Whigs and Tories, recovering from their united hostility to James, soon found themselves able to disagree and to provide, in a conflict of interests, the basis of the important invention of party government. A short account, then, seems desirable of the two parties, inheritors of Roundhead and

Cavalier traditions, and distinguished by opposed views on the subjects of Church and State.

Parties are a prominent and lively part of the Augustan scene, yet the first point about them is that they were far less organised and coherent than they have since become. The party system only very slowly became the basis of government; the King might choose his advisers regardless of their attachments, the ministries might have a mixed complexion, and a ministry of one party might coexist with a House of Commons predominantly of another. Party lines fluctuated and parties themselves were looked on as a temporary expedient, so that a pamphleteer like Defoe was not necessarily inconsistent in supporting first one side and then the other, a party-politician like Bolingbroke in arguing that parties might well be dispensed with, or a Government propagandist like Fielding in hoping, 'by these my labours, to eradicate out of our Constitution' the very idea of party (*The True Patriot*, No. 1, 5 November, 1745).

Yet Whigs and Tories did stand for recognisably opposed beliefs and they fought with particular fury in the early years of the century until George I and Walpole settled things firmly in the Whig interest. The Tories were, on the whole, strong Churchmen, rather uneasy acquiescers in the doctrine of Parliamentary supremacy, and landed gentry misliking William III's and Queen Anne's continental wars, the taxes for which bore considerably upon them. William they swallowed as King *de facto* (except for the 'Nonjuring' wing which refused the oath of allegiance), yet they felt that an aura of sanctity had vanished from the kingly office. They were happier under Anne, herself strongly of their legitimist faith, but George I, brought over in the pockets of the Whigs, was a heavy trial and put them into despondent but unavailing opposition. The Whigs on the other hand, though in a minority throughout the country as a whole, and though Swift chose to portray them as a rabble of Dissenters, anarchists and atheists, were more united and effective, with support mainly among merchants and the 'moneyed interest'. They were strong for the Protestant succession, opposed to the Tory-Anglican dislike of Dissent, and enthusiastic about the settlement of 1689.

Party enmity under Queen Anne was volcanic. The Whigs pressed on the war with France, and their prestige rose high with Marlborough's successes from 1704 to 1710, years which saw also Peterborough's Spanish campaign, Rooke's capture of Gibraltar, the union with Scotland, and the failure of an attempted Jacobite invasion in 1708. At first, it is true, there were Tories in the famous Godolphin ministry which achieved this constellation of triumphs; St. John (Bolingbroke) for instance, though he had entered Parliament in 1701 to assail the Whigs and promote peace, became Secretary for War himself in 1702 and changed his front. But the Tories were gradually squeezed out and from 1708 to 1710 there was, for the first time, a true Cabinet of one party backed by its majority in the Commons—a phenomenon which was to become the fundamental condition of party government. Yet the position was unstable; the Whigs were disliked by the Church and by that strong Churchwoman Anne, discredited by the Sacheverell fiasco (cf. p. 140) and by national war-weariness. In 1710 the Tories succeeded to four stormy years of office, marked by quarrels between their rival leaders Harley and Bolingbroke, the former a steady Churchman who wanted toleration, peace on good terms and George of Hanover as king, the latter an erratic Deist who wanted intolerance, peace on almost any terms, and James Stuart. The most vivid sense of this explosive situation comes from the pages of Swift: in *The Faggot* (1713) he tried to unite the Tories with the fable of the twigs which were broken only when not bound together, and to Stella he confided his troubles:

This kingdom is certainly ruined as much as was ever any bankrupt merchant. We must have *Peace*, let it be a bad or a good one, though nobody dares talk of it. The nearer I look upon things, the worse I like them. I believe the confederacy [the alliance against Louis XIV] will soon break to pieces; and our factions at home increase. The ministry is upon a very narrow bottom, and stand like an Isthmus between the Whigs on one side, and violent Tories on the other. They are able seamen, but the tempest is too great, the ship too rotten, and the crew all against them.

Journal to Stella, 4 March, 1711

In this confusion the century's gravest decision impended. The Queen's health was poor and the question whether Stuarts or Hanoverians were to succeed grew daily more urgent. The Whigs were all for George, to forestall a Jacobite succession, and George was well-disposed to them. The Tories were disunited, and strongly tinged with Jacobitism (indeed they angrily expelled Steele from the Commons on 18 March, 1714, for attacking them on this point in *The Crisis* and *The Englishman*), and Bolingbroke was negotiating with James. The Queen wanted James but she wanted Protestantism even more and the two were clearly incompatible. Suddenly she died, with the Tories still disorganised: the Whig members of the Privy Council invited George; and against all prediction the Hanoverian succession went smoothly. The Tories fell and Bolingbroke, (who soon fled to the Pretender in France), summed up mournfully to Atterbury—'The grief of my soul is this; I see plainly that the tory party is gone.'

This outline of hostility has been sketched not for its own sake but because it is the dark background to a good deal of literature. Swift's *Enquiry into the Behaviour of the Queen's Last Ministry* (written 1715–20, published 1765) declares that

the Hearts of most Men are filled with Doubts, Fears, and Jealousies, or else with Hatred and Rage, to a Degree that there seems to be an End of all Amicable Commerce between People of different Parties.
Political Tracts 1713–1719, ed. Davis and Ehrenpreis
(1953), 131

His *Four Last Years of the Queen* (written 1713, published 1758) speaks of 'universal mischief', 'false and scandalous libels' and 'political and factious libels', and indeed the fanaticism which should have died with the seventeenth century seemed ready to break out fatally again. Against that outlook we must judge the influence of Addison, and if his moderation now seems insipid that is because the stormy and dangerous passions into which it brought light and good humour are forgotten. At the height of the succession-dispute he lamented that 'these politicians of both sides have already worked the nation into a most unnatural ferment' (*The Spectator*, No. 556,

18 June, 1714), and by raillery or serious persuasion he worked for agreement. Fortunately,

> *George in pudding-time came o'er,*
> *And moderate men look'd big, Sir,*

though anger still crackled during the long years of Walpole's ministry while impotent but scandalised opponents fired accusations at him, or during the prosecution of Wilkes in 1763, or over the letters of Junius (1769-71), or the French Revolution and its English echoes.

Newspapers and pamphlets fuelled the excitement. Defoe's *True-Born Englishman* (1701) had nine authorised editions by 1704, as well as twelve unauthorised running to eighty thousand copies. Sacheverell's extravagant sermon on *The Perils of False Brethren* sold forty thousand in a few days (1709) and an answer to it by one Benson sixty thousand. Eleven thousand of Swift's *Conduct of the Allies* (1711) were disposed of in a month (five editions between 27 November and 31 December), and Steele's *Crisis* ran to forty thousand. Newspapers multiplied. Before 1701 there were hardly any in the provinces but by George I's death they were established in about twenty-five towns. Circulations were small—hand-presses could turn out only a few thousands of an issue, though at their peak some anti-Walpole organs like *Mist's Journal* and *The Craftsman* were said, probably exaggeratedly, to top ten thousand. But papers made up in violence what they lacked in distribution, and the last section of this chapter touches on the verbal prize-fighting without which the Augustan reader was apt to think his politicians insincere.

The lines of Whig and Tory division remain fairly constant throughout the century (Swift traces them, rather partisanly, in the 44th *Examiner*), but happily the graver aspects of quarrel gradually disappear—committals to the Tower, impeachments for treason, flights abroad and expatriate plottings. Most importantly, the deeper fissures were filled in so that the 1745 rebellion failed to find the Tory support it hoped for. In the long course of the Hanoverian settlement men learned that moderate government and moderate opposition were the thing. Notable voices called for harmony—those of Halifax the 'Trimmer', Defoe, Addison, Steele, Pope, Fielding and even Bolingbroke. Swift himself, strong as he was for Church and Toryism, admitted the folly of division:

> Let any one examine a reasonable honest man of either side, upon those opinions in religion and government which both parties daily buffet each other about, he shall hardly find one material point in difference between them.
>
> *The Examiner*, No. 16

Pope was in genial agreement (*Essay on Man*, iii. 303-6):

> *For forms of government let fools contest;*
> *Whate'er is best administer'd is best:*
> *For modes of Faith let graceless Zealots fight;*
> *His can't be wrong whose life is in the right.*

Since political questions were often linked with religious, the decrease of religious tension contributed to quieter politics, but that theme must be left to the next chapter. By Johnson's day men learnt to tolerate, even (like Burke) to value, a moderate opposition: as Goldsmith's pleasant essay on *National Concord* observes, 'opposition when restrained within due bounds is the salubrious gale that ventilates the opinions of the people'. It braces the government like a crew in a fresh breeze, provided that it is 'the jealousy of patriotism, not the rancour of party, the warmth of candour, not the virulence of hate'. To have learnt that lesson is a great Augustan achievement.

iii. MEN OF LETTERS AND SOME MAJOR EVENTS

I am glad to have it observed, that there appears throughout all my Verses a Zeal for the Honour of my Country: and I had rather be thought a good *Englishman*, than the best Poet, or greatest Scholar, that ever wrote.

M. PRIOR
Preface to *Solomon*, 1718

THE following samples of the interest certain writers took in certain critical episodes make no claim to be exhaustive. They show men of letters participating in historical events but no particular event can be shown as an historian would show it, nor can more than a few be shown at all. A brief miscellany must stand for the whole trend.

The first example concerns Ireland, and Swift in particular. In *A Short Character of His Ex[cellency] T[he] E[arl] of W[harton], L[ord] L[ieutenant] of I[reland]* (1711), Swift fiercely denounces the

arbitrary power and oppression ... whereby the people of Ireland have for some time been distinguished from all Her Majesty's subjects ... being now at its greatest height under his Excellency Thomas Earl of Wharton.

He followed this 'damned libellous pamphlet', as he cheerfully called it to Stella on 8 December, 1710, with another attack, but his main campaign for Ireland was fought in the 1720s. In the session of 1720–1, Parliament enacted a law to foster the English woollen industry and forbid the use of printed and dyed calicoes. This hit the Irish calico manufacture and Swift proposed a boycott of English goods—*A Proposal for the Universal Use of Irish Manufacture* (1720). The same year certain financial satires by Swift and his friends caused a proposed National Bank of Ireland to be rejected. Then came the great affair of Wood's halfpence. Ireland needed small coin to the value, Swift himself and later Archbishop Boulter estimated, of £10,000–£15,000. In July 1722 a commission to provide halfpence and farthings to the value of £100,000 was issued to William Wood of Wolverhampton, or rather to the Duchess of Kendal, the King's mistress, who sold it to Wood for £10,000. Wood struck some coin late in 1722, whereupon Swift, Archbishop King and others protested that it was too light. The Irish Parliament resolved against it, and Walpole promised an enquiry. This vindicated Wood's coinage (but only, said his enemies, on samples of an improved second issue) but recommended a reduction in quantity to £40,000. Meanwhile, an anonymous *Letter to the Shop-Keepers, Tradesmen, Farmers, and Common-People of* IRELAND ... *by M. B. Drapier* (1724) set the Irish aflame. A second letter followed, a third which asserted the Irish to be enslaved, and a fourth which brought into question the whole dependence of Ireland on England. Walpole had been learning caution and in August 1725 the Lord Lieutenant, Carteret, announced that Wood's patent was cancelled. Swift was a national hero, medals were struck in his honour, and 'The Drapier's Head' became a common inn-sign.

This was not all Swift's propaganda for his country. Later works like the *Short View of the State of Ireland* (1727) and the extraordinary *Modest Proposal* (1729) paint a horrible picture of national tragedy, and it has been argued that many of his Irish experiences went into the 'Voyage to Laputa'. In a lecture on *The Political Significance of Gulliver's Travels* (British Academy, ix, 1919), Sir Charles Firth detected a close analogy between England, in her treatment of Ireland, and the Flying Island of Laputa, which hovers over the subject land of Balnibarbi, keeps off the sun and rain and threatens to crush the people below. The 'Academy of Projectors' fits in with Swift's hatred of questionable schemes for Ireland; the conflagrations which prevent Laputa from descending to destroy Balnibarbi are perhaps his own inflammatory pamphlets. The Laputan book was the last of *Gulliver's Travels* to be written, about 1725, and Swift's mind was full of Ireland.

Irish affairs were never again so prominently before English eyes until, perhaps, the Wolfe Tone rebellion in 1798. Yet Burke, who deeply felt his countrymen's wrongs, tried persistently to secure for Ireland trade concessions and religious emancipation, and in 1778 he angered his Bristol constituents by supporting a bill for the partial liberation of Irish commerce. He explained his position in the two admirable *Letters to Gentlemen in the City of Bristol*: 'is Ireland united to the crown of Great Britain', he asked, 'for no other purpose than that we should counteract the bounty of Providence in her favour?' But the gentlemen of Bristol were not mollified and in 1780 they were so clearly bent on not re-electing him that he withdrew from the poll before the voting was over. Froude, who judges the absenteeism of Ireland's men of genius to have been worse than that of her landlords, suggests that had Burke stayed in the land of his birth he could have changed its history. But he gave his life to other concerns, and the Irish cause foundered on the rocks of English self-interest.

Concurrent with Swift's exertions for Ireland were those of various writers against Walpole. Through most of his long rule (1721–42) the Prime Minister was a natural though unruffled target —unruffled because his effective bribery disarmed the opposition. Corruption is, indeed, the theme of much Augustan political writing —of Swift's attacks on Wharton, Marlborough and Wood, of the South-Sea-Bubble furore, of Burke's animus against the East India Company, and so on, but of all targets Walpole's administration was the most persistently under attack. The question of Hanoverian corruption is more complex than it might appear, and it receives some comment below, but however it may be excused it provided those out of office with ammunition against those in. Gay's *Beggar's Opera* (1728) satirised 'Robin of Bagshot [the haunt of highwaymen], alias Gorgon, alias Bluff Bob, alias Carbuncle, alias Bob Booty', and the ignoble Peachum declares to Lockit the turn-key that thief-takers and statesmen alike live by treachery. Bolingbroke tried to combine discontented Whigs with both Hanoverian and Jacobite Tories against Walpole by means of *The Craftsman* (1726–36), helped by the editor Amhurst, Swift, Pope, Gay, Arbuthnot, Chesterfield, Lyttelton, Akenside and the Pulteneys. Savage derided the literary man who sold himself to the politician (*The Poet's Dependence on a Statesman*), and Thomson's *Liberty* deplored the shadier practices of government (v. 99–101, 209–10):

> *Unblest by* VIRTUE, *Government a League*
> *Becomes, a circling junto of the Great,*
> *To rob by law* . . .
> *Forbid it,* HEAVEN*! that ever I need urge*
> INTEGRITY IN OFFICE *on my Sons!*

Fielding assailed Walpole in *The Historical Register for 1736* (1737), *The Champion* (1739–41), and *Jonathan Wild* (1743; written, however, before Walpole's fall): as Bolingbroke had done in *The Craftsman*, he compared the criminal Wild and the statesman Walpole. In 1742 another Opposition organ, *Common-Sense* observed that two 'great men' had met their deserts, the one being hanged and the other dismissed. For twenty years the minister whose exasperated rivals could not see his greatness was the target of affronted virtue.

Even apart from him, however, the scene was seldom blank. Some topics were perennial, the daily small talk of political zeal, like the National Debt, Bubbles, the 'landed' or 'moneyed' interests, the increase or decrease of royal prerogative, the decadence or advance of the times, the dangers or benefits of luxury, the patriotic duty of urging wars with France and Spain if none were being waged, and of deploring them if they were. A larger incident like the 1745 aroused acuter concern. Fielding in particular denounced the Jacobite invasion, which outraged his Hanoverian loyalties. In October 1745 he produced *A Serious Address to the People of Great Britain* against the '*Popish Pretender*, advised and assisted with the counsels and arms of *France* and *Spain*'; in November appeared *A Dialogue between the Devil, the Pope and the Pretender*, an Unholy Trinity in the eyes of a Hanoverian Protestant; simultaneously he launched *The True Patriot* which ran until June 1746, to be followed in December 1747 by *The Jacobite's Journal*, whose first seventeen numbers were an ironic eulogy of Jacobitism. His sentiments, to quote Leslie Stephen, were those of 'a good old-fashioned English Whig, with an intense aversion to papists and foreigners, and a slightly superstitious veneration for trial by jury and Habeas Corpus'. *Tom Jones*, published in 1749, had been long a-writing, and its inception approximately coincided with the '45, which it calls 'the late rebellion'. Its crucial events—Tom's chase after Sophia, for instance—fall within the period of Prince Charles's exploit. The Jacobite Squire Western vows he'd rather be anything than 'a courtier, and a presbyterian, and a Hanoverian too' (VI. ii); Mrs. Western rejoices at good news from the North (VI. iv); Tom falls in with redcoats marching against the invaders and expecting to be commanded by 'the glorious Duke of Cumberland' (VII. xi), and argues with Partridge that 'the cause of King George is the cause of liberty and true religion' (VIII. ix). No special stimulus was ever needed to elicit Fielding's Roast-Beef-of-Old-England patriotism, but had any been needed the '45 would certainly have sufficed. It is by a happy chance that his greatest novel, the embodiment of Hanoverian England, was written when history was intensifying his patriotism and faith. The invasion finds other, and brilliant, reflections in Horace Walpole's letters, which follow with inimitable wit its episodes—the flurry in London society (whether well- or ill-disposed to the Pretender), the *débâcle* of Prestonpans, the capitulation of Carlisle, the entry into Derby and the immediate change of mood which marked the retreat. The letters to Horace Mann, written in August, 1746, on the trial and execution of the rebel lords, are among the most vivid of historical documents. In comparison, Shenstone's accounts to his friends, in letters of late 1745 and early 1746, have the modesty of small talk, yet they reflect the shadows of a great and tragic event.

The remaining glimpses of literary men and politics concern foreign affairs and Burke, in whom oratory became literature through its magnificent style. Above all it was on American, Indian and French matters that he made his mark, and in examining his dealings with these we may see his political philosophy, which radically revised the rationalism of Locke and transmitted to succeeding generations the lesson that reason in statecraft is not enough.

Britain's relationship to the American colonies was bound to be precarious. The colonies taxed themselves for internal needs and resented external control: yet British interests were continually tempted to organise colonial trade for their own benefit. While the colonies were ridden on a loose rein trouble was minimised—

'salutary neglect', as Burke called it, was sound policy. Sensible statesmen left a discreet gap between what Parliament wished and what was attempted; for instance Walpole's Molasses Act (1733) was passed in deference to West Indian interests (to direct colonial trade to the West Indies) yet little was done to enforce it.

In time, however, 'salutary neglect' began to yield before a wish to enforce the laws, and the Americans' free enterprise began to reject interference. Britain's victory in the Seven Years' War removed the danger of French invasion and so the need for caution; Grenville's Stamp Act (1765)—for the reasonable purpose of financing a standing army against the Indians—was an irritant; so too were lawful but untimely attempts to suppress the profitable contraband trade, and the Church of England's desire to establish American bishoprics. On the Stamp Act's passing the Americans flocked to town-meetings, seized stocks of stamps, boycotted British trade and protested to the King. Amidst these events Burke made his maiden speech (27 January, 1766) and won the admiration of Pitt, himself strongly opposed to any pedantic legalism about British 'rights'. Dr. Johnson told Bennet Langton that Burke had a greater success on his first venture than any man before. His second speech, also on American affairs, followed a week later, and the repeal of the Stamp Act in March 1766 brought a temporary calm.

The theme of these speeches is developed in *Observations on a Late Publication entitled 'The Present State of the Nation'* (1769), which discusses colonial trade, declares new impositions to be impracticable and praises the repeal of the Stamp Act. Then, on 19 April, 1774, after further attempts at taxation had led to the Boston Tea-party and the punitive closing of Boston harbour, came the great speech *On American Taxation*, which begged for honourable trust rather than penal legislation. The same arguments and a grander flow of feeling inspired the magnificent plea for conciliation with the colonies (22 March, 1775). Characteristically Burke looked on the colonies' wealth as a proof that a wise Providence prospers human affairs better than man's own short views can do:

When I contemplate these things; when I know that the colonies in general owe little or nothing to any care of ours, and that they are not squeezed into this happy form by the constraints of watchful and suspicious government, but that through a wise and salutary neglect a generous nature has been suffered to take her own way to perfection ... I feel all the pride of power sink, and all presumption in the wisdom of human contrivances melt and die away within me.

On Conciliation with the Colonies, in *Works*, World's Classics edition, ii. 183

(A year later, it will be remembered, Adam Smith's *Wealth of Nations* gave classic expression to the same belief in Providence's superiority to 'human contrivances'.) In the conclusion, all Burke's reverence for the spirit of political honour and of a free but united society expressed itself with unsurpassed dignity (*Works*, ii. 234–5):

My hold of the colonies is in the close affection which grows from common names, from kindred blood, from similar privileges and equal protection. These are ties which, though light as air, are strong as links of iron. ... As long as you have the wisdom to keep the sovereign authority of this country as the sanctuary of liberty, the sacred temple consecrated to our common faith, wherever the chosen race and sons of England worship freedom they will turn their faces towards you. The more they multiply, the more friends you will have; the more ardently they love liberty, the more perfect will be their obedience. Slavery they can have anywhere. It is a weed that grows in every soil. ... But until you become lost to all feeling of your true interest and your natural dignity, freedom they can have from none but you.

The great theme moves to its great close, in that paragraph which begins 'All this I know well enough will sound wild and chimerical to the profane herd of those vulgar and mechanical politicians who have no place among us', and then Burke lays, as he hopes, 'the first stone of the temple of peace' by moving six resolutions for conciliation. That these were lost is a matter of history; within a month, on 19 April, the first clash took place, in the elm-lined country roads of Massachusetts, between General Gage's men and the 'embattled farmers' of Lexington and Concord. But never did a lost debate have a more eloquent champion, or one better vindicated by later events. These speeches, and also the superb *Letter to the Sheriffs of Bristol on the Affairs of America* (1777), have the hallmark of greatness and are unrivalled in English oratory for understanding, range and wisdom.

As for India, space allows here only the briefest reference to Burke's passionate concern which raised his speech on Fox's East India Bill (1783) to the heights of power. The East India Company was notoriously corrupt, and after initial support Burke turned to uncompromising hostility. The background to his Indian interest is unfortunate, it is true, for even as he was prosecuting Warren Hastings for corruption (1788) he himself stood to gain from peculations in which, unknown to him, his kinsman William Burke was deeply involved. Moreover the prosecution itself arose largely from the uncritical zeal with which he swallowed accusations brought by Hastings's inveterate enemy Philip Francis. But ill-based as Burke's judgment in many ways was, his motives were always irreproachable, and he took on himself the task of speaking for justice and humanity. He was largely responsible, when the coalition of Fox, Lord North and the Duke of Portland briefly held power (January–December 1783), for a bill empowering the Commons to appoint the Company's governors; his great friend Fox threw himself into the fight and introduced the bill, and Burke spoke to the matter with wonderful breadth of humanitarian vision. Accusing the Company of exploitation worse than that of barbarian conquerors he launched an unforgettable onslaught on the irresponsible youths who made fortunes and returned as nabobs to debase the English society which supported their extortions:

> Animated with all the avarice of age, and all the impetuosity of youth, they roll in one after another; wave after wave; and there is nothing before the eyes of the natives but an endless, hopeless prospect of new flights of birds of prey and passage, with appetites continually renewing for a food that is continually wasting. Every rupee of profit made by an Englishman is lost for ever to India. With us are no retributory superstitions by which a foundation of charity compensates, through ages, to the poor for the rapine and injustice of a day. With us, no pride erects stately monuments

which repair the mischiefs which pride had produced, and which adorn a country out of its own spoils. England has erected no churches, no hospitals, no palaces, no schools; England has built no bridges, made no highroads, cut no navigations, dug out no reservoirs. Every other conqueror of every other description has left some monument, either of state or beneficence, behind him. Were we to be driven out of India this day, nothing would remain, to tell that it had been possessed, during the inglorious period of our dominion, by any thing better than the ourangoutang or the tiger.

Mr. Fox's East India Bill, in *Works*, iii. 79

No wonder John Morley wrote that this is to be found in every book of British eloquence. The whole speech pulses with life, and the tribute to Fox with which it concludes is, considering the ultimate quarrel between the two men, of extraordinarily moving power. Almost as magnificent is the speech on the Nabob of Arcot's debts (1785), and even more famous is the campaign against Warren Hastings, culminating in the historic trial which Fanny Burney brilliantly describes in her *Diary* (beginning 13 February, 1788). Her pages are so vivid that no analysis here can do them justice, but they are a worthy record of a most dramatic episode. Hastings was rightly acquitted, but the nation's eyes were opened to the general evils of corruption, and the duty of imperial power towards a subject territory had been stated in terms of true responsibility.

The last event to be mentioned—the French Revolution—is so vast that it can be introduced merely to point to two other topics. The first is the growth of radicalism, and the second Burke's own philosophy. The two are related as thesis and antithesis and they make the end of the century particularly rich in political importance.

Society was rapidly changing, whereas the revolution of 1688 had at least one unhappy consequence, that of putting a premium on the established order. *Quieta non movere* was Walpole's motto, and his century easily adopted it. The remedy was noise and protest. Social evils gained more publicity as consciences began to awake; Fielding's *Amelia* (1751) comments sombrely on them, and so does a series of novels up to and beyond Godwin's *Caleb Williams*

(1794) and *St. Leon* (1799). They are paralleled by protests such as Paine's *Rights of Man* (1791), Mary Wollstonecraft's *Vindication of the Rights of Women* (1792), George Dyer's *Complaints of the Poor People of England* (1793), and Godwin's *Political Justice* (1793). The conservatives however were not idle: Mathias's *Pursuits of Literature* (1797) is a set of verse satires on progressive ardours, often in a pamphleteering way amusing and effective, and George Canning contributed parodies to the *Anti-Jacobin* (1797-8) which have survived better than their originals (Southey's well-intentioned but slightly ridiculous verses *The Soldier's Wife* and *The Widow*). To the radical, everything was wrong with society: to the conservative, as Canning said in *The Soldier's Friend*, radicalism was

> *Reason, Philosophy, 'fiddledum diddledum',*
> *Peace and Fraternity, higgledy piggledy,*
> *Higgledy piggledy, 'fiddledum diddledum'.*

Canning was a brilliant parodist and *The Soldier's Friend* and *The Needy Knife-Grinder* are famous. But not much reading in social history is needed to discover evils worse than 'fiddledum diddledum'.

Late eighteenth-century political literature is quite interesting. When radical, it features Rousseauistic idealists, natural philosophers, noble savages living in primal sociability, valiant proletarians magnanimously triumphant over corrupt aristocrats, and honest men applying to society the uncompromising solvents of Godwinian Reason and Justice. There is some nonsense in this but there is much one can admire, invective against inhumanity, idealism about fraternity, and a knowledge of the lives the poor actually live. Radicalism finds in Godwin its most methodical and in Shelley its most inspired exponent. Godwin's *Political Justice* is a most remarkable book because it surveys politics by the light of unmitigated reason. At this stage (though he is less austere later) Godwin rejects the irrational ties, the traditional affections of human nature, and even family attachments; every action is to be rational, and every convention not based on strict 'justice' between men jettisoned. Wordsworth, like many others, fell under the spell of these

MEN OF LETTERS AND SOME MAJOR EVENTS 119

> *speculative schemes*
> *That promised to abstract the hopes of Man*
> *Out of his feelings, to be fixed henceforth*
> *For ever in a purer element*
> *The Prelude*, xi. 224–7

though he soon found that man cannot live by thought alone. Shelley rose from *Political Justice*, he told Godwin, 'a wiser and a better man': Hazlitt in *The Spirit of the Age* describes the impact of its Olympian intellectualism. It aimed at strict moral objectivity, 'seeing everything in its true light and estimating everything at its intrinsic value' (i. 337). The defects such a scrutiny revealed in the privileged classes, selfish politics and 'unreasonable' religion of the existing order were fundamental. Godwin's work is still impressive despite its unbending rationalism for its clear style and majestic iconoclasm; it seems to herald the dawn, and what it could mean to the poetic idealist is shown in the fourth act of Shelley's *Prometheus Unbound*, that vision of overthrown churches, crowns, bigots and warmongers. Godwin's faith that 'Truth is omnipotent: the vices and moral weaknesses of men are not invincible: man is perfectible' (3rd edition, 1798, i. 86) was then, and is still, a trumpet which sings to battle for the zealots of progress.

But overthrowing crowns and churches did not appeal to all tastes. An outlook such as Johnson's distrusted indeed far smaller degrees of political change. His *False Alarm* (1770) argues that to rationalise a system of government is probably to destroy it:

> Governments formed by chance, and gradually improved by such expedients as the successive discovery of their defects may happen to suggest, are never to be tried by a regular theory. They are fabricks of dissimilar materials, raised by different architects upon different plans. We must be content with them as they are: should we attempt to mend their disproportion, we might easily demolish and difficultly rebuild them.

It is the position of Burke, whose beliefs it is now time to discuss. They have been mentioned already as supplementing Locke's rational, unitary, political man by a sense of political communities rich in tradition and moved by ancient loyalties. He has been called the Bossuet of politics because of his impassioned sense of custom and his veneration of established habit. But it was Montesquieu whom he particularly admired, because of the theme of the *Esprit des Lois* that governments arise organically from the whole character of their time and place. Burke hated drastic change; 'we compensate, we reconcile, we balance' was his reply to the ardour of revolutionaries. In the *Appeal from the New to the Old Whigs*, as we have seen, he spurned the brave new world of 1789 and attested his loyalty to 1688, to the ancient liberties of England, to what he once called (in a phrase that almost parodies himself) 'the generosity and dignity of thinking of the fourteenth century'. Man's moral and political duties result not from rational argument but from age-old inheritance. Nothing starts afresh, as the radicals proposed it should:

> Men come [as children] into a community with the social state of their parents, endowed with all the benefits, loaded with all the duties, of their situation.... Our country is not a thing of mere physical locality. It consists, in a great measure, in the ancient order into which we are born.... The place that determines our duty to our country is a social civic relation.
>
> *Appeal from the New to the Old Whigs*, in *Works*, v. 94

This social civic relation may comprise injustice or traditions based on injustice, yet even these have become almost sacred through long habit. In the *Reflections on the French Revolution* he vents his scorn on the Duke of Bedford and the Earl of Lauderdale, both supporters of the Revolution: wiser men are more conservative:

> We fear God; we look up with awe to kings; with affection to parliaments; with duty to magistrates; with reverence to priests; and with respect to nobility. Why? Because, when such ideas are brought before our minds, it is *natural* to be so affected.
>
> *Reflections on the Revolution in France*, in *Works*, iv. 94-5

With such a philosophy, Burke might be expected to follow Bolingbroke in propounding national unity under a wise king and statesmen above the schisms of party. He did not, for good reasons. One, no doubt, was that the customs of politics were against it. A second was that George III and Lord North tried something of the sort from 1770 to 1782, to the national dismay. A third was that being himself nearly always in what he called 'a tedious, moderate but practical resistance' to the ministry he appreciated the value of an opposition and knew too much of political affairs to think that they would thrive better under any simpler scheme than the curious one of British parliamentary government. Intricacy was in the nature of things (*Reflections*, in *Works*, iv. 67):

> The nature of man is intricate; the objects of society are of the greatest possible complexity; and therefore no simple disposition or direction of power can be suitable either to man's nature or to the quality of his affairs. ... The simple governments are fundamentally defective, to say no worse of them.

It was a belief that the years strengthened; during the French Revolution it stiffened into dislike of almost any reform however small, though even at the end of a furious diatribe in *Thoughts on French Affairs* (1791) he could turn upon himself (Matthew Arnold called this one of the finest moments in literature) and admit that when history needs a great change the minds of men move inexorably towards it and opposition seems merely petulance in the face of Providence. His French Revolution pamphlets are a disturbing part of his work; prescient though they are, they have nevertheless a fury, a possession, that for some purposes may be good political intuition but is not good political thinking. His distrust of rational enquiry was certainly excessive; political societies cannot be preserved without it. Much of Burke's rhetoric about 'the whole chain and continuity of the commonwealth' is mere sound and fury:

> we have consecrated the state [he declares] that no man should approach to look into its defects or corruptions but with due caution ... that he should approach to the faults of the state as to the wounds of a father, with pious awe and trembling solicitude.
>
> Ibid., in *Works*, iv. 105

Often it seems that nothing should be done about the wounds of a father other than persuading oneself that they are signs of health.

Yet Burke's influence has not been solely spent in buttressing reactionaries. By understanding the psychology of men in communities, and particularly the nature of British liberty, so paradoxical in its union of self-assertion and discipline, he wonderfully deepened the percipience of political philosophy. It is the triumph of something deeper than logic that in the middle of the twentieth century Britain should be united under a hereditary monarch supported by the strange conventions of constitutional rule, by the ceremonies of an Established Church and (from time to time) by the loyal services of a Socialist government, and should moreover, despite every probability to the contrary, still be the centre of widely diverse countries owing allegiance, if not all to the Crown, at least to the political traditions of the British inheritance. Nothing less reasonable by Godwinian standards can be imagined, and Burke, hating as he did the foursquare simplicities of theoretical reason, would surely approve these developments, dictated as they have been by remarkable practical instinct and a disregard for logic which arouses the derision but also the uncomprehending admiration of much of the world.

This account of Burke, as of every other topic raised here, is inadequate. He does, however, appropriately balance Locke, who had a century before so finely clarified political issues and expounded that balanced constitution which Burke so deeply revered. He honoured Locke, yet he marks the different late eighteenth-century climate, so much more aware of man's intuitions than the late seventeenth century with its new-found rationalism had been. His philosophy embodies the admission, which moralists and poets also were making, that human nature has every right to its complexities and irrational instincts.

iv. PARLIAMENT

Know that no man can make a figure in this country but by Parliament.
    LORD CHESTERFIELD
        Letters to his Son, 11 February, 1751

BURKE was not a great parliamentarian, in the sense of one who succeeds in the political game. Horace Walpole calls him 'a very indifferent politician', and others echo the verdict. But his respect for Parliament as the centre of national life was profound, and his admiration for it almost strains credulity. From Swift the following eulogy would have been ironic; from Burke it is entirely serious:

> we know that the British House of Commons, without shutting its doors to any merit in any class, is, by the sure operation of adequate causes, filled with everything illustrious, in rank, in descent, in hereditary and in acquired opulence, in cultivated talents, in military, civil, naval, and politic distinction, that the country can afford.
>   *Reflections*, in *Works*, iv. 47-8

Is this, one asks, that hotbed of corruption, that progeny of rotten boroughs and tyrannical landowners, which supposedly comprised the Augustan Commons? 'I am afraid', Dr Johnson wrote in 1773 to his namesake the Reverend Dr Johnson of Connecticut, 'the next General Election will be a time of uncommon turbulence', and that is indeed the idea the Hanoverian hustings bring to mind. If the drunken revelry of Hogarth's 'Election' cartoons, or the corruption of Fielding's *Pasquin* (in which Lord Place and Colonel Promise for the Court party outbribe Sir Harry Fox-chase and Squire Tankard) are typical, could Parliament deserve such praise?

The truth lies between the extremes. Not all M.P.s were such shining examples as Burke in the flush of his anti-Gallican propaganda makes them out to be. On the other hand the Commons were not a corrupt rabble or elections merely an indecent farce. Corruption itself was not new; it was recognised as evil yet was not unnatural, for a governing class always makes provision for its own safety, and much 'corruption' was nepotism inherent in an age which recognised no ladder of promotion other than personal influence. A seat in Parliament might be costly to achieve and was often used to recoup expenses and indeed make a profitable career. Moreover there was no real party discipline: party lines wavered, and party government needed some means of cementing its majority. This was why Horace Walpole justified bribery in a letter to Horace Mann of 5 May, 1782:

> Esteem is no principle of union. When men are paid, they must vote for what they are bidden to vote. They will have a thousand vagaries when at liberty to vote for what they fancy right or not.

This method gave his father twenty-one years of power, and that may be counted a virtue. The twentieth century controls party loyalties by party discipline, the eighteenth century by *douceurs*.

Indeed, for most of the century no great principle was at stake. Corruption let one group rather than another enjoy power and place but did not subvert a fundamental unity. The anger of honest men, it is true, creates the contrary impression, and bribery certainly spread down from Parliamentary levels, where both sides waged equal battle, to many aspects of daily life where merit was neglected while folly bought success. But at the Parliamentary level bribery was not disastrous and Parliament was not disabled from functioning well. No-one defended bribery as a moral principle but many accepted it as a practical necessity, and in his *Structure of Politics at the Accession of George III* (1929) Sir Lewis Namier concludes that it was 'not a shower-bath from above, constructed by Walpole, the Pelhams or George III, but a water-spout springing from the rock of freedom to meet the demands of the people'.

What was Parliament like? Only a restricted class might reasonably hope for a seat, but for that class election was not difficult, and the accessibility of Parliament was a political stimulant. Certain types took their place almost automatically—the eldest (and sometimes younger) sons of politically-active peers, and country gentlemen who owned seats and occupied them to gain prestige. High army and naval officers often entered politics; so did lawyers, merchants and bankers. On the whole the social standing of M.P.s was fairly high: in 1761 more than half of the Commons were among the peerage and baronetage and the rest were nearly all gentry. These categories more or less coincide with the classes Burke mentions as the glory of the House. Though unrepresentative, Parliament was not without sources of strength. In the first place it allowed young men to grow up in public life acquiring the shrewdness of political experience. In the second, members with a landowning or mercantile background were used to public duty and the management of men. In the third—and this is what Burke felt—a predominantly aristocratic body, if it still remains in living contact with the nation's interests, attracts to itself a good deal of respect, and represents a continuity from the past into the future. And in the fourth, the worst electoral trickery was confined to certain boroughs where a few voters might turn the scale; the county constituencies with fairly numerous voters were far from being always successfully bought and sold.

All this is not a clean bill of health. Nevertheless men of ability did enter Parliament, and once there it was up to them to make their way. Government was not a closed oligarchy and even influential men like the Duke of Newcastle did not in fact control many seats. Members could rise high by their abilities, and though Burke held no prominent office that is partly because his erratic judgment aroused anxiety and partly because his party was mostly in opposition. The House imposed its own standards; within the Chamber it was a man's capacity which counted. Even the existence of rotten boroughs could be defended—and was, by Burke—on the ground that M.P.s represent not particular places but the country as a whole. That is the burden of his *Speech to the Electors of Bristol* (1774), a short but famous statement of the principle that a member of Parliament is a member of Parliament, not a delegate of his constituents. Burke went further in the *Reflections*, and argued that the actual inequality of representation was 'perhaps the very thing which prevents us from thinking or acting as members for districts' (*Works*, iv. 208).

So with all its faults Parliament, newly growing up to its emergent system of responsible Cabinet with majority government and constructive opposition, was viewed with complacency. Henry Brooke's *Fool of Quality* (1766) contemplates the British constitution almost ecstatically; Helenus Scott's *Adventures of a Rupee* (1782) assured its readers that Britain was 'a glorious instance of the blessings that freedom bestows'; Goldsmith's Chinaman observed that the British system combined the strength of the oak and the flexibility of the tamarisk (*Citizen of the World*, letter L), and Paley's *Moral and Political Philosophy* (1786) was equally complimentary:

> When a wise council [*sic*] or beneficial regulation is once suggested it may be expected, from the disposition of an assembly so constituted as the British house of commons is, that it cannot fail of receiving the approbation of a majority.
>
> (Bk. VI, ch. vii)

Without being so uncritical, without forgetting such high-handedness as the attack on Defoe's *Shortest Way*, or the Wilkes election (1769) or the repression of radicals from 1792 onwards, we may conclude that the Augustan Parliament did on the whole what was required of it, that its members were often able watchdogs of the nation's interests and sometimes of its conscience (as with Oglethorpe or Wilberforce), and that members could earn the success to which merit was the passport. There are vivid pages in Moritz's *Travels* showing the Commons in action and capturing the spirit of magnanimous debate as Fox speaks on a motion of gratitude to Admiral Rodney. The ambition 'from heights sublime Of patriot eloquence to flash down fire', as Cowper put it in *The Task*, made this a noted age of oratory. Bolingbroke declared that no man could have a greater honour than that of caring for the public good, and (in a burst of rant) that neither Montaigne, Descartes, Burnet nor Newton 'felt more intellectual joys than he feels who is a *real patriot*'. This, from the *Letter on the Spirit of Patriotism*, is high-flown stuff: the ordinary politician felt few intellectual joys. Yet within normal human limits Parliament stimulated the knowledge of statecraft; at home and abroad it grappled with policy; and it represented the characteristic tone and temper of Hanoverian England.

v. POLITICS AND LITERATURE

There is scarce any Man in *England*, of what Denomination soever, that is not a Free-thinker in Politicks, and hath not some particular Notions of his own, by which he distinguishes himself from the rest of the Community. Our Island, which was formerly called a Nation of Saints, may now be called a Nation of Statesmen.
ADDISON
The Free-Holder, No. 53

POLITICS, then, stamped its impress on the nation's mind. The fifth of Goldsmith's *Citizen of the World* letters describes 'the singular passion of this nation for politics', the 'leaf of political instruction' served up with morning tea, and the politician morning noon and night scurrying from coffee-house to tavern in chase of the news. It is a familiar jest. But was there anything, apart from this mania for news, which particularly affected the writer's outlook?

In the first place, many writers were drawn directly into political affairs. Prior, son of an artisan, became secretary in the Paris embassy; Addison's pro-Marlborough *Campaign* bore fruit in an under-secretaryship of state; Defoe and Swift, Rowe and Parnell, however different their views, worked for Harley, who was perhaps the first statesman to make the press a regular instrument of policy. Gay and Steele were rewarded for political services, and a flock of writers took part in the struggle for and against Walpole. As the century wore on the influence of literary men perhaps declined; literature was in the front line of political struggle until the failure of the 1745; thereafter, in the stability of Hanoverian order, and until the French Revolution, it is rather an onlooker than a participant. Hume, Smollett, Johnson, Goldsmith and Horace Walpole intervened on occasion but they left to politicians like Burke or

'Junius' the close attention which had been characteristic of Swift, Defoe, Prior, Steele, Thomson and Fielding. Sheridan, a dramatist who embarked on politics, belonged to both camps but kept the two distinct. It was in the early half of the century that politics most directly affected the writer, that Addison's *Cato* upheld Whig principles, that the press rained pamphlets on the Hanoverian succession, that Swift championed the Irish, or undermined Marlborough with *The Conduct of the Allies*, and that Bolingbroke united his friends to oppose Walpole. Yet throughout the century politics was generally felt not to be far away, for the whole matter had become (as it was not before Parliamentary government) the daily concern of all men, carried on not in the mysterious sanctum of a Court but by elected representatives whose debates could not (despite Parliament's efforts) be excluded from the newspapers.

In the second place, the constitutional system created a mood of confidence. There was indeed some pessimism—Swift's and Fielding's over corruption and vice, Horace Walpole's lament to Horace Mann (26 July, 1745) that he was 'one of the *ultimi Romanorum*', living at the end of England's greatness, or, on 30 March, 1784, that 'we shall fall into all the distractions of a ruined country'. There was hypochondria in the 1750s, of which John Brown's *Estimate of the Manners and Principles of the Times* (1757) is the mournful monument, and prophets of doom were never lacking. Yet underlying all this was the sense of living under a comprehended system of freedom and loyalty. Personal rights were assumed to be safe, and on the whole they were so.

In the third place, the political system was moderate. Men's ambitions, not their frenzies, ruled the country, and after the conflicts of Anne's reign political passions were kept more or less within bounds. An agreeable *sang-froid*, indeed, often prevailed, as in Pope's idea that only fools contest for forms of government, or in Bubb Dodington's well-considered *Ode* which begins

> *Love thy Country, wish it well,*
> *Not with too intense a care,*
> *'Tis enough, that when it fell,*
> *Thou its ruin didst not share,*

or in John Byrom's characteristic praise of *Careless Content*:

> Of Ups *and* Downs, *of* Ins *and* Outs,
>   *Of* They're i'th'Wrong, *and* We're i'th'Right,
> *I shun the Rancours, and the Routs,*
>   *And wishing well to every Wight,*
> *Whatever Turn the Matter takes,*
> *I deem it all but Ducks and Drakes.*

Not everyone was so nonchalant, but the fact that politics had, as Locke showed, a reasonable basis, that men agreed on fundamentals, that the dismissed minister went into the Opposition or the country rather than the Tower or France, and that in general the nation prospered, meant a world of assurance. The representative writer, then, like Addison, Steele, Defoe, Prior, Green, Pope, Fielding or Johnson reflected an active yet stable world. Pope for instance knew about political vicissitude, for Bolingbroke was his friend, yet his work implies a steady beat in the national pulse: under the brilliant details of social folly there exists a sturdy body on which the follies are only superficial blemishes. In the *Essay on Man* he explained how 'Poet or Patriot' taught the doctrine of unity (iii. 289–301):

> *Taught Pow'r's due use to People and to Kings,*
> *Taught nor to slack, nor strain, its tender strings,*
> *The less, or greater, set so justly true,*
> *That touching one must strike the other too;*
> *'Till jarring int'rests, of themselves, create*
> *Th'according music of a well-mix'd State.*
> *Such is the World's great Harmony, that springs*
> *From Order, Union, full Consent of things;*
> *Where small and great, where weak and mighty, made*
> *To serve, not suffer, strengthen, not invade,*
> *More pow'rful each as needful to the rest,*
> *And, in proportion as it blesses, blest,*
> *Draw to one point, and to one centre bring*
> *Beast, Man, or Angel, Servant, Lord, or King.*

Such an idea, the Augustans felt, was attainable by persuasion, and the British constitution was the natural medium for its realisation.

Pope, it will be noticed, brings political co-operation into harmony with something deeper—that 'Order, Union, full Consent of Things' which the study of nature was confirming as far beyond human contrivance. There is a *mystique* even in rational good sense. Bolingbroke sees the Patriot King achieving this 'full Consent' and arousing in his subjects transports of joy like those Plato describes as arising from the vision of ideal beauty, and Mallet's Bolingbrokean *Truth in Rhyme* finds the prophecy realised in that 'Patron of all worth and truth' George III. The *mystique* involves the belief that political order, as established in 1688 and expounded by Locke, has divine approval behind it, and that that approval is for something traditional as well as reasonable. In his *False Alarm* Johnson argues that no patriot can support a man like Wilkes, since patriotism cannot 'tend to the subversion of order and let wickedness loose upon the land by destroying the reverence due to antiquity'. The phrase is significant; to destroy settled forms is 'wickedness', since the reverence due to antiquity has gathered around them. The argument is weakened by its prejudice: the pamphlet breathes inflexible antipathy to Wilkes and unquestioning support of Parliament's interference. But the deep feelings Johnson expresses are important and emerge again in Burke's claim that the state has been 'consecrated' by antiquity.

This *mystique*, no doubt, made less imaginative appeal than did the earlier political philosophies of Tudor and Stuart England. Both political and natural philosophy were more prosaic than in the Renaissance and both inspired a lot of verse but little poetry. In *The Seventeenth Century* (1929) Professor G. N. Clark describes how scientific method affected political thought; the collection of evidence, the correlation of facts, and the compiling of statistics, all passed over from natural science into 'political arithmetic'. Facts were the thing, instead of the moral-theological concepts by which the Middle Ages sought to legislate for life. Politics itself, it appeared, might be a science (indeed, two centuries had passed since Machiavelli shocked the orthodox by treating it as such). In the 'Voyage to Brobdingnag' Gulliver excuses the King's disdain of Europe because the Brobdingnagians are behind the times, 'not having reduced politics to a science, as the more acute wits of Europe have done'. Later one of Hume's *Essays Moral Political and Literary* (1741) was entitled 'That Politics may be reduced to a Science', and Johnson's *False Alarm* prophesied that

> causeless discontent and seditious violence will grow less frequent and less formidable, as the science of Government is better ascertained by a diligent study of the theory of Man.

Politics, it is true, is far from a pure science and Burke was to protest against the 'geometrical spirit' which treats men as counters. Nor was a scientific theory of politics in the minds of squires, merchants, courtiers and journalists as they negotiated Parliamentary business. But in the general conception of what politics is for, and the fundamental beliefs which support it, the new order was less nourishing to the imagination. Tudor and Stuart politics, for instance, believed in a divinely-appointed hierarchy of powers in the State and a religious reverence for Divine Right. This faith promoted deep feelings about social relationships, as Shakespeare and Hooker show. After Locke the faith was cooler; the 'science of government' and the 'diligent study of the theory of Man' might intoxicate the idealist like Burke, Godwin, or Shelley but to most minds was a prosaic practical thing. The rationalisation of politics led that strong politician Swift indeed to claim it as merely common sense, accessible to all men:

> I have been frequently assured by great Ministers, that Politicks were nothing but common sense.... God hath given the Bulk of Mankind a Capacity to understand Reason when it is fairly offered; and by Reason they would easily be governed, if it were left to their Choice. Those Princes in all Ages who were most distinguished for their mysterious Skill in Government found by the Event that they had ill consulted their own Quiet or the Ease and Happiness of their People.
> *Free Thoughts upon the Present State of Affairs*, in *Political Tracts 1713–1719* (1953), 77

As fact and common sense advanced, imagination and poetry retreated.

One kind of divine sanction, then, gave way to another. God's approval of strong authority, of kingliness haloed by a richly-poetic aura, yielded before God's approval of reasonable men rationally obeying a reasonable constitution. That approval, the century felt, was a very real thing, and to speak of politics as completely secularised would be wrong. But the tone of the Hanoverian settlement is more prosaic, as is that of natural science as compared with the rich jumble of Plinyan natural history and pre-Copernican astronomy which went into the Elizabethan world-picture. God was only just behind the political philosophy of Queen Elizabeth, Shakespeare and the Stuarts (and indeed of Cromwell and Milton), as he was just behind their science, whereas he was a long way behind the politics and science of the Hanoverians. He was still there, as a Prime Mover, but he worked through remote control; the metaphysical element is not absent but it is much less prominent except, perhaps, in the rich amalgam of Burke's thought where it produced a fervour of imagination not seen since the seventeenth century.

Hanoverian politics consequently tended to a sober though approved philosophy. The major questions were settled and even Johnson's Jacobite sympathies did not persuade him to regret Charles Stuart's failure at Culloden, 'so fearful was he', says Boswell, 'of the consequences of another revolution on the throne of Great-Britain' (*Life of Johnson*, 14 July, 1763). Yet the simple formula of prosaic stability needs some modifying, for political language could still be vehement. Some of the vigour of Augustan prose came from the robustness of political argument and the defiant tempers of pamphleteers; there is a good deal which is not formal or Addisonian. The Elizabethan pamphleteers had had their swelling style; so had Milton and his antagonists. Some of the best Restoration prose is in a swingeing mood, fired by the energy of dispute; Sir Roger L'Estrange's *Observator* papers, for instance, are downrightly and picturesquely abusive of Dissenters, and particularly of Oates and the Popish Plot. They have the concrete force of seventeenth-century controversy, graphic and short-rhythmed, and since they are not easily accessible a sample is reprinted (in all its typographical variety) at the end of this chapter, together with a few other passages. Such qualities persist: Halifax's *Maxims* (1693) crack like nutshells:

> That a wise *Prince* will not oblige his *Courtiers*, who are *Birds* of *Prey*, so as to disoblige his *People* who are *Beasts* of *Burden*.

> That *Parties* in a *State*, generally, like *Free-Booters*, hang out *False Colours*; the pretence is the *Publick Good*; the real *Business* is, to catch *Prizes*; like the *Tartars*, where ever they succeed, instead of improving their *Victory*, they presently fall upon the *Baggage*.

Such writing must be as vivid as possible; each stroke must thwack on an adversary's shoulders or at least make enough noise to keep the listener awake. Strong emotion, concrete images and short rhythms are the means to this end, and the earlier Augustans did not disdain a battery of italics. Here is part of Sacheverell's ferocious sermon on *The Communication of Sin*, preached at Derby on 15 August, 1709; its theme is that the duty of not participating in sin either actively or passively makes it necessary to suppress schismatic doctrine:

> He that *Propagates*, or *Publishes*, any pernicious *Writings*, or *Tenets*, knows not how far their *Poyson* will reach, or where the *Deadly Contagion* will stop. It is an *Epidemical Evil*, a *National Calamity*, an *Ever-lasting Plague*, that has slain its *Thousands and its Ten Thousands*, that in the name of that *Destroying Angel* the *Devil* can *taint* whole Families and Kingdoms, and transmit its venom down to Posterity, and continue *Spiritual Death* to the End of the World.

Therefore, it continues, not only heretics such as Socinus and Arius, Hobbes and Spinoza, are to be condemned, but also all the Dissenters'

> *Wild, Latitudinarian, Extravagant Opinions*, and *Bewitching False Doctrines*, the *Impudent Clamours*, the *Lying Misrepresentations*, the *Scandalous* and *False Libels*, both upon the *King* and the *Church*.

Defoe's style, though not so angry, has a similar short-rhythmed energy and cudgelling vigour: Swift's, if often lither, has great resources of vernacular force, the force not of formal composition but (especially in the Irish pamphlets) of the actual speech he would use in hammering his views into his hearers' heads. That is the true style of pamphleteering; as a correspondent wrote to *The Freeholder's Journal* (No. xxxv, 22 August, 1722).

The Expectations of Readers run so high, that unless you *Journalists* now and then cut a bold Stroke, they give you over; cry you are grown insipid, or what is worse turn'd *Pensioners*; and have not one Grain of *Spirit*, *Wit* or *moral Honesty* left.

By Fielding's time the blows were less swashing and the italics fewer, yet Fielding himself has fire and force, less subtle than Swift's but not much less powerful. This is from *The Champion* of 17 June, 1740:

If we desire to preserve our Constitution, if we are willing to propagate Children who shall not have Reason to curse us for giving them Being; if we are ambitious to retain the name of a strong, vigorous and warlike People, let us treat the Doctor [Walpole, under the figure of a quack], his *Zanys* and his *Nostrums* with the Contempt they deserve. Let us cultivate the Temperance and plain Diet of our Ancestors, and shun that luxurious Way of Living, which hath been of late introduced among us, and which may incline us to fly to the *Aurum Potabile* for a short and palliative Relief, since we may be assured of this, that all such Medicines, tho' they may give us a little present Ease, will be attended with a bitter and fatal Consequence, will demolish our Nerves, slacken our Sinews, and in the End totally destroy our Constitution.

And later there was 'Junius', with more finesse and venom, attacking the Duke of Grafton, the usual strong wit being whetted by a rapier-sharp precision of form (the point of assault is the illegitimacy of the first Duke, a natural son of Charles II):

The Character of the reputed ancestors of some men has made it possible for their descendants to be vicious in the extreme without being degenerate. Those of your Grace, for instance, left no distressing examples of virtue, even to their legitimate posterity, and you may look back with pleasure to an illustrious pedigree, in which heraldry has not left a single good quality upon record to insult or upbraid you. You have better proofs of your descent, my Lord, than the register of a marriage, or any troublesome inheritance of reputation. There are some hereditary strokes of character by which a family may be as clearly distinguished as by the blackest features of the human face. Charles the First lived and died a hypocrite. Charles the Second was a hypocrite of another sort, and should have died upon the same scaffold. At a distance of a century we see their different characters happily revived and blended in your Grace. Sullen and severe without religion, profligate without piety, you live like Charles the Second, without being an amiable companion, and for aught I know may die as his father did, without the reputation of a martyr.

Letter XII, 30 May, 1769

Crossing the general stability, then, there is a hard-hitting vitality. The settled order was not neutral or negative; it expressed a creative force. Political writing could be proud of its rational philosophy and yet retain an energy which came of strong feeling. Policies and personalities were vulnerable, and were attacked by manful assurance and a pungent style. Carefully considered, Hanoverian politics abounds in human interest and displays a world in whose basic reasonableness and daily skirmishes the ordinary man could fully participate.

APPENDIX: EXAMPLES OF CONTROVERSIAL PROSE

(*a*) Sir Roger L'Estrange: *The Observator*, 11 February, 1684/5. The paper is the first of the third volume:

Trimmer: Thou art a Man of a *Strange Confidence*; to be *Launching-Out* into *Another Volume*, upon such a *Juncture* as **This** is! Why thou mightst as well Undertake to make a *Main-Sail* for a *First-Rate-Frigat*, of a *Pocket-Handkercher*, as to furnish *Matter* for a *Third Tome* : **Squabbling** and **Controversy** *Apart*.

Observator: Prethee Hold thy self Contented *Trimmer*. Either the People I have had to do withall, **Will** be *Quiet*, or they will **Not** be *Quiet*. If they will **Not** there's Work enough *That* way Cut out, Ready to my Hand: But if they **Will** be *Quiet*, I have as large a Field before me

T'other way: And I shall be as *Ready* to Celebrate the *Miracle* of their *Loyalty*, and *Conversion*, as ever I was to set forth the History of their *Ingratitude*, and *Disobedience*.

(*b*) E. Ward: *Hudibras Redivivus*, 'Apology Added to the Second Edition' (1708):

If the Fanaticks, Dissenters, Moderators, Whigs, Low-Church-men, Saints, Reformers, or whatsoever new Denomination they are pleas'd to rank themselves under, the better to disguise their old base Principles, as well as Practices; should, thro' their great Zeal to the Interest of their Party, think it a Hardship upon the several Tribes, to have some of their obliterated Villanies trump'd up a-fresh, in such a pious Age too, when the wonderful Effects of their pretended Reformation, has made it so very difficult for an honest Man to distinguish a howling Wolf from a Shepherd, or a modern Saint from a Knavish Hypocrite; I desire they could accept of the following Reasons, as a short Apology why I have taken upon me to expose some of their old Madness, Folly, Perfidy and Cruelty, as well as their present Craft.

(*c*) 'Caleb D'Anvers' (Nicholas Amhurst): *The Craftsman*, 3 April, 1736:

As Perfidy is the basest of all Vices, on one Side, so nothing is more grating to human Nature, on the other, than being made *Dupes*, or *Bubbles*. This is so odious in private Life that the Vilest of Criminals are ashamed of it, and often chuse to suffer an ignominious Death, rather than betray their Companions—But when it is practised in Publick Life, by *one* Court against *another*, it is call'd *Policy*, and generally look'd upon as a Mark of political *Wisdom*; though in Truth it is only a bastard Kind of it, and substituted in the Room of superior Abilities; for there is certainly a wide Difference between *Sound Policy*, which is founded upon a *comprehensive Knowledge of Affairs*, and the mean Arts of *Trickery* which require only a *False, Deceitful Heart*, and a little *Cunning*. . . . But when *such base Arts* are put in practise by a *Minister* against the People of his *own Country*, it is still more infamous and provoking; for what may be esteemed only *State-Craft* and *Fair Play* against another Nation (which hath perhaps used *Him* in the same Manner) is downright *Treachery* and *Breach of Trust* against Those in whose Service he is retained.

(d) *Common Sense; or, the Englishman's Journal:* 8 October, 1737:

Excepting a late Imitation of *Horace*, by Mr. *Pope*, who but seldom meddles with publick Matters, I challenge the Ministerial Advocates to produce one Line of *Sense*, or *English*, written on their side of the Question for these last Seven Years. Has any one Person of distinguish'd eminency, in any one Art or Science, shown the least Tendency to support or defend 'em?—Has there been an Essay in Verse or Prose, has there been even a Distich or an Advertisement fit to be read on the Side of the Administration?—But on the other Side, what Numbers of Dissertations, Essays, Treatises, Compositions of all Kinds, in Verse or Prose, have been written, with all that Strength of Reasoning, Quickness of Wit, and Elegance of Expression, which no former Period of Time can equal?— Has not every body got by heart Satires, Lampoons, Ballads and Sarcasms against the Administration? And can any body recollect or repeat one Line for it?

IV. RELIGIOUS LIFE

i. AN ACTIVE INTEREST

We know, and what is better we feel inwardly that religion is the basis of civil society, and the source of all good and of all comfort.
BURKE
Reflections on the Revolution in France, in *Works*, iv. 98

FOR several decades the reputation of Augustan religion has been rising. Where the Victorians saw on the whole only apathy and even cynicism, their successors have found that the sober good will, rising at times to a luminous devotion, which characterises much Hanoverian worship still makes an appeal. At first sight, indeed, there is little colour or spectacle in the Hanoverian panorama, except where it displays the Methodist or Evangelical revivals (themselves protests against apathy), or certain great but exceptional volumes like Law's *Serious Call to a Devout and Holy Life* (1728), Butler's *Analogy* (1736), and the works of Berkeley. Even these, standing out against an apparently widespread unbelief, seem to witness rather to the strength of the tide against which they strain than to any general faith. It is true that certain merits have long been recognised; since Leslie Stephen's *English Thought in the Eighteenth Century* (1876) and Abbey and Overton's *English Church in the Eighteenth Century* (1878), the Church has been vindicated from intellectual sloth and indeed found rich in controversial distinction, and the publication of ecclesiastical records and biographies is weakening the charge of spiritual sloth. Yet even the better Churchmen and Dissenters, with a few exceptions, seem to lack spiritual poetry, and prompt us to accept the Victorian judgment. How far was that judgment true?

This chapter aims not at epitomising Augustan religious history but at discovering how religion influenced writers and their public. Whatever apathy there may have been, men of letters were greatly concerned about religion and many of them, including some not usually credited with spiritual interests like Waller and Roscommon in the Restoration years and Pomfret and Prior among the Augustans, tried their hands at religious themes. Prior indeed is characteristic; brilliant in social verse, he yet looked on *Solomon* (1718) as his most important poem. The public too was interested: 'there is not any where, I believe, so much Talk about Religion as among us in England' *The Guardian* (No. 65) asserted in 1713. Three decades later Young's *Night Thoughts* echoed the comment—'Few ages have been deeper in dispute about Religion than this' (book vi, preface). As Swift put it in *Thoughts on Various Subjects*, 'we have just enough Religion to make us hate, but not enough to make us love one another', and Defoe's *True-Born Englishman* mocked at disputants fertile in dogma and barren in charity:

> *In their Religion they are so unev'n,*
> *That each Man goes his own By-way to Heaven.*
> *Tenacious of Mistakes to that degree*
> *That ev'ry Man pursues it sep'rately,*
> *And fancies none can find the Way but he.*

Hanoverian religion was anything but unbroken torpor: a Churchman, in the eyes of a Methodist or 'freethinker', was a Laodicean; a Methodist, in the eyes of a Churchman or freethinker, was a fanatic; and a freethinker, in the eyes of a Churchman or Methodist, was a coxcomb.

The appetite for polemics and morality was remarkable. Addison's Saturday lay sermons in *The Spectator* were widely read (though Berkeley's 'grave discourses' in *The Guardian* were not so popular), Butler's austere *Analogy* went into three editions in its year of publication (1736), and Young's *Night Thoughts*, almost ten thousand lines of inexpressible tedium, had ten editions in five years. Sermons flowed from the printers: controversies filled the land with gesticulating contestants. Leslie Stephen once observed that nobody could recall the causes of the eighteenth century's wars save examinees whose knowledge had not yet had time to leak out, and the same is true of its religious quarrels. Yet in their own day, as Johnson said of the Bangorian affair, they 'filled the press with pamphlets, and the coffee-houses with disputants' (*Life of Savage*). A fertile press and reverberating coffee-houses are unmistakable signs of popular interest.

The Bangorian controversy exploded from a sermon by Hoadly, Bishop of Bangor, in 1717, alleging that no earthly institution (such as an organised church) properly represents the spiritual kingdom of Christ. From a bishop this was a startling doctrine and the consequences were violent; it has been reckoned that fifty-three writers fired off two hundred pamphlets on the subject, and forty years later Goldsmith in *The Bee* (17 November, 1759) complained that clergymen were still bemusing their long-suffering congregations with it. Another storm arose over the Arian doctrines of William Whiston, Newton's successor in the Lucasian professorship at Cambridge, who was deprived of his Chair in 1710 for disbelief in the Trinity. Incidentally he also held that clergymen should marry once only, and it was the Vicar of Wakefield's devotion to this doctrine that jeopardised his son's marriage, since the bride's father was about to take a fourth wife. On Arianism and Deism something will be said later.

When tempers were fired with political as well as religious fuel the blaze was particularly fierce. This was evident in the famous trials of Sacheverell and Atterbury. The former so immoderately denounced the toleration of Dissenters that he was impeached by Parliament in 1709 and to the accompaniment of anti-Dissenter riots found guilty in 1710. If the pillory, said Defoe in *A Hymn to the Pillory*, held all who deserved it,

> *There would the Fam'd* S[achevere]ll *stand*
> *With Trumpet of Sedition in his Hand,*
> *Sounding the first* Crusado *in the Land.*
> *He from a Church of* England *Pulpit first*
> *All his Dissenting Brethren curst:*
> *Doom'd them to Satan for a Prey,*
> *And first found out* the shortest way

(an allusion to Defoe's own parody of High-Church fury, *The*

Shortest Way with the Dissenters, which had landed him in the pillory). Yet Sacheverell's sentence was so light as to seem a moral victory and to be wildly celebrated by his Tory friends and the hotheaded citizenry.

The trial of Atterbury, Bishop of Rochester, was not dissimilar, though the Whigs now won outright. Found guilty of Jacobite intrigues he was exiled in 1723 and died abroad in 1732. As at Sacheverell's trial tumults broke out in his favour, and both affairs illustrate the dangers of religious inflammation, which blazed at intervals until the Gordon riots of 1780 provided a tragic climax.

Polemics can flourish while spirituality decays. Yet spirituality if often absent from these disputes was not always so. Law's first work arose out of the Bangorian turmoil and Butler's out of his criticism of Deism, the *Analogy* being its culmination. And in non-controversial matters there was steady respect for religion sometimes deepening into real devotion. Burke throws an unexpected light on this in commenting on a custom—the Grand Tour—not often associated with faith. Youths on their travels, he says, have clergymen-tutors

> not as austere masters, nor as mere followers, but as friends and companions of a graver character, and not seldom persons as well born as themselves. With them, as relations, they most commonly keep up a close connection through life. By this connection we conceive that we attach our gentlemen to the church; and we liberalize the church by an intercourse with the leading characters of the country.
>
> *Reflections*, in *Works*, iv. 109

On a deeper level Burke often asserts with earnest passion the integral nature of religious reverence to the whole organism of Church and State. The Augustans were often enough worldly, but they often also encouraged devotion, sometimes prosaic but reliable as with Parsons Cole and Woodforde, sometimes complacent yet genuine, as with Addison, sometimes troubled as with Butler, Johnson and Cowper, and sometimes passionate and joyful as with Berkeley and Law.

ii. MODES OF FAITH

In the Shops and Warehouses the prentices stand some on one side of the Shop and some on the other (having Trade little enough) and there they throw *High Church* and *Low Church* at one another's Heads like battledore and shuttlecock.

DEFOE
Reasons Against the Succession of the House of Hanover (1713), 5

For modes of faith, Pope thought, only graceless zealots could fight. Two centuries of anger had taught the folly of dissension. Yet dissension itself reflected the importance attaching to faith, and Burke's pronouncement that religion was the basis of civil society would have been echoed by each of the three main parties—Churchmen, Papists and Dissenters. The lines of eighteenth-century division must now be drawn, with the proviso that they grew gradually less harsh.

Over the Roman Catholics it is unnecessary to linger. Excluded by the Test Act of 1673 from civil and military office they were suspect of Jacobitism and drew as little attention to themselves as possible. 'I had my beginnings among men of a proscribed religion', Pope told Joseph Spence, and he spoke of his private boyhood and youth. Popular distrust was always simmering; the Monument (which, Pope wrote in the third *Moral Essay*, 'like a tall bully lifts its head and lies') bore an inscription that Papists had caused the Great Fire; the '15 and '45 rebellions threatened a Stuart restoration; and even Horace Walpole smelt Papal machinations in a most improbable quarter—'the Methodists', he surmised, 'are secret Papists and no doubt they copy, build on, and extend their rites towards [Rome]' (*Memoirs of the Reign of George III*, 1894, iii. 35). A Relief Bill in their favour caused an upheaval in Scotland (1778) and the still more violent Gordon Riots in England (1780), when London had a week's reign of terror and the mob besieged Parliament, menaced the Bill's promoters, and burnt Papist chapels and the formidable Newgate Prison. Yet the frenzy died away; another Relief Bill became law in 1791 and granted a fair measure of toleration. All in all, the Roman Church loomed in English eyes (with some reason) as a bogy, but its adherents were a small and peaceable minority.

The relations of Church and Dissent were more intricate. The two were not always in sharp antithesis, any more than were the two ill-defined political parties, and as with the political parties the split of allegiances was accepted with some dismay. Before the Restoration the main division—between Episcopalians and Presbyterians—had been within the Church, between the advocates of prelacy, ritual and temperate reform, and those of presbyterianism (organisation by presbyteries of clergy and people), austerity and thorough change. The Act of Uniformity (1662), however, caused a break by enforcing episcopal ordination, and drove from the Church those who 'dissented'. Even so, the more Latitudinarian Churchmen, towards the end of the seventeenth century, hoped for renewed comprehension within a tolerant Church, and this hope is interestingly presented in Dr. Carpenter's *Thomas Tenison* (1948). Because it failed, many able men were lost to the Church, universities and crown offices, though with corresponding benefit to chapels, trade and industry.

Within the Church there was much variety. On one wing came the Non-Jurors like Archbishop Sancroft, Bishop Ken, Thomas Hearne and Jeremy Collier, loyal to the divine right of James II, unprepared to swear allegiance to William and Mary, and the centre of vigorous pamphlet polemics. Colley Cibber's comedy *The Non-Juror* (1718) is a stoutly Whiggish view of 'the stiff Non-Juring Separation Saint' Sir John Woodvil, seduced by a 'vile Non-juring Zealot' Dr. Wolf, and reclaimed by a sensible son. This, it need hardly be said, is a caricature of a devoted body of men faithful to a lost cause. Apart from this small minority (gradually lost to view as time passed) there were the High- and Low-Church parties which prompted Swift's High- and Low-Heel satire in 'Lilliput'. The former upheld Caroline traditions of Church power and prerogative, the latter the Latitudinarian rationalism which played down dogma and privilege and preached mainly a reasonable faith and the social virtues. The 'men of Latitude' found their programme in Locke's *Letters Concerning Toleration* (1689–1706) and *The Reasonableness of Christianity* (1695), and their leader in Archbishop Tillotson. Their faith seems now to have an ethical rather than a religious flavour, yet it was then a matter of high humanity and of Christian charity, certainly not the less admirable for seeing Christian faith in the light of divine mercy and human brotherhood. From the time of the Cambridge Platonists through the eighteenth century and into the nineteenth it diffused a spirit, at best of extensive charity, at worst of prosaic reason, which was the best possible antidote to sectarian strife.

Of Dissent it is harder to generalise. Strictly speaking, one needs to distinguish, as Tenison's *Argument for Union* (1683) says, between

> Presbyterians, Arians, Socinians, Anabaptists, Fifth-Monarchy Men, Sensual Millenaries, Behmenists, Familists, Seekers, Antinomians, Ranters, Sabbatarians, Quakers, Muggletonians [and] Sweet Singers.

Ignoring these niceties of fission, the main divisions were between Presbyterians, Independents and Baptists. All went back to Elizabethan times or the early Stuarts. The Presbyterians had cherished from the later sixteenth century the idea (triumphant in Scotland) of a national Church organised not under bishops but under the more democratic system of presbyteries, and had for a while in Commonwealth days accomplished their dream. The Independents, descended from Elizabethan Separatists, had also known their hour of glory as Cromwell's strongest supporters, but unlike the Presbyterians they looked not for a national Church but for independent congregations gathered by the magnetism of direct religious experience. The Baptists, originating in the early seventeenth century, prizing adult baptism as the hallmark of the true Christian, were fired with a zeal which later brought many of them into sympathy with Methodism. Theirs is the credit of having introduced the eighteenth century's great innovation in worship—the supplementing of metrical psalms by congregational hymns, and the establishment thereby of a profoundly important body of popular poetry.

Such was the main, original, constitution of Dissent. Fewer but increasingly influential were the Quakers and Unitarians. The latter, followers of Arius or Socinus in denying Christ's equality with the Father ('silver-tongued anti-Christs', John Wesley called them), gained ground gradually as 'the reasonableness of Christianity' encroached on dogmatic faith; Milton, Newton and Locke were touched with Arianism, and Samuel Clarke and William Whiston imbibed it deeply. The most notable of eighteenth-century Unitarians were Richard Price the minister of Old Jewry whose radicalism provoked Burke into his *Reflections on the French Revolution*, Joseph Priestley the chemist-philosopher, and Josiah Wedgwood. Like the Quakers they were a small sect but comprised an intelligent and public-spirited body of Dissent, and their ethical Christianity bore fruit out of proportion to their numbers, in England and New England alike.

Methodism has hardly yet been mentioned, for though it is now perhaps the most characteristic example of Nonconformity it was not, originally, Dissent. It arose long after the dissenting sects of 1662, it was frowned on as hysterical by many Hanoverian Dissenters (now sober citizens), and its founders did not mean to secede from the Church, which they wished only to revitalise. Yet in effect Methodism became a form of Dissent, casting its spell on thousands whom the Church did not touch, and the greatest religious movement of the time fell largely outside the Establishment.

There are few greater Englishmen than John Wesley, and to compress his achievement into a paragraph is like trying to see the world in a grain of sand and eternity in an hour. From his father's High-Church devotion and from William Law's religious passion he and his brother Charles drew a spirit which instilled into England and the American colonies a profound emotion, breaking up ignorance and apathy and bringing their followers the most personal sense of religious experience. Churchmen and Dissenters had every excuse for suspicion; convulsions and apocalyptic frenzies seized the early congregations as if with a consuming fire. Yet there was hardly any other channel for the sense Methodism brought—that of the soul's condition—and fortunately this happened on the whole not (as it might have done) under the severity of Calvinism but under the charity of Arminianism, which preached salvation to all men. The Wesleys' hymns will be considered later; their spirit recalls Blake (influenced by them) when, to the question whether he did not see the sun like a disk of fire, he answered 'O no, no, I see an innumerable company of the heavenly host crying: "Holy, Holy, Holy is the Lord God Almighty!"' George Whitefield, it is true, was a Calvinist, and it was the Calvinistic side of Evangelicalism which so afflicted Cowper, but the Wesleys announced the comforting faith of salvation for all, and their influence is perhaps the most remarkable social phenomenon of the later eighteenth century. Yet the movement was not entirely their doing; there was evangelicalism apart from and indeed prior to Methodism, as in Cornwall under Samuel Walker of Truro; men like John Berridge of Everton, John Newton (Cowper's friend), William Wilberforce and Charles Simeon at Holy Trinity, Cambridge, were moved by an independent though similar spirit. By the end of the century Evangelicalism both within and without the Church united Churchmen and Nonconformists in that powerful religious emotion which meant so much to the future.

Though sympathy between the different denominations grew by degrees it was not very conspicuous in the early years of the century. The controversial violence of Queen Anne's reign is reflected in Swift's *Journal to Stella* and *Examiner* papers, in Defoe, and in his adversary Ned Ward's *Hudibras Redivivus*. The more vehement sectarians entertained feelings such as Blake was to epitomise in *The Everlasting Gospel:*

> *Both read the Bible day and night,*
> *But thou read'st black where I read white.*

Swift and Defoe represent this state of affairs, though not in an extreme form. Swift held by a consolidating Toryism of Church and State; most Englishmen, he thought, were for uncompromising churchmanship and the belief that

the Church of England should be preserved entire in all Her Rights, Powers and Priviledges; all Doctrines relating to Government discour-

aged which She condemns; all Schisms, Sects and Heresies discountenanced and kept under due Subjection . . .; Her open Enemies (among whom I include at least Dissenters of all Denominations) not trusted with the smallest Degree of Civil or Military Power; and Her secret Adversaries, under the Names of Whigs, Low-Church, Republicans, Moderation-Men and the like, receive no Marks of Favour from the Crown, but what they should deserve by a sincere Reformation.
Free Thoughts Upon the Present State of Affairs, in *Political Tracts 1713–1719* (1953), 88

He was strong for unity round a reverenced Church and Crown; like the Vicar of Bray in his Tory phase,

> *Occasional Conformists base*
> *[He] damn'd, and Moderation;*
> *And thought the Church in danger was*
> *From such Prevarication.*

When 'faction' is suppressed and 'things return to the old course', he says in the 43rd *Examiner*, then 'mankind will naturally fall to act from principles of reason and religion'. That reason could lead rather to dissent than to assent was a thing he apparently could never understand; though far less extreme than many Churchmen he stood stoutly to the right of centre and thought all virtue stood with him.

He loathed Dissent and tolerant cosmopolitan Whiggery:

These men take it into their imagination that trade can never flourish unless the country becomes a common receptacle for all nations, religions and languages. Such an island as ours can afford enough to support the majesty of a crown, the honour of a nobility, and the dignity of a magistracy; we can encourage arts and sciences, maintain our bishops and clergy, and suffer our gentry to live in a decent hospitable manner; yet still there will remain hands sufficient for trade and manufactures.
The Examiner, No. 22

It is an illiberal passage in some ways, prompted by fear of an influx of European Protestants if the Whigs were allowed to admit them, but its basis is an emotional attachment to the poetry of Church and

State shared, in different ways and without Swift's limitations, by Shakespeare, Johnson, Burke and Coleridge.

It was not shared, however, by Defoe, patriotic though he was, for his attachments were to Dissent, toleration and trade. No more than Swift does he show any real religious experience—each is devoted rather to religious politics, Anglican or nonconformist. But his devotion, like Swift's, was sincere, and though he gave Harley some time-serving advice on the way to discourage Dissent he remained a Dissenter himself for his soul's good. In face of High-Church fury he and his fellows robustly cried down the High-flyers and Jacobites, and naturally they provoked their enemies:

> *They made a fearful Acclamation,*
> *And loudly cry'd up Moderation . . .*
> *The Low-Church are Prevaricators,*
> *Proud of the Name of Moderators:*
> *By subtle Arts made factious Tools,*
> *In short, they're the Dissenters' Fools.*

So did Ward's *Hudibras Redivivus* deride them. But Defoe's pleas for toleration and his support of the Low-Church and Hanoverian parties were anything but fractious. In a group of pamphlets—*An Answer to the Question, 'What if the Queen should Die?'*, *What if the Pretender should Come?*, and the ironical *Reasons Against the Succession of the House of Hanover* (all 1713) he campaigned against Jacobitism, as in *The Storm* he had turned the tempest of 1703 into a divine judgment on intolerance. These quarrels are remote now, but then they were matters of life and death—men convicted on religious grounds could die in the pillory, and an attempt was made to assassinate Defoe's friend William Colepepper. The reign of Anne cannot be understood without a knowledge of the violent winds still blowing from the storm-centres of the seventeenth century.

Yet the Augustans gradually learned the middle way. Defoe's fine apologia for his propagandist work—*An Appeal to Honour and Justice* (1715)—sounds a note of reconciliation:

It is and ever was my Opinion, that Moderation is the only Vertue by which the Peace and Tranquillity of this Nation can be preserv'd. I think I may be allow'd to say, a *Conquest of Parties* will never do it! *A Ballance of Parties* MAY.

The mob was sometimes dangerous, but reason slowly prevailed. The old prepossessions, it is true, survived in a modified form; Johnson was a Tory and a Churchman and thundered against the American colonists for their dissidence, while Burke was a Whig and admired the Protestantism of the Protestant religion which animated them. Yet Burke and Johnson were warm friends, and the latter was even sympathetic, late in life, with the new evangelicalism. In the 1790s, unfortunately, a chasm opened between rationalist Dissenters and the great body of Churchmen and others, on the subject of radical politics; in this case Burke who had moved to the right stormed against radical Dissent as an ally of 'atheism'. But during most of the eighteenth century the lessons of forbearance were learned, and antipathies brought within reasonable bounds.

iii. ATTACK AND DEFENCE

My friend Sir Roger told them, with the air of a man who would not give his judgment rashly, that much might be said on both sides.
ADDISON
The Spectator, No. 122

MODERATION, however, may look like apathy; it may originate less in charity than in carelessness. Was religion apathetic, heedless and dull? Is the indictment correct which condemns the Church as sycophantic and complacent, Dissent as drab or hysterical, and the public as ignorant and irresponsible? The devil's advocate must be heard, though with the proviso that most of what he says comes from worried clerics who were anything but advocates of the devil.

The first objection might be that dull preaching went on in dull churches. Postponing the question of preaching, one may admit that many people find neoclassic buildings less rich in religious emotion than mediaeval or even pseudo-mediaeval, and indeed often as pagan as the fashionable chapel which Pope describes in the *Epistle to Burlington* (141–8):

> And now the Chapel's silver bell you hear,
> That summons you to all the Pride of Pray'r;
> Light Quirks of Musick, broken and uneven,
> Make the Soul dance upon a Jig to Heaven.
> On painted Cielings you devoutly stare,
> Where sprawl the Saints of Verrio or Laguerre,
> On gilded Clouds in fair expansion lie,
> And bring all Paradise before your eye.

Gothic churches are taken to symbolise ages of faith, classical churches nothing but humanism. We see too clearly in these well-lit, symmetrical structures. Like Milton we may prefer 'storied windows richly dight'; like Gray, we desire 'the long-drawn aisle and fretted vault'; like Burke, we feel that the clear and the sublime do not go together. And the services in these buildings were, we deduce, too prosaic: mediaeval murals had disappeared under a coat of whitewash, and poetic faith under that of plain reason.

To these objections there are reasonable answers. The church had become an auditory for hearing the service rather than a setting for ritual, a development influenced perhaps by Inigo Jones's St. Paul's in Covent Garden, a simple rectangle with galleries to provide more seats. Wren planned his churches similarly, so that each worshipper could actively participate in the whole service. The spatial unity emphasised the unity of priest and people, and the intention was far from one of pagan pomp—it was the desire that the act of worship should be felt intimately by each person. The best study of these questions (Addleshaw and Etchells's *Architectural Setting of Anglican Worship*, 1948) describes the better churches as 'a perfect expression of eighteenth-century Anglicanism, its lucidity, its classical view of life, its freedom from cant and humbug, its objectivity'. The Augustans' religious emotions were different from ours but not necessarily inferior, and they found a style congruous to their needs, spacious, dignified and thoughtful. Berkeley likened St. Paul's Cathedral to the whole spirit and purpose of Anglicanism (*The Guardian*, No. 70):

> The Divine Order and Œconomy of the one seemed to be emblematically set forth by the just, plain and majestick Architecture of the other. And as the one consists of a great Variety of Parts united in the same regular Design, according to the truest Art and most exact Proportion; so the other contains a decent Subordination of Members, various sacred Institutions, sublime Doctrines, and solid Precepts of Morality digested into the same Design, and with an admirable Concurrence tending to one View, the Happiness and Exaltation of Human Nature.

Speaking of the happiness and exaltation of human nature Berkeley is not making humanity self-sufficient; as little as anyone in his age did he forget spirituality, and it is a religious happiness and exaltation he has in mind. Defoe too found St. Paul's 'the beauty of all the churches in the city, and of all the Protestant churches in the world', and correlated its dignity with the plainness of Protestant doctrine (*Tour*, i. 336). St. Paul's, it is true, is the masterpiece of English classical buildings but its idiom is the language of the time and the Augustans found it abundantly reverent, as indeed it is. Nor did Dissenters think their meeting-houses too prosaic, those plain brick boxes or severe stucco-and-Doric-columned halls for the direct service of God, such as still placate the eye in country towns and indeed, though sadly grimed, in most industrial cities.

The twin-objection, of dull services, must be admitted to be more valid. Latitudinarianism was the spirit of prose. Swift found the normal Anglican preacher tedious, and by contrast exhibited an abnormal Anglican ('little parson Dapper', *i.e.* Joseph Trapp, High-Church-and-Sacheverell partisan) and a Dissenter (Daniel Burgess of Covent-Garden Meeting-House), both famous for their vehemence (*The Tatler*, No. 66). Church services, Wesley complained, were perfunctory, and Goldsmith even lamented the vogue of Tillotson's much-praised style, under whose influence 'the spruce preacher reads his lucubration without lifting his nose from the text and never ventures to earn the shame of an enthusiast' (*The Bee*, 17 November, 1759). Dissenting sermons were not always better; in mid-century both Church and Dissent were respectable, and generally dull. The evangelical revival of course made a difference; on 30 July, 1763, as Johnson and Boswell sailed down to Greenwich and talked of preaching styles, Johnson praised the Methodists and Scots Presbyterians for their vivacity, as 'the only way to do good to the common people', and in 1764 Goldsmith's essay *On the English Clergy and Popular Preachers* contrasted the polite tedium of the one party with the zeal of the other. In extenuation one might plead that Church and Dissent by forfeiting some poetry had acquired more reason, that clerical duties were often done well, and that dull sermons are not one age's monopoly. But that hardly refutes the persistent charge.

There remains, however, a worse accusation—that of worldliness. Some accounts show the clergy as worse than worldly: Swift drew his vicar-schoolmaster in the 71st *Tatler*, a coarse figure who sometimes played bowls while his curate conducted his services, and sometimes slept 'sotting in the desk on a hassock' while the curate preached. Crabbe was mordant about the sporting parson in *The Village* who scorned a pauper's funeral, or the reprobate in *Inebriety* (177–82):

> *The reverend wig, in sideway order plac'd,*
> *The reverend band, by rubric stains disgrac'd,*
> *The leering eye, in wayward circles roll'd,*
> *Mark him the pastor of a jovial fold,*
> *Whose various texts excite a loud applause,*
> *Favouring the bottle, and the good old cause.*

Fielding has his repulsive Trulliber in *Joseph Andrews* and Thwackum in *Tom Jones*, Hogarth his grotesques in *An Election Entertainment* and *The Sleeping Congregation*, and Churchill his 'Atheist Chaplain of an Atheist Lord'. In actual life there were men like Churchill himself, the strongest satirist between Pope and Byron, and drawn by Hogarth as a bear in clerical bands grasping a club and a tankard of ale—a hit at his dissipations. Sterne, consumptive and of an electrical sensibility, was not perhaps strictly accountable for his dubious morals, but *Tristram Shandy* is a Rabelaisian novel for a clergyman and it is not surprising that Warburton came to think him 'an irrevocable scoundrel' and that Wesley, as he told Sophie von la Roche, hoped 'never to have a Sterne amongst the seven hundred clerics of his community'. Less erratic but still hardly praiseworthy were easy-going men like Edmund Pyle, royal chaplain and prebendary of Winchester, who remarked that 'the life of a prebendary is a pretty easy way of dawdling away one's time; praying, walking, visiting, and as little study as the heart could wish', or Cornwallis, a man of the world whose lavish entertainments were reproved by George II as 'levities and vain dissipations' yet who became Archbishop in 1768. As for men like Swift, Hoadly and Warburton, those characteristic Augustan figures, though they clearly felt they were doing their duty by the Church they conceived it to lie rather in controversy than in spiritual enlightenment.

The higher preferments were part of politics, and Whig and Tory alternation swayed the bench of bishops this way and that, a condition which, when the Whigs established something like a monopoly, Johnson described as 'no better than the politics of stockjobbers and the religion of infidels'. Behind this partisanship there was something religious—a concern for the Church's honourable estate on the Tory side, and for liberalism towards Dissent on the Whig. But in the foreground these decent motives were hidden by opportunism. A striking instance of religious politics was the help Walpole received from his Whig bishops in 1733, when in two critical divisions twenty-four of the twenty-five bishops who voted supported him, giving him victory by a single vote. Such a performance might conceivably reflect a conscientious conviction but it could also look remarkably like venality.

Preferment was unsystematic, with favouritism on one hand and neglect on the other. Hoadly, by propagating the principles of 1688, flattering George I, and taking a strong line against Atterbury, garnered from successive Whig ministries the sees of Bangor (1715) which he never visited, Hereford (1721), Salisbury (1723) and the valuable Winchester (1734). More remarkable was the career of Brownlow North, younger half-brother of Lord North who was

Prime Minister from 1770 to 1781, and as Lord North was a Tory it cannot be said that only the Whigs took their responsibilities lightly. Brownlow became a canon in 1768 at twenty-seven, Dean of Canterbury at twenty-nine, and Bishop of Coventry at thirty. Even an unsqueamish age was surprised at this, and Lord North is said to have rejoined that Brownlow was indeed rather young but that if he were kept waiting he might no longer have a Prime Minister for his brother. Lord North in fact conveniently held on to office and continued his fraternal care: Brownlow was translated to Worcester in 1774 and in 1781 to Winchester, the wealthiest see after Canterbury and Durham, where his income of £5,000 was worth in modern terms about four times as much. Surviving there for thirty-nine years he netted in all, in modern values, well over £750,000. Happily he was a good and generous man; he founded charities and raised large sums for church building. But no more than Lord North was he averse from favouritism; he made his elder son master of St. Cross Hospital, his younger son prebendary of Winchester, and the latter's son (another Brownlow) registrar of the diocese (a sinecure) at the somewhat remarkable age of seven.

At the other extreme there were poor curates, poor parsons, and even poor bishops. In the 22nd *Examiner* Swift spoke of the clergy as 'groaning everywhere under the weight of poverty, oppression, contempt and obloquy' until Queen Anne's bounty relieved them. Soon afterwards *The Guardian* (No. 65) felt compelled to ask

How is it possible for a Gentleman under the Income of fifty Pounds a Year, to be attentive to sublime Things? *Power and Commandment to his Ministers to declare and pronounce to his People* is mentioned with a very unregarded Air, when the Speaker is known in his private Condition to be almost an Object of their Pity and Charity.

Curates received in general from £30 to £40 a year—Fielding's Abraham Adams has £23 for himself, his wife and six children. Even benefices were often miserable: in the early eighteenth century more than half were under £50 a year. Goldsmith's parson in *The Deserted Village* is, we recall, 'passing rich on forty pounds a year', and the Vicar of Wakefield holds one living of £35 and then moves to another of £15 which he supplements by farming. Churchill spoke of himself in *The Author* (347–50) as

> *Condemn'd (whilst proud and pamper'd sons of lawn,*
> *Cramm'd to the throat, in lazy plenty yawn)*
> *In pomp of* rev'rend beggary *to appear,*
> *To pray, and starve, on forty pounds a year.*

Poor stipends had often to be raised by the holding of pluralities, but the normal Augustan cleric remained in moderate position at best, respected in the varying degrees which his own worth merited and the civility or boorishness of his parishioners prompted. The ordinary clergy were truly a part of their times, not markedly above their fellows in social standing, somewhat superior in learning and conduct but, for both evil and good, little separated from the mass of the people. They fished, shot, hunted, farmed and marketed with their neighbours, and on Sunday assumed a degree of extra dignity and preached to them. They were often ill-paid or ill-qualified, but if not always invested with the reverence which the nineteenth century thought proper (and which prevailed in Scotland from the days of John Knox) yet they included many good parish priests and Dissenting ministers, and an unspecialised relationship of church and people has its merits.

The clergy, on the whole, spread a touch of civilisation: is it not a good thing, Swift asks ironically in the *Argument Against Abolishing Christianity*, 'to have one literate man in each parish?' Thomas Percy, famous for the *Reliques of Antient English Poetry*, observed to Johnson that one could tell 'whether or no there was a clergyman resident in a parish by the civil or savage manner of the people', and Johnson quoted the remark to a discouraged young parson who sought his advice. 'A clergyman's diligence', Johnson added, 'always makes him venerable' (Boswell, *Life of Johnson*, 30 August, 1780). The 112th *Spectator* is a pleasant picture of social civility; the villagers, 'with their best faces and in their cleanliest habits', meet every Sunday 'to converse with one another upon indifferent subjects, hear their duties explained to them, and join together in adoration of the Supreme Being'. Country Sundays have changed but little. Sir Roger de Coverley's clergyman is the true shepherd of such a flock, sensible, sound in scholarship, handy at backgammon, and judicious in choosing his sermons from the published works of eminent divines. Good instruction is what he purveys, with no nonsense about original composition. The Vicar of Wakefield is equally companionable with his parishioners, and when he moves from his first to his second cure the neighbourhood comes to greet him, 'dressed in their finest clothes and preceded by a pipe and tabor'. In actual life diaries such as William Cole's, of Bletchley, and Parson Woodforde's, record honest lives devoted to their country charges; and Pastor Moritz describes a Sunday at Nettlebed in Oxfordshire in words which recall the life of Hardy's Wessex (*Travels*, 1924, 135–6):

> The service was now pretty well advanced, when I observed some little stir in the desk; the clerk was busy, and they seemed to be preparing for something new and solemn; and I also perceived several musical instruments. The clergyman now stopped and the clerk said, in a loud voice, 'Let us sing to the praise and glory of God, the forty-seventh psalm'. I cannot well express how affecting and edifying it seemed to me, to hear this whole, orderly and decent congregation, in this small country church, joining together, with vocal and instrumental music, in praise of their Maker. It was the more grateful, as having been performed not by mercenary musicians, but by the peaceful and pious inhabitants of this sweet village. I can hardly figure to myself any offering more likely to be grateful to God.

Through Augustan worship there runs the feeling which still rules in quieter districts, a steady element in normal life, not unworldly or intense, but taken naturally and for granted. It has its limitations, admittedly, as Parson Adams found when he questioned the innkeeper about salvation. 'Faith, master,' replied the host, 'I never once thought of that; but what signifies talking about matters so far off?' (*Joseph Andrews*, II. 3). The answer, however distressing to Adams, is as natural as any that Hardy's countrymen might give; it reflects a religious life as normal as the process of the crops, and sunshine and rain in due season.

Yet this sensible religion, it may be objected, omits everything of importance; it impresses neither those to whom religion means much nor those to whom it means little. Neither hot nor cold, like the Laodiceans it knows not that it is 'wretched, and miserable, and poor, and blind, and naked'. Was Georgian religion mere complacency?

It did certainly anticipate Talleyrand's warning against zeal, but stability was newly-won and still precarious. 'Enthusiasm' did indeed seem, in Bishop Butler's phrase to Wesley, 'a horrid thing, a very horrid thing', and Samuel Butler and Abraham Cowley, those forerunners of the Augustans, flayed the extremists, the former in the Puritan Hudibras, the latter in *The Character of a Holy Sister*. So did Dryden, and so did Addison, denouncing 'false zealots in religion', including those whose zeal was for atheism (*The Spectator*, Nos. 185–6). Fielding, through the mouth of Adams, equated 'nonsense and enthusiasm'; John Shebbeare's *Letters on the English Nation* (1756) denounced 'swivel-headed bigots or fallacious free-thinkers'; and Johnson deplored Milton's polemics, wrote of Puritan fervour in the *Life of Butler* as an almost incomprehensible thing, and in the *Dictionary* defined enthusiasm as 'a vain confidence of divine favour or communication'. Some of this was regrettable but all of it was natural; to be moderate was not to shirk but to seek the truth. William Law was anything but a Latitudinarian, yet he like others lamented that sectarian zeal split the Church (*Address to the Clergy* 1764, 58):

> Christendom, full of the nicest Decisions about Faith, Grace, Works, Merits, Satisfaction, Heresies, Schisms, &c., is full of all those evil Tempers which prevailed in the Heathen World.

Latitudinarian tolerance seemed the dawn of a saner age, purged only of the inessentials of faith. The Augustans were often self-satisfied in their beliefs, but the terms in which such men as Swift, Fielding (in his anti-Stuart *Champion* and *Jacobite's Journal*) and Burke (in the *Reflections* and the *Speech on the Army Estimates*) defend their position are those of confident men to whom extremes, not moderation, were wretched, miserable, poor, blind and naked aberrations.

One more charge must now be considered, that Hanoverian religion suffered from widely-testified spiritual anaemia and stands convicted by its own defenders. Swift's *Argument Against Abolishing Christianity* is a virtuoso's exercise in irony, but its tenour cannot, one feels, be entirely discounted. Swift does not intend, he explains, to advocate real Christianity—that would be 'a wild Project'; it would 'destroy at one Blow all the Wit, and half the Learning, of the Kingdom'. He pleads only for nominal Christianity, which deters no-one from his vices and even heightens their relish by the sauce of hypocrisy. Religion keeps the masses obedient, gives free-thinkers an easy butt and gratifies our Continental allies; surely this convenient veneer is worth preserving? This is ironic but its diagnosis is not reassuring. The 21st *Guardian* speaks of a 'prevailing Torrent of Vice and Impiety', and Berkeley's *Principles of Human Knowledge* (1710) of 'the absurdities of every wretched set of Atheists' (section xcii). John Byrom told his sister Phoebe, in February 1729, that he had bought Law's *Serious Call* but that 'Mr. Law and the Christian Religion . . . are mightily out of fashion at present'. And Bishop Butler's 'Advertisement' to the *Analogy* (1736) is a sombre comment:

> It is come, I know not how, to be taken for granted, by many persons, that Christianity is not so much as a subject of enquiry; but that it is now at length discovered to be fictitious. And accordingly they treat it as if, in the present age, this were an agreed point among all people of discernment, and nothing remained but to set it up as a principal subject of mirth and ridicule, as it were by way of reprisals, for its having so long interrupted the pleasures of the world.

In 1737 Butler's friend Secker became Bishop of Oxford, and it is hardly coincidence that his first charge to his clergy (1738) is almost an echo of these words. Butler's own charge to the clergy of Durham in 1751 speaks of a positive zeal for infidelity, 'truly *for* nothing, but *against* everything that is good and sacred amongst us'.

These protests sound serious, but any age might be proved irreligious with no more trouble than has gone to the collecting of them—that is, with very little trouble at all. Was spiritual decay then unduly prominent? On the whole, the ordinary man at any time is neither very religious nor very irreligious, and one would expect this to be so with the Augustans also. In his *Evidences of Christianity* (1794: pt. iii, ch. vii) Paley sensibly remarks that religion is a private thing and

> operates most upon those of whom history knows the least; upon fathers and mothers in their families, upon men-servants and maid-servants, upon the orderly tradesman, the quiet villager, the manufacturer at his loom, the husbandman in his fields.

Among such people the variations from age to age will not be spectacular. The trouble lay not in the middle levels but on the lowest and the highest: two classes were perceptibly at fault.

One was the very poor. Developing a social conscience as they did, the Augustans came to realise the brutal misery in which the destitute lived: Wesley found the Kingswood colliers 'one remove from the beasts that perish'. In such circumstances religious ignorance was natural, and the century's awakening to the consequences of poverty is not to its religious discredit.

The other class was that of the social sophisticate, sometimes but not always identical with the 'freethinker'. Polite society is seldom very religious, and as polite society under the Georges was prominent its indifference was a source of concern. In the 6th *Spectator* Steele declares that 'the affectation of being gay and in fashion has very near eaten up our good sense and religion'. Law writes the *Serious Call*, he avers, because 'this polite age of ours' has scared men away from devotion, and Swift's *Letter of Advice to a Young Poet* speaks of the current distaste for anything so unmodish as faith, for 'our Poetry of late has been altogether disengag'd from the narrow Notions of Virtue and Piety'. Young's *Night Thoughts* (book viii) also recommends the orthodoxy of 'sense' as against the heterodoxy of 'wit', though making much heavier weather of it than Swift.

The polite world being supercilious, religion had to be presented in terms it might understand. It might appear, for instance, as a matter of good taste—as it does in Steele's *Christian Hero* (1701), his and Addison's periodicals, and Shaftesbury's *Characteristicks* (1711). *The Guardian* (No. 21) recalls that the infallible Tillotson had found the Bible's style better than Virgil's, and No. 86 raises *The Book of Job* above the classical epics, and anticipates the day

> when it shall be as much the Fashion among Men of Politeness to admire a Rapture of St. *Paul*, as any fine expression in *Virgil* or *Horace*; and to see a well-dressed young Man produce an Evangelist out of his Pocket and be no more out of Countenance than if it were a Classick printed by *Elzevir*.

The connoisseur might read his Bible without harm to his taste.

Religious and moral truths, moreover, were to be conveyed by the politest of means, urbane ridicule of irreligion. Shaftesbury advocated this manner and Addison followed him. The heretic would be bantered into faith, the profligate reformed through laughter. So, said Addison in *The Spectator* (No. 445), 'I have set up the immoral man as the object of derision.' Ridicule, it is true, was a weapon the infidel could use too, and Mandeville, Hume and Gibbon did so with disturbing skill. 'The truth' was not a monopoly. But the store set by ridicule was the sign both of less vehement tempers and of the civilised taste which preferred rapiers to cudgels. And if it were fashionable to be a sceptic, it was still a fashion with drawbacks even in worldly terms; Chesterfield himself, the virtuoso of the graces, was severe upon infidelity and polite towards religion, though in suavely ambiguous terms which relegated it rather to the status of a social guarantee (*Letters*, 8 January, 1750):

> Depend upon this truth, That every man is the worse looked upon, and the less trusted, for being thought to have no religion; in spite of all the pompous and specious epithets he may assume, of *esprit fort*, freethinker or moral philosopher; and a wise atheist (if such a thing there is) would, for his own interest and character in the world, pretend to some religion.

Despite the tone of this, we need not conclude that Chesterfield is merely recommending hypocrisy as the tribute vice pays to virtue; he is also urging a serious truth in language attuned to the man of society. Social irreverence was not widely approved, though it was current enough to seem dangerous, and was to be laughed out of its presumption.

As troublesome as the atheist was the 'freethinker', a polymorphous nightmare. The 'Advertisement' to Berkeley's *Alciphron, or the Minute Philosopher* (1732) undertook to consider him 'in the various Lights of Atheist, Libertine, Enthusiast, Scorner, Critic, Metaphysician, Fatalist and Sceptic'. Almost any accusation could hit so large a target, and the whole matter reflects the difficulty of replacing dogma by a 'reasonable' faith. The main freethinkers were Deists, who tried to determine the elements of religion independently of the Bible and Revelation, since a benevolent Deity would surely not have concealed the great truths from all but a small proportion of mankind. There were pre-Augustan Deists but the main trouble came with Toland's *Christianity not Mysterious* (1696), Wollaston's *Religion of Nature Delineated* (1724), Tindal's *Christianity as Old as the Creation* (1730), and Chubb's *The True Gospel of Jesus Christ* (1738). Despite the references to Christianity in these titles the Deists were devising not Christian apologetics but proofs that unaided reason could find out the essentials of faith.

There is no room here for detail but Deism naturally shocked the orthodox, who rallied strongly, and whose reaction is reflected in the Vicar of Wakefield's outburst—'No freethinker shall ever have a child of mine'. Law's *Case of Reason* is an answer to Tindal, Berkeley's *Alciphron* is intelligent satire, and Butler's *Analogy* replies to Deism though without mentioning it. That 'free thought' should venture to discuss faith seemed impertinence; Addison reprimanded 'bigoted infidels' who spread scepticism (*The Spectator*, No. 185), Horace Walpole listened to the Parisian *philosophes* and then told George Montagu, on 22 September, 1765, that there is 'as much bigotry in attempting conversions from any religion as to it', and Burke, infuriated by the radicals, wrote in the *Reflections* that 'if our religious tenets ever want a further elucidation we shall not call on atheists to explain them' (*Reflections*, in *Works*, iv. 99). Deists were not, indeed, atheists; they believed in a benevolent God. But their rejection of Revelation and their universalising of religious belief seemed tantamount to atheism. When Herbert Croft was gathering materials for the *Life of Young* Johnson passed him information about Tindal, Young's dialectical adversary at All Souls. 'Don't forget that rascal Tindal, Sir,' he would vociferate, 'Be sure to hang up the Atheist' (A. Chalmers's *English Poets*, 1810, xiii. 341 fn.). Such was the general sentiment. The Deists were raked (though not without effective reply) by guns far heavier than their own. The orthodox blazed away with all they could muster—Swift, Berkeley, Addison, Steele, Law, Butler, Warburton, Fielding, Johnson, Young and Burke. Through the reigns of Anne, George I and George II there were intermittent tremors, with a quake of exceptional force in 1754 when Mallet published the works of Bolingbroke. These, said the 9th *Connoisseur*, gave new life and spirit to free thinking, and Garrick thrust a strongly anti-Bolingbroke stanza into his poem on Lord Pelham's death. Deism caused long-lasting concern—indeed, in 1760 Goldsmith had to suggest that it was time to give up the controversy for something fresher (*On the English Clergy and Popular Preachers*).

But the dispute passed away or changed gradually into different forms. Despite the outcry against infidelity, Johnson told Boswell on 14 April, 1775, 'there are in reality very few infidels'. 'Who now reads Bolingbroke?' Burke asked in the *Reflections*, 'Who ever read him through?' (*Works*, iv. 98). The new alarm centred rather on the scepticism of men like Hume and Gibbon and the rationalism of the radicals. Johnson frowned when the name of Priestley was mentioned, and walked out of company when Richard Price entered it. But the monument to the late-Augustan phase of the battle is not Johnson's but Burke's. With deep emotion the *Reflections* upholds the fundamental connection between Christianity and national life; Church and State are connected in a sacramental bond and the commonwealth is 'consecrated' by the Church establishment. All who minister in Church and State, therefore, have 'high and worthy notions of their function and destination', and an eye

not to the paltry pelf of the moment, nor to the temporary and transient praise of the vulgar, but to a solid, permanent existence, in the permanent part of their nature, and to a permanent fame and glory, in the example they leave.

Britons are conservative by nature, Burke explains, and prefer rather to maintain an imperfect religion than to tinker with it:

> there is no rust of superstition with which the accumulated absurdity of the human mind might have crusted it over in the course of ages that ninety-nine in a hundred of the people of England would not prefer to impiety.
>
> Reflections, in Works, iv. 99

Allowing for rhetorical fervour that was largely true. 'Freethinkers' and radicals argued an unpopular case and extended the horizons of thought; they were grossly misrepresented and their courage deserves gratitude. But the ordinary man held by his ordinary notions, whether in church or chapel, and sympathised with the old rather than the new.

The 'truth' about Hanoverian religion will not go in a sentence, but the more that religion is understood the less it need be broadly condemned. Its weaknesses were recognised then as they are now. Yet neither Church nor Dissent should be judged merely by its defects; if they were prosaic and cautious they were served by many labours of worth and devotion. Vulnerable to attack, and sometimes despondent about their influence, their defence still evoked from the ablest men of the age more passion than was shown on any other subject.

iv. 'AN INWARD CHEARFULNESS'

> *Whether amid the gloom of night I stray,*
> *Or my glad eyes enjoy revolving day,*
> *Still Nature's various face informs my sense*
> *Of an all-wise, all-pow'rful Providence.*
>
> GAY
Contemplation on Night, 1–4

THE characteristic Augustan belief is in the mercy of God and the duty of beneficence in man. This, though no new invention, is markedly different in tone from the characteristic belief of the century before, which had produced so much emotion. Individuals like Cowper, convinced of their sins by apparent revelation, could still suffer as excruciatingly as Bunyan had done, but in general the age was, like Johnson's hermit in *Rasselas*, 'cheerful without levity'. It felt in its faith not so much the ecstatic joy that Cowper felt when he thought himself saved as the steady joy of descrying God's beneficence displayed at large. Religion, Thomson assures us in *Liberty*, has now become a thing of joy and confidence:

> *Nor be Religion, rational and free,*
> *Here pass'd in silence, whose enraptur'd eye*
> *Sees Heav'n with Earth connected, human things*
> *Link'd to divine; who not from servile fear,*
> *By rites for some weak tyrant incense fit,*
> *The God of Love adores, but from a heart*
> *Effusing gladness.*
>   (iv. 561-7)

The stars, in Addison's hymn, sing in their God-given paths, and their bright constancy betokens a divine assurance.

The new spirit encouraged a new optimism: God, as Locke said, was actively interested in his creatures' happiness. This faith, too, was anything but a new discovery; the Christian tradition has cherished love as often as it has feared judgment. But so much stress on happiness was novel; so well-designed a universe must have good ends, and what end better than universal happiness? Shaftesbury followed Locke: so did Addison: Pope declared happiness (rather than, though certainly not instead of, salvation) to be 'our being's end and aim': the preface to Akenside's *Pleasures of the Imagination* (1744) celebrated 'the benevolent intention of the Author of Nature in every principle of the human constitution', and introducing William King's *Origin of Evil* (1731) the Reverend John Gay, an early Utilitarian, said that man's happiness is 'the criterion of the will of God'. The old fears might still be felt—the names of Law, Butler, Johnson and Cowper remind us that orthodoxy could still oppress the believer. But characteristically it was optimism which the Augustans cherished, optimism not without precedent but increasingly dominant over the fear of God, and expressing itself in the soul's calm sunshine and the heartfelt joy.

Perhaps the belief that the universe was ruled not by an autocrat but by a constitutional monarch observing the comprehensible laws of reason was not an unmixed blessing, since it might remove God to a distance, as a power working not directly as a First Cause but indirectly through natural laws, second causes discoverable by science. 'Philosophy that lean'd on Heav'n before', Pope observed as a symptom of impending intellectual night, 'Shrinks to her second cause and is no more' (*Dunciad*, iv. 644), and Berkeley protested against this shrinking, this loss of the sense of the numinous, by which the very uniformity God observes in presenting the universe to our minds is misread as the mere mechanical working of physical laws (*Principles of Human Knowledge*, sec. xxxii):

> This consistent, uniform working, which so evidently displays the goodness and wisdom of that governing Spirit whose will constitutes the laws of Nature, is so far from leading our thoughts to him, that it rather sends them a-wandering after second causes.

Yet in many cases, perhaps most, an enlargement of mind and elevation of spirit followed the scientific 'proof' of what Addison calls 'the exuberant and overflowing goodness of the Supreme Being whose mercy extends to all His works' (*The Spectator*, No. 519). It did so in Berkeley's own case; for him, man's steady sense of the external world is the mark of God's unwearying creative care. Asking how an immaterial mind can know the material universe Berkeley answers that all perceptions (including the evidence the senses seem to give of the world around) are directly presented to the mind by God, who perpetually creates our world for us in its beauty and order. The ironic result is that men take this very order as the sign of an automatic universe; only in calamities and interruptions of order (what insurance companies unfortunately call 'acts of God') do they see evidence of divine power. For Berkeley God is manifested not so much in prodigies as in the perpetual stability of things, in the fact that every time the eyes look in a certain direction they see a certain tree, and every night is succeeded by the following morning. The passages in which Berkeley praises this divine dispensation, this spiritual motivation, this unremitting fostering care, are among the finest prose of the century. Other writers too, without Berkeley's almost mystical intelligence, found reason for joy. Gay and Thomson have been quoted; Shaftesbury, following the Cambridge Platonists, spoke of man's duty to be in the 'sweetest' disposition whenever he thinks of spiritual things, and Addison recurrently echoed the advocacy of happiness:

> I cannot but look upon it [a cheerful mind] as a constant habitual gratitude to the great Author of Nature. An inward chearfulness is an implicit praise and thanksgiving to Providence under all its dispensations. It is a kind of acquiescence in the state wherein we are placed, and a secret approbation of the divine will.
> *The Spectator*, No. 381

Eccentric beliefs therefore were not only unorthodox but a forfeiture of happiness. Freethinkers, it was argued, must be morose because they reject a personal God and lose the believer's truest joy, which only a sense of guilt and atheism (Addison thinks) can banish. Berkeley's 27th *Guardian* speaks of 'those gloomy Mortals who by their Unbelief are rendered incapable of feeling those Impressions of Joy and Hope'. It was a retort to the claim that wit and confidence were the marks of free thought and sourness and gloom those of faith. When Methodism brought back the introspection of an earlier age Churchmen could still claim that they were the happy ones and only 'enthusiasts' miserable (an idea the Wesleyans would fervently have rebutted)—Goldsmith has a pleasant *Citizen of the World* paper (No. 111) relating how the new sect 'weep for their amusement and use little music except a chorus of sighs and groans', and how lovers 'court each other from the Lamentations'. It need hardly be said that an Irish imagination is at work here, but at least the stress put on the happiness of the accepted faith and the misery of deviations from it is significant.

To imply that for no orthodox person was the world a vale of tears would be absurd: moods are controlled by temperament and circumstances as well as by the trend of the time. Butler's *Analogy* is shadowed with the darkness of life, which reason interprets no better than revelation; it speaks of 'the present state of vice and misery', and admits that neither religion nor reason can afford satisfaction, since 'satisfaction in this sense does not belong to such a creature as man' (*Works*, ed. W. E. Gladstone, 1896, i. 364). Johnson too felt the mood of religious dread, and reviewing Soame Jenyns's *Free Inquiry into the Nature and Origin of Evil* (1757) he demolished the argument that because pain and evil seem to be ordained by God man should pretend they are a form of good. Young too was gloomy; most of the earth, he declared, is savage wilderness, a symbol of fallen man (*Night Thoughts*, i. 285). And when in 1750 London experienced a combination of storm, earthquake, and Aurora Borealis (acts of God in the popular but not Berkeleyan sense), the citizens forgot that the Deity was the Prime Mover of an Age of Reason, and gathered in the fields expecting the doom of Sodom and Gomorrah, just as if Enlightenment had not dawned.

Yet an earthquake is one thing, and normal life another. At ordinary times men paid a reasonable obedience to moral duty, cheered by a sense of God's approval and that 'sweet contemplation' of which Gay speaks (*Rural Sports*, i. 107–20):

> *Now night in silent state begins to rise,*
> *And twinkling orbs bestrow th'uncloudy skies . . .*
> *Millions of worlds hang in the spacious air,*
> *Which round the sun their annual circles steer;*
> *Sweet contemplation elevates my sense*
> *While I survey the works of Providence.*
> *O could the muse in loftier strains rehearse*
> *The glorious author of the universe,*
> *Who reins the winds, gives the vast ocean bounds,*
> *And circumscribes the floating worlds their rounds,*
> *My soul should overflow in songs of praise,*
> *And my Creator's name inspire my lays.*

Such sentiments were typical of their time, and they inspired, if less of earnest passion than did the sense of mystery and dread, both personal serenity and an expansive goodwill towards others.

V. RELIGION AND LITERATURE

A reasonable life, and a wise use of our proper condition, is as much the duty of all *men*, as it is the duty of all *Angels*, and *intelligent* beings. These are not *speculative* flights, or *imaginary* notions, but are *plain* and *undeniable laws*, that are founded in the *nature* of rational beings, who as such are obliged to live by reason, and glorify God by a continual right use of their several talents and faculties.

WILLIAM LAW
A Serious Call to a Devout and Holy Life (1728), 77

How then did the muse 'rehearse The glorious author of the universe'? Was literature influenced by the instinct for faith?

To ask this is to ask whether writers were affected by some of the themes that most deeply concerned them, and the answer must clearly be that they were, that in this supposedly indifferent age religion provided a standard of judgment and a mode of expression both consciously and subconsciously important. Tillotson and *The Guardian*, we have seen, showed even the venerated classics to be 'faint and languid' by the side of the Bible. Familiarity with the Bible did as much as anything, even familiarity with Shakespeare, to nourish the imagination. This influence was partly rhythmical (no other source could so have affected Law and Burke, for instance), and partly concerned with diction and imagery, with a willingness to break through the 'polite' modes and be passionate and elaborate. Its effect on Thomson was described by an early editor, Patrick Murdock, as follows:

It is certain he owed much to a religious education; and that his early acquaintance with the sacred writings contributed greatly to that *sublime*, by which his works will be for ever distinguished. In his first pieces, the *Seasons*, we see him at once assume the majestic freedom of an Eastern writer, seizing the grand images as they rise, cloathing them in his own expressive language, and preserving throughout the grace, the variety, and the dignity, which belong to a just composition, unhurt by the stiffness of formal method.

Works of James Thomson (1762), introduction, iv

In particular it was hymnody which showed this influence, and the eighteenth century, rapidly developing the congregational hymn, was 'the Century of Divine Songs' (the phrase is from George Sampson's *Seven Essays*, 1947). This is not the place to compete with Sampson's admirable discussion or with Bernard Manning's *Hymns of Wesley and Watts* (1942), yet even a brief inspection must see in the better hymns a range of feeling and wealth of imagery which other poems of the time hardly approach. The hymn as we know it is the child of Dissent and its first great writer —Isaac Watts—a Congregationalist. It partakes, then, of the fervour of early Dissent and it amplifies this enormously when the Wesleys set to work. Methodist hymns are often thought to be gloomy and even morbid, but this strain (with a few exceptions) belongs rather to the Calvinist than the Arminian side, which delights to celebrate divine mercy. William Law speaks of the joys of psalm-singing, and these joys the Wesleys preserve in their hymns, Charles in particular abounding in images of spacious, radiant and infinite things like oceans, rivers, water, fire and light, and commanding too a concise, firm utterance, strongly observant of line and rhyme, which is part of his Augustan inheritance. Unlike the polite connoisseur the hymn-writer needed no prompting to admire the Bible; the force of its contents impressed upon him its vigour, its concrete and picturesque phrasing, its lyrical and dramatic power. From it there flowed an oriental wealth of colouring, into hymns like Watts's 'We are a garden wall'd around' or Newton's 'Glorious things of thee are spoken', or a passion of joy, in Byrom's 'Christians, awake!' (which shows what the heroic couplet could do besides satire), Olivers's 'The God of Abraham praise', Doddridge's 'Hark the glad sound', Perronet's 'All hail the power of Jesus' name', and many hymns by Watts and the Wesleys, Newton and Cowper. Others were grave, like Toplady in 'Rock of Ages', or confident, like Addison in 'The spacious firmament' and 'When all Thy mercies, O my God'.

This is a sparse account of a large topic, and it ignores—an inviting theme—the question whether literary criteria are relevant to the judgment of hymns. Still, amenable or not to literary criticism, the hymn reveals a good deal about its time, and its character extends into other poems not themselves hymns, which include Watts's vehement *Ode on the Day of Judgment* (the most passionate sapphics in English) and pre-eminently Smart's *Song to David*, which peals like the clash of bells, or organs played at a thanksgiving. Smart is often spoken of as *sui generis*, and so he is in the degree in which his imagination rises, his verse throbs with excitement and his images have a Biblical majesty. But his poem is only the crown of a flourishing mode and nothing in it is surprising except its genius.

In less directly Biblical ways religion enriches literature with a sense of values which writers and readers were readier to recognise than some conceptions of the age might suggest. Sophisticated breakfast-tables, one might imagine, would hardly welcome in their periodicals such things as versified Biblical texts, Addison's and Watts's hymns, and Pope's *Messiah* (which Steele introduced as being 'by a great genius who is not ashamed to employ his wit in the praise of his Maker'—*Spectator*, No. 378). Yet *The Spectator* did not hesitate to print these and other religious compositions. The journals abounded in lay sermons and moral discourses, and Addison in particular made it his business to promote religion. For this above all Swift and Pope praised him, Somervile asserted that 'presumptuous Folly blush'd and Vice withdrew' before him (*To Mr. Addison*), and Tickell, in verses *To the Supposed Author of The Spectator*, averred that as a result

> *the rash fool who scorn'd the beaten road*
> *Dares quake at thunder, and confess his God.*

The essays which produced this gratifying effect are not all palatable, but some are still persuasive and dignified. They plead the social virtues—good nature, benevolence, forbearance—and the Christian virtues—faith, hope, charity. The 413th *Spectator*, for example, one of Addison's 'Pleasures of the Imagination' series, takes on a characteristic illumination of religious gratitude. God encourages man to explore the universe by giving him pleasure in novelty, makes the sexes mutually attractive, and inspires a general enjoyment of beautiful things, in order

that he might render the whole creation more gay and delightful. He has given almost everything about us the power of raising an agreeable idea in the imagination, so that it is impossible for us to behold his works with coldness or indifference, and to survey so many beauties without a secret satisfaction or complacency.

Such themes recur—themes of the soul's improvement, of divine beneficence, and of immortal happiness. Berkeley too rises to admirable eloquence by religious meditation, by his faith that 'all the choir of heaven and furniture of the earth, in a word all those bodies which compose the mighty frame of the world' are thoughts in the mind of God (*Principles of Human Knowledge*, section vi), and in Law there coexist the religious senses of sin and ecstatic happiness:

If any one would tell you the shortest, surest way to all happiness, and all perfection, he must tell you to make a *rule* to yourself, to *thank and praise God for every thing that happens to you.* For it is certain that whatever seeming calamity happens to you, if you thank and praise God for it you turn it into a blessing. Could you therefore work miracles you could not do more for yourself than by this *thankful spirit*, for it *heals* with a word speaking, and turns all that it touches into happiness.
Serious Call, 279

In such writing there is a particular dimension, that of a scale of supramundane values. It is the background against which Swift pillories hypocrisy in the *Argument Against Abolishing Christianity*, and it inspires that underthrob of rhythm which brings Addison's Westminster-Abbey *Spectator* (No. 26) to an end. It appears gravely in Cowper, in his sense that the world is being weighed in the balance of religion and that its cares—commerce, politics, diversion —distract man from his fundamental search. It develops in Johnson's criticism a magnificence of evaluation which convinces him that neither criticism nor literature is the most important thing in life—nor, indeed, are the daily experiences of life itself. The most important thing for Johnson goes beyond criticism and literature;

it is that man's real concern is religious. Divine themes, he declares, are indeed often too high for poetry; in the *Life of Waller* he speaks of the poet's difficulties when faced with higher subjects than poetry can attain. In the *Life of Young* he accounts for the failure of Young's *Last Day* on the grounds that its very subject 'makes every man more than poetical' and inspires 'a general obscurity of horrour that disdains expression'. *Paradise Lost*, however, he admits to have risen to the height of its great argument, and his emotions on its theme are expressed in a passage which rings with something of the seventeenth century's power and shows what resonance could be sounded in the eighteenth by the enormous prospect of religious beliefs:

We all, indeed, feel the effects of Adam's disobedience: we all sin like Adam, and like him must all bewail our offences; we have restless and insidious enemies in the fallen angels, and in the blessed spirits we have guardians and friends; in the Redemption of mankind we hope to be included; in the description of heaven and hell we are surely interested, as we are all to reside hereafter either in the regions of horrour or of bliss.

One of his finest meditations is the end of the last *Idler*, in the Holy Week of 1760. It is one single magnificent sentence which must be quoted despite its length; indeed, in its length sustained by its majestic deliberation lies its very quality:

As the last *Idler* is published in that solemn week which the Christian world has always set apart for the examination of the conscience, the review of life, the extinction of earthly desires and the renovation of holy purposes; I hope that my readers are already disposed to view every incident with seriousness, and improve it by meditation; and that, when they see this series of trifles brought to a conclusion, they will consider that, by outliving the Idler, they have passed weeks, months and years which are no longer in their power; that an end must in time be put to everything great, as to everything little; that to life must come its last hour, and to this system of being its last day, the hour at which probation ceases and repentance will be vain; the day in which every work of the hand, and imagination of the heart, shall be brought to judgment, and an everlasting futurity shall be determined by the past.

Nothing in Johnson's journalism became him like the leaving it; the commonplace idea rises into fresh power in that stately gravity which relates the recurrence of daily work to the passage of time and the imminence of eternity.

That same sense of great significance sounds throughout the century. In Berkeley, Law, and Goldsmith's earnestness as he composes Dr. Primrose's sermon (*The Vicar of Wakefield*, ch. 29), the age's reason rises into something of poetry, which comes not as an overtone of fear but from a desire that men shall realise their spiritual selves. This desire in this degree could come only from a religious sense of life (though not necessarily an orthodox or even a Christian one), and whether coloured by the gloomy dignity of Bishop Butler or Johnson, the rapture of Berkeley or Law, or the various tones of Cowper and the hymn-writers it reveals a dimension of life of which the Augustans are too often thought heedless.

In Law this dimension is particularly prominent; life for him is consecration. In the *Address to the Clergy*, finished just before his death in 1761, he speaks earnestly of 'the *one Thing* needful, the one Thing *essential* and only *available* to our Rising out of our fallen State'—that is, participation in the divine spirit. He rejects creeds 'not wholly built upon this *Supernatural Ground*' but based wholly on human reason, and denies that his spiritual zeal is gross 'enthusiasm' (*Address to the Clergy*, 2nd ed. 1764, 89):

> Poor miserable Man! that strives with all the Sophistry of human Wit, to be delivered from the immediate continual Operation and Government of the Spirit of God, not considering that where God is not, there is the Devil, and where the Spirit rules not, there is all the Work of the Flesh, though nothing be talked of but Spiritual and Christian Matters. I say talked of: for the best ability of the natural Man can go no further than Talk, and Notions and Opinions about Scripture Words and Facts; in these he may be a great Critic, an acute Logician, a powerful Orator, and know everything of Scripture except the Spirit and the Truth.

The *Serious Call* reclaimed Johnson from being, as he put it to Boswell, 'a lax *talker* against religion': picking it up casually at

Oxford, and 'expecting to find it a dull book (as such books generally are)' he found himself outmatched by Law's passion and reason. To include the *Serious Call* in the province of literature as well as of religion is not stretching the point, for in a lucid and supple style it conveys the true illumination of the time, the high value given to reason as man's distinctive faculty, the alliance between reason and intuition, and the sense of life as a perfecting of man's better qualities (*Serious Call*, 75):

If we had a Religion that consisted in absurd superstitions, that had no regard to the perfection of our nature, People might well be glad to have some part of their life excused from it. But as the Religion of the Gospel is only the refinement, and exaltation of our best Faculties, as it only requires a life of the highest Reason, as it only requires us to use this world as in reason it ought to be used, to live in such *tempers* as are the glory of intelligent beings, to walk in such *wisdom* as exalts our nature, and to practise such *piety* as will raise us to God; who can think it grievous to live *always* in the spirit of such a Religion, to have *every part* of his life full of it, but he that would think it much more grievous, to be as the Angels of God in heaven?

If Law's 'vigorous mind', said Gibbon judiciously in his *Autobiography*, had not been 'clouded by enthusiasm, he might be ranked with the most agreeable and ingenious writers of the times'. One might safely go further; Law shows that the 'reason' to which his age appealed was not always mere intellectual abstraction but could be (as with the Cambridge Platonists in the seventeenth century) a faculty of spiritual light.

The Augustan writer, then, gained from religion an emotion which no other subject so strongly inspired. Even on themes not specifically religious he benefited from what was, despite controversy, a stable frame of accepted values. In Fielding, for instance, there is little about religious fundamentals though much about clergymen good and bad, deists and (in *Amelia*) moral conduct; yet his characteristic air of assurance owes much to the settled Hanoverian Protestantism which enabled him unquestioningly to 'place' these debatable matters. Much the same is true of Pope, though he was by birth a Roman Catholic and by friendship a

Deist. He shows little sense of personal religion, or indeed of ability to philosophise deeply for himself, yet the current metaphysical certainty enables him to feel at home in life and to answer its problems, impregnable in ultimate conviction. Johnson, though sombre where Pope is confident, trusts no less in the established 'truths'; *Rasselas*, with little explicit reference to religion, is a deeply religious book. And Gray's *Elegy*, though its ostensible theme is the lot of the poor, has behind it the acceptance of Augustan faith, a ceremonial of feeling which unrebelliously submits to the settled order. With few exceptions the Augustans show as little uncertainty over fundamentals as architects did over style; whether orthodox or not they know the right solutions.

Did literature, finally, gain or lose in passing from seventeenth- to eighteenth-century religious feeling? As the emotional temperature dropped something precious was indeed lost. 'They say miracles are past', Shakespeare's Lafeu had already complained in *All's Well*,

> and we have our philosophical persons to make modern and familiar, things supernatural and causeless. Hence is it that we make trifles of terrors, ensconsing ourselves into seeming knowledge, when we should submit ourselves to an unknown fear.

Ensconsing itself into seeming knowledge the eighteenth century sometimes found the world too intelligible. If, with Pope, one thought all discord harmony not understood, all partial evil universal good, it was a cause for satisfaction but it denied the convictions of human experience. One could be blinded by excess of light. For great poetry a sense of the tragic is nearly essential, a sense of the mystery of things without too much of that 'irritable reaching after fact and reason' which Keats deplored in Coleridge. From Chaucer to Yeats and Eliot the finest poetry has come from those who have recognised evil as firmly as good. Among the Augustans the real poetry came from those in whom optimism wore thin (as with Pope), or was missing entirely (as with Johnson), or alternated with melancholy (as with Gray's *Elegy*, Goldsmith's *Deserted Village*, Cowper and Crabbe), or was eclipsed by a variety of moods outside the rational vogue (as with Smart, Collins, Burns and Blake). In much Augustan writing, despite its competence, good sense and good taste, we miss the sense of the numinous. Feeling may not be lacking, yet it often fails to move us; the *Hymn* Thomson appended to *The Seasons* is not without passion and clearly Thomson was full of exultation and awe, yet the awe arises from the thought of a universe designed to awaken man's unmitigated admiration, and the exultation inspires only a heavy rhetoric. Parnell's *Night-Piece on Death*, with tomb-stones, shrouded spirits, croaking raven and similar apparatus, has a theme that would have stirred the seventeenth century to an emotional crisis, yet it is a calm discourse reproving death for frightening men instead of seeming a natural state in the transition to heaven. Young is equally calm about the great mysteries (*Night Thoughts*, ix. 2049–50):

> *What's* Vice?—*Mere want of compass in our thought.*
> Religion *what?*—*The proof of* Common-Sense.

Religion was too often the proof of common sense; it was so for the Deists ('I banish all hypotheses from my philosophy', Toland observed); it was so for Pope's *Essay on Man* and for rationalistic divines like Bishop Watson of Llandaff, who rejected 'dark disquisitions concerning necessity and liberty, matter and spirit' in favour of what he thought the plain contents of the Bible (*Anecdotes of the Life of Richard Watson*, 1817, i. 15).

As in architecture, order and clarity were prevailing over complexity and mystery: such a process is valuable especially after an age of dispute. The Augustan simplification reduced but did not nullify the emotional nourishment which literature drew from religion, just as the rational order of Augustan church architecture did not mean an absence of religious feeling though its feeling was less complex than that of preceding ages. The rational order of Augustan faith made the intimacy and variety of the seventeenth century's faith unattainable, yet it inhibited neither the tenderer moods nor the expression of deep and steady belief. Of the former kind there are, for instance, Isaac Watts's *Horae Lyricae* (1706), *Hymns and Spiritual Songs* (1707–9), and *Divine Songs* (1715),

Charles Wesley's verses for children, and, supremely, Blake's *Songs of Innocence* (1789). Poems like *The Lamb*, *The Little Black Boy*, *Holy Thursday*, *The Divine Image* and *Night* are exquisitely 'innocent', and touched with mystical penetration. Blake it is true differed profoundly from current fashion; there is in him no lack of mystery, which haunts *The Tyger*, *Jerusalem* and the prophetic books. He was a law to himself. Yet he had his religious affiliations within the century (Smart's *Jubilate Agno* is a striking anticipation of his 'possessed' manner and rapt perception), referred warmly to Methodism, and was affected by the mystical element in Evangelicalism. Not everything in Georgian religion was plain and orderly.

And even when it was plain and orderly, it might not lack in feeling. A verse in the *Dies Irae*, Mrs Thrale relates, would reduce Johnson to tears. The verse was that weighty one:

> *Quærens me, sedisti lassus;*
> *Redemisti, crucem passus;*
> *Tantus labor non sit cassus!*

Cowper too experienced and expressed both the agony and the devotion of belief, and John Newton was redeemed from slave-trading to share in writing the Olney hymns. Religion inspired dignified and reverent styles and a tone of steadiness and gravity. Its preference for the settled order prolonged injustices and it too easily assumed a divine sanction for remediable evils. Yet against this may be set the labours of many who from religious motives fought against injustice at home and abroad. If they were not revolutionary it was because they saw no reason to be so; stability was too recent a gain, the mob (as France was to prove) was too easily inflamed, and reforms could come quietly.

The religious background, then, was characteristically English, in the earnest dignity of the old order (conservative Anglican or Dissenting) and the fervent conscientiousness of the new (Evangelical). There is much to praise in it. As the last example of its quality let Tickell furnish some lines of his poem *On the Death of Mr. Addison*, which express its union of the personal and the social, a control and decorum which do not obscure the genuine emotion, and which foreshadow Gray's *Elegy*:

> *Can I forget the dismal night that gave*
> *My soul's best part for ever to the grave?*
> *How silent did his old companions tread,*
> *By midnight lamps, the mansions of the dead;*
> *Through breathing statues, then unheeded things,*
> *Through rows of warriors, and through walks of kings.*
> *What awe did the slow solemn knell inspire,*
> *The pealing organ, and the pausing choir;*
> *The duties by the lawn-rob'd prelate pay'd;*
> *And the last words, that dust to dust convey'd!*
> *While speechless o'er thy closing grave we bend,*
> *Accept these tears, thou dear departed friend.*

That, as much as anything in English, has the moving solemnity of the ceremony of death. Its quality is hardly imitable in any other period, and as clearly as *The Guardian*'s praise of St. Paul's it indicates that the Augustans were not deficient in religious feeling.

V. PHILOSOPHY MORAL AND NATURAL

i. THE NEW TEMPER

> There is no part of history so generally useful as that which relates the progress of the human mind.
>
> JOHNSON
> *Rasselas*, chapter xxix

THE titles of philosophical works may lead us to the heart of their age, and this is strikingly true of the eighteenth century. Instead of Hooker's *Lawes of Ecclesiastical Politie* (1594), Hobbes's *Leviathan, of the Matter, Forme and Power of a Commonwealth* (1651), or Milton's *De Doctrina Christiana* (circa 1655), a new temper prompts a new kind of title. As 'enlightenment' brightens on the horizon it warms man's interest in his fellow-men as social and rational beings, and the result is Timothy Nourse's *Nature and Faculties of Man* (1686), Locke's series of *Letters Concerning Toleration* (1689–1706) and the *Essay Concerning Human Understanding* (1690), Shaftesbury's *Characteristicks of Men, Manners, Opinions, Times* (1711), Francis Hutcheson's essays on *The Original of our Ideas of Beauty and Virtue* (1725) and *The Nature and Conduct of the Passions and Affections* (1728), and Pope's *Essay on Man* (1733). No trend of course is absolutely regular; Bacon's *Advancement of Learning* and Hobbes's *Leviathan* in some ways look forward to the eighteenth century as, in some ways, Warburton's *Divine Legation of Moses* (1737–41) looks back to the seventeenth. But the prevailing tendency is there, and by a general consensus 'enquiries' into Virtue, Morals, the Understanding and the Nature of Man are increasingly numerous. Tudor and Stuart England had their analyses of 'the passions'—often under French influence—and their interest in melancholy and in social conduct, but nothing as methodical as Hume's *Treatise of Human Nature* (1739), *Philosophical Essays Concerning Human Understanding*

(1748) or *Principles of Morals* (1751), Hartley's *Observations on Man* (1749) and Adam Smith's *Theory of Moral Sentiments* (1759).

Readers were interested in all this; England, in Hume's words, was a country 'where all the abstruser sciences are studied with a peculiar ardour', and the philosopher could contemplate addressing, as did Samuel Clarke the rationalist Dean of St. Paul's, 'any man of ordinary capacity, and unbiassed judgment, plainness and simplicity'. The public for Addison's *Spectator*, that is to say, was also the public for the philosopher, who spoke in general not as a specialist but as a reasonable man talking to reasonable men. One of the century's best features is the social tone, the sensible and mellow humanity, which civilise its philosophy.

Instead of the passionate religious conflicts of the preceding age men turned their attention to the nature of reason and the passions, the goodness or badness of 'natural' impulses, the relations between individual and community, and the origins of society whether in fear or friendship. They sought a credible and if possible creditable social psychology; they founded morality, as Christians, on love of God and charity towards men; as 'intellectualists' (a term explained later) on universal moral law to be obeyed through reason; and as believers in 'moral sentiment', on the affections of the heart. Few of their ideas were novel: Hooker for instance often anticipates them, as for instance in his stress on man's happy and sociable nature (in *Ecclesiastical Politie*, I. x, xi), and was himself drawing on long tradition. But the full emergence of these ideas into the dominant mood of the time is the notable thing; though Christianity had long preached man's unity with his fellows in a bond of religious love it was the Augustans who rationalised this doctrine to the light of common day and presented it less to Christians than to Christian gentlemen. Not the doctrine but the idiom is new; the flavour has changed in the degree to which Addison differs from, say, Jeremy Taylor.

There is a new temper in natural as well as moral philosophy. The practical bias of the time extends to the methods of intellectual enquiry; with a new perception of what science could do there comes a lively confidence in man's mental powers and a scorn for the intellectual methods of the past. This too was nothing new, for Bacon and Hobbes had already laid down the lines of advance, pointing out the failures of scholasticism and defining the ways in which thought could deal effectively with the world. Yet the Augustans inherited not only these revolutionary ideas but also the scientists' practical vindication of them, and could therefore congratulate themselves on their 'new philosophy'.

Hobbes decisively defined the aims and methods of thought:

> The Light of humane minds is Perspicuous Words, but by exact definitions first snuffed, and purged from ambiguity; *Reason* is the *pace*; Encrease of *Science* [knowledge] the *way*; and the Benefit of man-kind, the *end*.
>
> *Leviathan* (1651), 21–2

Consequently the new interest concentrated shrewdly on 'real' things rather than on what Bacon called 'vain imaginations, vain altercations and vain affectations'—on physical phenomena and the nature of mankind as deduced from observation. It was keenly concerned too with definitions: Bacon had warned against 'the false appearances that are imposed upon us by words' and had advised that we 'imitate the wisdom of the mathematicians in setting down in the very beginning the definitions of our words and terms'. Hobbes too is always raising such topics as 'the right ordering of names in our affirmation', or the search for 'precise truth' and 'true knowledge'. He scorns scholasticism and its logomachies, '*entity, intentionality, quiddity,* and other insignificant words of the school'. Locke is equally concerned for 'the original, certainty, and extent of human knowledge', 'the grounds and degrees of belief, opinion and assent', and 'the discerning faculties of man'. As Bacon had distinguished under the name of 'idols' the prejudices which prevent clear thinking, so Locke in book III of the *Essay* analyses the reasons for confused discussion. Like Bacon, Hobbes, Cowley and others he particularly blames the schoolmen for 'learned ignorance' which 'did no more but perplex and confound the signification of words'.

The new philosophy, then, meant the mind's impartial examination of 'fact'. It is generally spoken of as rationalism, and so it was in its perpetual recommendation of reason, but what is important is not its use of reason as such but the uses to which it put reason. The scholastic philosophies, after all, have abundance of reason; Bacon himself recognises in them 'their great thirst of truth and unwearied travail of wit [intellect]'. Not the use of reason, then, but the working of reason on 'things' is the mark of the new method, that working 'according to the stuff' of the world that Bacon spoke of, and not the working 'on itself' which 'brings forth cobwebs of learning'. It is that reason which, in Bacon's famous phrase, 'doth buckle and bow the mind into the nature of things'. It means distinguishing 'dreams', 'fancies' and other delusions from the truth of 'fact'; it means the rejection of superstition—Hobbes's 'kingdom of fairies and bugbears': it means the scepticism Theseus upholds—

> *I never may believe*
> *These antique fables nor these fairy toys.*
> *Lovers and madmen have such seething brains,*
> *Such shaping fantasies, that apprehend*
> *More than cool reason ever comprehends.*
>   *A Midsummer Night's Dream*, V. i. 2–6

To lovers and madmen Hobbes and Locke would add any fantasy-shapers, while applauding the antithesis of 'seething brains' and 'cool reason'.

This poise of mind and rejection of dogma fostered a tolerant spirit. Hooker had deplored the 'tedious prosecuting of wearisome contentions' and the tragedy of bringing disputes 'to one only determination, and that of all other the worst, which is by the sword' (*Ecclesiastical Politie*, Preface, ix. 3, and book I, x. 14). The Civil Wars reinforced this warning, and there was growing agreement with Benjamin Whichcote the Cambridge Platonist that 'the longest Sword, the strongest Lungs, the most Voices, are false measures of Truth' (*Moral and Religious Aphorisms*, 1703, No. 500), that 'there is nothing more unnatural to Religion, than *Contentions* about it' (No. 756), and that 'Charity of universal Extent is better than Truth of particular Application' (No. 1164). The lesson was not learnt at once; strong lungs if not long swords abound in Augustan controversy. But the evolution of the time tended towards moderation in philosophical argument, which went with unity on fundamentals and a sociable disposition. Men were ready, indeed, not only for toleration but for expansive and benevolent readings of human nature. Thomson's *Liberty* concludes in an effusion of optimism not altogether unlike Shelley's in *Prometheus Unbound*: liberty frees men's minds and fits them for society (v. 608–11)—

> *instead of barren heads,*
> *Barbarian pedants, wrangling sons of pride,*
> *And truth-perplexing metaphysic wits,*
> *Men, patriots, chiefs and citizens are form'd.*

For anyone like Thomson it was bliss to be alive in the dawn of rational daylight.

ii. LOCKE AND THE ENLIGHTENMENT

> The authority of this great man is doubtless as great as that of any man can be.
>
> BURKE
> *The Sublime and the Beautiful*, IV. xiv

To give the true perspective of Locke's thought would need more space and philosophical equipment than can be mobilised here. These few pages take his ideas not in their historical derivation but as the Augustans received them from him; they run the risk of crediting him with more originality than he possessed but that risk must be accepted, for his achievement was so to organise the requisite philosophy that the century hardly needed to look beyond him.

At the outset of the *Essay Concerning Human Understanding* we sense the excitement of new enquiry. The 'Epistle to the Reader' breathes the bracing air of mental independence: the man who seeks truth for himself, not trusting 'scraps of begged opinions', will find 'the hunter's satisfaction' and 'every moment of his pursuit will reward his pains with some delight'. But the pursuit will capture no game if it follows the wrong traces, and the first thing is to establish how the mind works, what it can deal with, and what are its pitfalls. 'To let loose our thoughts into the vast ocean of being' is useless until we know the way it works and what it can understand. Like Bacon Locke concedes that the mind is imperfect but believes it sufficient 'for the Conveniences of Life and the Information of Virtue' (*Essay*, I. i. 5): we must neither over- nor underestimate it. 'Our Faculties of Discovery are suited to our State' (II. xxiii. 12), and God gives understanding to lead through the study of his world to the worship of himself. The study of the mind is a preliminary to the study of nature and the praise of God's beneficence.

We have already seen Locke (like Bacon and Hobbes) concerned with language and definitions: understanding depends on words used clearly and with reference to something 'real'. Locke's enquiry moves among the mind's thoughts and ideas, how they are acquired and how they are to be expressed. With all his discussion of intellectual matters there is, significantly, little said of the emotions, those troublesome intruders on anyone trying to think clearly. Admittedly Locke's interest is in 'discourse', not in feelings, and to point out that he neglects something outside his subject may seem unfair. But the fact remains that Locke is reserved about the use of language for emotive or poetic purposes (he disparages poetry in the *Thoughts Concerning Education*): his interest is in discussion, where the lack of 'distinct ideas' leads to ambiguity (III. x. 26, 29). Men cannot, he admits, always express exact ideas in exact words or talk of nothing but what they can define clearly, but speaking in the best interests of language that is what they should do (III. xi. 2). Such is the conclusion to which his dislike of cobwebs leads him, and such is the direction in which the mind is to advance. Characteristically Locke stresses the use of language as 'the great Bond that holds Society together' (III. xi. 1); whatever impairs it acts against social union. The latter portion of book III consists of proposals to clarify discussion; one, for instance, is a scientifically-compiled dictionary to give exact definitions of physical things.

The world was ill-supplied with such tools of knowledge until the eighteenth century was well advanced, which is why it so highly esteemed dictionary-makers and encyclopedists. If this project were too expensive, Locke proposes instead a dictionary with 'little draughts and prints' of picturable things, especially of foreign or unusual words. Swift's sages of Laputa indeed improve on this; they abolish words altogether and rely on gesticulation and the display of innumerable objects carried around in sacks. Locke's more modest plan has carried the day: as Molière observes,

> La parfaite raison fuit toute extrémité,
> Et veut que l'on soit sage avec sobriété.

Locke prompts the mind, then, clearly to discriminate and compare ideas. Hobbes had distinguished between 'wit' (or 'fancy') and 'judgment', as the faculties which respectively see resemblances and differences, and had declared judgment to be a valuable faculty even without wit, but wit without judgment to be 'one kind of madness' (*Leviathan*, I. viii). Locke follows him, with rather less readiness to admit that 'wit' may rightly predominate in great poetry. Wit (which resembles but is narrower than our 'imagination') is in Locke's eyes suited mainly to the agreeable titillations of make-believe while judgment does the serious work. It makes up 'agreeable visions in the fancy', whereas judgment 'lies quite on the other side, in separating carefully, one from another, ideas wherein can be found the least difference', so protecting us from delusions. Wit makes up poetic figures and charms by its 'entertainment and pleasantry' but its delights are specious and lack ultimate 'truth':

> The Mind, without looking any farther, rests satisfied with the agreeableness of the Picture, and the gaiety of the Fancy; And it is a kind of affront to go about to examine it by the severe Rules of Truth and good Reason; whereby it appears that it consists in something that is not perfectly conformable to them.
>
> (II. xi. 2)

Alas for the vain deluding joys; the mind's true discipline consists in those 'severe rules of truth and good reason'.

If Locke's characteristic vocabulary is analytic, his characteristic tone is reasonable: here is the honest enquirer sharing his thoughts with his sensible fellows. Hobbes never achieved quite the authority of Locke with the Augustans, despite his admirable style and shrewd mind, because they preferred not to accept the conclusions he urged, of materialism and political absolutism. Locke's was the level acceptable voice which persuaded them into confidence in man's reasoning power and God's rational benevolence, and the persuasion was still more effective when its prosaic flavour had been sweetened by Addison and made luscious by Thomson.

The mind, Locke asserts, begins as 'white Paper, void of all Characters, without any *Ideas*' (II. i. 2), and its contents enter it originally through the senses alone. Human nature it is true has certain natural faculties and inclinations; it perceives things, prefers pleasure to pain, and so on. But of intellectual knowledge and moral or religious beliefs it has none by nature, and only acquires such as experience and reasoning bring to it. Our senses are the means by which we communicate with the world, and they provide the impressions which are the basis of all we know. Naturally we use reason and memory about what we gather—it does not remain a myriad disconnected fragments. We compare, deduce, and (unless we are mad) combine ideas into a coherent notion of the world around, but the raw materials are the sense-impressions which the nerves convey to the brain. For this operation Locke uses the simile of a small hole opening into a dark room: the understanding is enlightened only by the rays entering from the outside world and creating images. The process is suggested by the optical devices of the time, the camera obscura or chamber and lens, by which scientists were investigating light and perception and which led Berkeley to compose his major work under the title of *A Theory of Vision*.

The 'white paper' simile was no more original than most things in Augustan thought. The idea itself seems obvious and unremarkable. Yet its consequences were important, for by greatly simplifying the constitution of the mind, by stripping off notions of inherited reverences, prejudices, and beliefs supposedly grounded in its very nature, by clarifying what had seemed a complex so involved as to defy analysis, Locke enabled 'the science of man' to stand forth as an intelligible subject of knowledge. Moreover he undermined tradition; each mind being a fresh creation makes a fresh start. Furthermore, if men are what they are because of their experiences, an improvement in their experiences (that is, their controlling circumstances) will make them better. And the last consequence is that by insisting on the passive nature of perception Locke undervalued (and led the Augustans to undervalue) the imagination as an active creative power. The main distinction he draws between a human mind and a camera obscura is that the former can and the latter cannot store its images. In fact, the mind not only stores but is active in selecting and ordering images. Yet though Locke recognises that individual minds have an almost unlimited power to transform sense-data he gives little credit to the creative act by which the mind makes an individual vision of what it sees and he would indeed, like the eighteenth century, deplore more than the minimum of subjective interpretation. That extension of insight awaited the age of Wordsworth, Coleridge and Lamb: Locke's limited theory is part of the Baconian process whereby the mind is buckled to the stubborn data of 'reality'.

One other of Locke's tenets is important—that good and evil are the same as pleasure- and pain-producing actions. For previous ages the good was what led to salvation, the bad what led to damnation, and morality was religious ordinance backed by eternal consequences. Admittedly Heaven and Hell were, in the highest degree, sanctions of pleasure and pain; the Augustans, however, managed to localise the pleasure and pain on this earth and make them essential in their social philosophy. In Locke's view, God has ordained that in obedience to moral law man most completely achieves his own happiness and that of his fellows. This is not to say that the pursuit of pleasure is obedience to the moral law. But God, as Locke conceives him, has designed a universe as harmonious in the moral as the physical sphere, where the law of each thing's being is for its own advantage and that of the whole also, and where, if each man follows his truest (not his most immediate) happiness he finds himself promoting that of other men. It is an argument to which Adam

Smith's economic theory is a parallel. Virtue becomes no lonely thing, no solitary worship of God, no hermit-like renunciation, no agonised striving for purity and salvation; it is obedience to those arrangements by which a kindly Deity has linked together the happiness of all his Creation.

To be morally good, then, is willingly to obey any law, divine or human, meant for man's welfare. The highest law is the divine, revealed in the Bible and also through reason, the light of nature; obedience to it means eternal happiness. Other laws though inferior to this work in the same way: civil laws are meant for society's good, and obedience to them produces benefits and happiness. Social laws (the rules of conduct) bring esteem to him who observes them and contempt to him who does not. A selfish hunt for pleasure has no virtue in it, but if we understand where our happiness truly lies—in obedience to God, in observance of the civil and social laws of society—we shall have the best of both worlds and find the true fulfilment of our being.

This was an encouraging doctrine. 'Utilitarianism', the belief that happiness is our being's end and aim, and that the greatest happiness of the greatest number is that aim in its highest purity, became the characteristic moral doctrine of the century. Here again Locke was by no means its inventor; the earliest extended statement of it in England is perhaps Richard Cumberland's *De Legibus Naturae Disquisitio Philosophica* (1672), translated in 1727 as *A Treatise of the Laws of Nature*. Cumberland, Bishop of Peterborough, was trying to vindicate man's nature against the aspersions of Hobbes. Locke's authority, however, gave the doctrine its full prestige and it was announced again and again. Hutcheson's *Original of our Ideas of Beauty and Virtue* (1725) originated the phrase 'the greatest Happiness of the greatest Number' (III. viii); then there was the Reverend John Gay's *Fundamental Principles of Virtue* (1731), Pope's *Essay on Man* (1733), Godwin's *Political Justice* (1793), and, most insistently, Bentham's *Principles of Morals and Legislation* (1789). 'Utilitarianism' is a dreary and misleading label for a movement that stirred men to widespread benevolence, and the 'happiness' championed by Locke, even if in the well-to-do it led to complacency, was a nobler aim than the name suggests, being a state God intended for all men, and a goal towards which the Augustans started on a long pilgrimage.

iii. DISCOURSE OF REASON

> The names *Man* and *Rationall*, are of equall extent, comprehending mutually one another.
>
> HOBBES
> *Leviathan* (1651), pt. i, ch. iv

THE eighteenth century, everyone knows, was 'The Age of Reason'. This deplorably simple formula creates the impression, still strong in undergraduate essays, that by some psychological freak three or four generations of Britons grew up colour-blind to the emotions: a common greyness sobered everything. The world was all before them yet they retired to garrets to write 'rational' essays and couplets on practical matters of town life.

Those who think of the century as phlegmatic must presumably be surprised when they find evidence of feelings not only frequent but effusive. 'At many public solemnities', as sensible a man as Addison informs us, 'I cannot forbear expressing my joy with tears that have stolen down my cheeks' (*The Spectator*, No. 69). The admission would sound sentimental in a modern essayist, and it suggests that if the Augustans spoke so much of reason it was not because their emotions were weak but because on the contrary they were strong. The effusions of sensibility were never far away, and many Augustan thoughts did not by any means lie too deep for tears. It is true that literary fashion required moderation in the expression of feeling, and philosophical fashion required the importance of reason to be asserted. But there is still abundant feeling in Augustan life, though in literature sometimes it must be detected by smaller signs than in 'romantic' work and sometimes (as with Thomson's or Akenside's raptures for science) it has lost its appeal. The relations between reason and feeling need tactful definition.

If we start with reason, it is because that faculty recommended itself first, chronologically speaking, to the Augustan attention. Reason had produced the seventeenth century's intellectual triumphs, though reason not as abstract intellect but as a measuring-rod of the 'real' world. The seventeenth century was of course not the first to see the universe as order; classical and oriental antiquity, the Middle Ages and the Renaissance had observed the working of a macrocosmic plan. Hooker for instance has a magnificent paragraph on the 'obedience of creatures unto the law of nature' which guarantees the harmony of things (*Ecclesiastical Politie*, I. iii. 2). Nor was it true that God's existence and ways had hitherto been thought inscrutable and were now found demonstrable by reason; the schoolmen had held that reason could prove the existence of God and deduce therefrom an elaborate theology, and Locke's 'rational' religion was within the tradition. What did impress the Augustans was that after the sectarian violences of the Reformation, with their terrible stress on damnation, predestination and a vengeful Deity, Christianity seemed to become reasonable and 'not mysterious', and that after ages in which the mind grappled with but did not understand the universe science had found, through one type of reason, a method of study which yielded satisfying fruit. Reason, then, had produced the triumphs of Newton and Boyle, and the quieter temper of politics and religion after years of tumult.

Leaving until later the question of science, let us consider how reason worked for the Augustans in the sphere of moral philosophy. Its prestige, in the first place, produced an enviable air of confidence; the dawn was dispelling the mists of night and error. In the second place it evolved a curious kind of moral geometry which generated what is called the 'intellectualist' school of ethics, and this is so characteristic that we may respectfully disinter it for a moment from its resting-place among dead-and-gone philosophical fashions, though all we may notice is the rattle of dry bones.

When in Fielding's *Tom Jones* the hypocritical Deist Square (significant name) champions virtue against the equally hypocritical Churchman Thwackum, he does so by invoking 'the unalterable rule of right and the eternal fitness of things'. This curious phrase was then familiar as the slogan of the thorough-going rationalists.

It meant that just as there was a perfectly co-ordinated physical order, which scientific reason could understand, so too there was a similar moral order which moral reason could understand. There was in fact a science of morality, and good behaviour meant the exact concordance of one's actions to this moral order, the nature and details of which were discoverable by pure reason. With their insistence on duty and obedience to moral imperatives the 'intellectualists' (as they came later to be called) were virtually Stoics, though their first representatives were the Cambridge Platonists, whose noble religious spirit was far better than mere rationalism. In their view we perceive by spiritual insight such qualities as Goodness, Truth and Beauty (which really exist and are not subjective or relative), and should harmonise with them through our noblest faculty, reason. Man is by nature good, not sinful, and his reason can keep him so. Vice, said Benjamin Whichcote,

is contrary to the Nature of Man, *as Man*; for it is contrary to the order of Reason, the peculiar and highest Principle in Man; nor is any thing *in itself* more unnatural or of greater Deformity, in the whole world, than that an Intelligent Agent should have the Truth of Things in his *Mind*, and that it should not give Law and Rule to his *Temper, Life* and *Actions*.
Moral and Religious Aphorisms, No. 212

By his best spiritual and intellectual perceptions man understands what his moral duties are, and by reason working on his normally virtuous disposition he obeys them.

This faith, optimistic about man's nature and originally spiritual in its quality, retained its optimism in the eighteenth century but became more coolly rational and therefore more rigidly theoretical —which is why Fielding satirised it in the pedantry of Square. Spirituality dwindled into argumentation. The impoverishment is obvious in Samuel Clarke, a devoted Newtonian and the leading English metaphysician of the early eighteenth century. He would have become Archbishop of Canterbury, Voltaire relates, had not Bishop Gibson of London told Queen Anne that his great intelligence and honesty were marred by one thing: he was not a Christian. He was in fact all but an Arian—not a strong qualification for the episcopate. His fame depended largely on two sets of Boyle lectures —*A Demonstration of the Being and Attributes of God* (1704) and *The Unchangeable Obligations of Natural Religion* (1705)—in which the Platonists' spiritual reason degenerates into Square's chop-logic.

His argument would hardly need outlining were it not that it is the kind of thing that gained the 'Age of Reason' its name and was influential up to the time of Godwin. The universe to Clarke is a moral jigsaw (as to the scientists it was a physical jigsaw), in which, if everyone performs exactly those duties which 'the nature of things' requires, the harmony of moral law will be attained and God's intention fulfilled. The great evidences of God's goodness are the exquisite interdependence and regularity of natural processes, and since this is so in physical law a similar interdependence must obtain in moral law. As a general doctrine this is acceptable enough; what is not acceptable is Clarke's drily demonstrative manner. Voltaire called him 'une vraie machine à raisonnements', and that is precisely his character: his arguments are not false so much as innutrient, with their methodical deductions quite lacking in the inspiration of poetry.

Other 'intellectualists', despite their good intentions, are no more palatable. Tindal's *Christianity as Old as the Creation* (1730) is characteristic in its lack of succulence, and its second chapter heading is an adequate sample of its manner. It runs:

That the Religion of Nature consists in observing those things which our Reason, by considering the Nature of God and Man, and the Relation we stand in to him and one another, demonstrates to be our Duty: and that those Things are plain: and likewise what they are.

Other men prolonged the same strain and it is not surprising that Hume was soon to reject the supremacy of reason altogether, that the main stream of ethics soon abandoned this flat and dusty bed for the deeper channel of 'moral sentiment', and that the torrent of Evangelicalism with its tumbling life-giving waters was soon to wash into men's minds the idea that there was more to life than this thin grasshopperlike scratching.

Yet the sovereignty of reason had a sudden restoration before the end of the century in the thought of the radicals and above all in Richard Price and William Godwin. Price's *Review of the Principal Questions and Difficulties in Morals* (1757) foreshadowed Kant in establishing absolute moral imperatives to which reason must impel us. Moral rectitude is 'a universal law; the whole creation is ruled by it; under it men and all rational beings subsist' (p. 178). Price is an absolutist with his imperatives understood by reason and conformed to by will; the occasion for passions and appetites, he avers (p. 124),

arises entirely from our deficiencies and weaknesses. Reason alone (did we possess it in a higher degree) would answer all the ends of them. Thus there would be no need of the parental affections were all parents sufficiently acquainted with the reasons for taking upon them the guidance and support of those whom nature has placed under their care, and were they virtuous enough to be always determined by those reasons.

In Godwin such uncompromising rationalism achieved its fullest expression, seeking to make reason supply the place of passion and instinct. Virtue is to him—at least in his early rigorous phase— entirely a matter of right reason and will, whereas vice 'depends for its existence upon the existence of error' (*Political Justice*, 1793, i. 4). The vicious man, that is, has either worked out his moral sum wrongly or has not squarely faced the result of his calculation. Life's true governor, in thought and action, must be the mind; all action must be voluntary, deliberate, and based on reasoning from first principles. Truth, the 'real' state of things, wins allegiance if it is properly understood, for man cannot stand against the conviction of reason. So did the century's confidence reach its peak, in a challenge to man to conquer error and become perfect. It is true that Godwin himself came to see that he had underrated feeling: prefacing *St. Leon* (1799) he admitted that 'for more than four years' (that is, we may assume, since he was first attracted by Mary Wollstonecraft) he had regretted dismissing 'domestic and private affections inseparable from the nature of man and from what may be called the culture of the heart'. But it was *Political Justice* (particularly its uncompromising first edition) rather than *St. Leon* that braced the young radicals with the sense that the dawn was breaking, and transmitted not only to politics but to ethics also the clarifying objectivity of (moral) science. This dramatic culmination of eighteenth-century rationalism in nineteenth-century radicalism is one of the outstanding events of intellectual evolution.

iv. REASON DEPOSED

> Reason is, and ought only to be the slave of the passions, and can never pretend to any other office than to serve and obey them.
>
> **HUME**
> *Treatise of Human Nature*, bk. ii, pt. iii, sec. iii

REASON did not however rule unchallenged, and it is time to prelude the theme which was fundamental even in the eighteenth century, that of 'the passions'. Godwin himself, as we have seen, came to admit 'the culture of the heart', and Wordsworth after 'Dragging all precepts, judgments, maxims, creeds, Like culprits to the bar' (*The Prelude*, xi. 294-5) under Godwin's influence found his spirit breaking and turned for salvation to the life of feeling. But long before Wordsworth there were protests against too much reason, and fortunately it was not only the rationalists who could invoke great names. If Newton and Locke showed reason's triumphs, Shakespeare showed those of inspired unreason—indeed, it was critical orthodoxy to elevate the impassioned creators like Homer and Shakespeare over the men of judgment like Virgil and Jonson. The Augustans were not so blind to life as not to know that feeling is the major and reason the minor component of man. Only the strictest rationalists could hold that men live by unimpassioned thought: the general and natural conclusion was that 'the passions' are the force of life and that reason, far from impelling life on its course, can at most guide it. Pope wrote a remarkable *Spectator* (No. 408) arguing that men's actions 'can never proceed immediately from Reason', and that the Passions 'are to the Mind as the Winds to a Ship', which may perhaps destroy it but without which it cannot move at all. To extinguish the passions in the supposed cause of virtue would be, he said, 'putting out the light of the Soul', and the attempt to do so by means of education 'certainly destroys more good Genius's than it can possibly improve'. In the *Essay on Man* he put these ideas more pithily (ii. 101–10):

> *In lazy Apathy let Stoics boast*
> *Their Virtue fix'd: 'tis fix'd as in a frost;*
> *Contracted all, retiring to the breast;*
> *But strength of mind is Exercise, not Rest;*
> *The rising Tempest puts in act the soul,*
> *Parts it may ravage, but preserves the Whole.*
> *On life's vast ocean diversely we sail,*
> *Reason the card, but Passion is the gale;*
> *Nor God alone in the still calm we find,*
> *He mounts the storm, and walks upon the wind.*

It is Hume, however, not Pope, who most brilliantly reduces the prestige of reason. He does not scorn reason as an instrument of discussion—indeed his greatest work, the *Treatise of Human Nature* (1739), is a most intently-conducted piece of argument. But he denies the almost divine efficacy attributed to reason by the intellectualists; he points out how fallible it is and how mistaken even the simplest deductions may be, and he argues the theoretical necessity of scepticism about all the evidence of sense or mind (though he candidly agrees that in practice one takes life as it seems to be and deals effectively with it). He admits a dilemma—to distrust reason is to incur fantasy and unreality; to rely on reason is to find nothing ultimately certain and to fall into an abyss of scepticism. This dilemma makes him alternately desert philosophy in despair and resume it from irresistible curiosity.

Having shown reason to be a pretender, Hume prepares to enthrone passion. Philosophic convention may hold that virtue lies in obedience to reason but, he says (*Treatise*, bk. ii, pt. iii. sec. iii),

> I shall endeavour to prove *first*, that reason alone can never be a motive to any action of the will; and *secondly*, that it can never oppose passion in the direction of the will.

Reason deals with logic and moves in a different sphere from passion; it compares and judges but cannot initiate feeling or action.

We think it capable of restraining us, when restraint is necessary, but what does restrain us is something we mistake for reason because it is of a quiet and temperate nature—in other words, passion of a subdued kind, 'certain calm desires and tendencies'. To take a modern parallel, reason no more makes a man embark on or desist from action than his reading of a road-map makes his car start or stop. From the map he judges the route to his destination: the motive power comes from the engine, and the brakes which provide control are only a negative form of that power.

As for moral judgments, they are a kind of feeling. Virtue arouses an agreeable, vice a disagreeable sensation. We like beneficent actions because we feel for the good of men in general, and it is sentiment not reason that prompts us to such liking (*Treatise*, bk. iii, pt. iii, sec. i):

> The approbation of moral qualities most certainly is not derived from reason, or any comparison of ideas; but proceeds entirely from a moral taste, and from certain sentiments of pleasure and disgust, which arise from the contemplation and view of particular qualities or characters.

'To have the sense of virtue', Hume says elsewhere, 'is nothing but to feel a satisfaction of a particular kind from the contemplation of a character'.

The argument is an intricate and brilliant one and penetrates much deeper into the springs of behaviour than did the intellectualists. The *Treatise of Human Nature*, it is true, made no stir at first. But others also were undermining reason: Hutcheson as well as Pope had spoken up for 'passion', and in his posthumous *System of Moral Philosophy* (1755) he maintained like Hume that reason judges the means but not the ends of action, which are what the emotions desire. Adam Smith's *Theory of Moral Sentiments* (1759) holds the same view of moral judgments (VII. iii. 1):

> If virtue therefore pleases for its own sake, and if vice as certainly displeases the mind, it cannot be by reason, but immediate sense and feeling, which reconciles us to the one and alienates us from the other.

Burke in politics was soon to show himself as distrustful of reason, and as devoted to instinct and emotion, as any philosopher of 'sentiment'. It is time to consider the deposition of reason less negatively, less as the demotion of reason and more as the promotion of feeling.

V. THE CULTURE OF THE HEART

> There has been a controversy started of late concerning the general foundation of MORALS: whether they are derived from REASON, or from SENTIMENT; whether we attain to knowledge of them by a chain of argument and induction, or by an immediate feeling and finer internal sense.
>
> HUME
> *Enquiry Concerning the Principles of Morals* (1752), i

AUGUSTAN philosophy is often mellower in tone and more benevolent in mood than we might expect, and the predominant reason for this is the influence of Shaftesbury. Of his elder contemporaries Locke (whose pupil he was) had preached a benevolent God and the duty of benevolence among men; the Platonists, whom he admired, had thought well of human nature; and Latitudinarian divines were holding forth from the pulpit on Christian charity and the social virtues. From such roots, from an ardent love of classical philosophy, and from his sanguine temperament, sprang Shaftesbury's trust in man's natural goodness; he had a generous quality of mind and feeling which was ready to credit mankind with instincts for good. If Locke set 'clear and distinct ideas' ringing down the century, Shaftesbury bequeathed it that no less important concept 'the moral sense', together with his engaging air of urbane humanism.

The *Characteristicks* (1711) has been called a landmark in English thought because it studies man not in his rational nature but by introspection into his mind and feelings (*Encyclopedia Britannica*, 'Shaftesbury'). Seventeenth-century moralists and physiologists had dissected the emotions, but Shaftesbury was the first to base his ethics entirely on good feeling. Against Hobbist and Puritan disparagements he upheld a benevolent enlightenment, enriching English ethics with a benign current of Greek thought more potent than that Christianized by the Platonists, in a style tempered by cool reason and warm emotion, popularising 'moral sentiment' as the basis of social relationships. The certainties in man are his feelings (*Inquiry Concerning Virtue*, ii. 2 *ad fin.*):

we cannot doubt of what passes within ourselves. Our passions and affections are known to us. *They* are certain, whatever the objects may be on which they are employed.

Wordsworth could not speak more clearly. These passions and affections are generous and social; human nature tends towards sympathy, expanding outward from the family by wider and wider circles throughout humanity. As Pope was to write,

> *Self-love but serves the virtuous mind to wake,*
> *As the small pebble stirs the peaceful lake.*
> *The centre mov'd, a circle strait succeeds,*
> *Another still, and still another spreads;*
> *Friend, parent, neighbour first it will embrace,*
> *His country next, and next all human race:*
> *Wide and more wide, th' o'erflowings of the mind*
> *Take ev'ry creature in, of ev'ry kind.*
> *Essay on Man*, iv. 363–70

Man fulfils the law of his being in exercising the social virtues and benevolent emotions. Descartes' *Cogito ergo sum* yields in Shaftesbury to a self-awareness of feeling, though the good life imposes its own discipline in a selection of impulses, the cultivation of charity and elevation of mind, and the suppression of their opposites. Shaftesbury as a champion of feeling has a benevolently patrician air not shared by Blake or D. H. Lawrence.

He gave his time what, on the whole, was good for it. The new spirit of warm and effusive emotion spread through life and letters and became still more popular through those 'overflowing feelings of a tender compassionate heart' which Patrick Murdock signalised in prefacing Thomson's poems in 1762. For Thomson was the most distinguished poetic disciple of Shaftesbury, whose name he joins with those of Bacon, Boyle, Newton and Locke as his favourite philosophers: he praises the 'inward rapture, only to be felt', evoked by benevolence (*Summer*, line 1646), and in *Spring* (556ff.—'Hail, Source of Being!') he versifies Shaftesbury's remarkable Nature rhapsody in *The Moralists*. Gradually the intellectual climate becomes milder and sunnier; literature glows with moral sentiment; the sharpness of satire and the chill of sovereign reason yield before the claims of feeling, as country gardens forsake geometry and soften into the outlines of natural grace. No book represents this better than Hutcheson's *Inquiry into the Original of our Ideas of Beauty and Virtue* (1725), which plays variations on the 'moral sense' (that is, the instincts of moral approval or disapproval). Why, Hutcheson asks, do we feel for or against others even in remote times and places, who cannot affect us personally? Why rate virtue higher than success? Why lose with honour rather than win with dishonour? Such preferences are not reasonable—they arise from moral sense or sentiment, an intuition untrammelled by calculations of advantage.

Human feelings, of course, are more numerous than the qualities (whether rational or instinctive) involved in the special task of moral judgment. But as philosophy begins to consider even moral judgment to be a matter of feeling or sentiment, as it stresses the fraternal emotions which should link mankind, so there unfolds a willingness in ways unconnected with moral behaviour to admit the primacy of feeling, to value the intuitive and indeed irrational impulses, to feel sympathy for living things and awe at the strangeness of Nature. Hutcheson increases the senses far beyond the traditional five, to include 'Public Sense' or sympathy, the 'Moral Sense', the sense of honour, and imagination—'the pleasant perceptions arising from regular, harmonious, and uniform objects'. Burke's *Inquiry into the Origin of our Ideas of the Sublime and Beautiful* (1757) enriches aesthetics as Shaftesbury had enriched moral philosophy. 'The influence of reason in producing our passions', it asserts, 'is nothing near so extensive as it is commonly believed' (I. xiii), and it examines such emotions as sympathy, and the awe aroused by sublimity (Burke is here under the strong influence of Longinus). Sublimity itself is a notable theme, for it transcends the region of the clear and comprehensible for that of mystery and dread. The beautiful, Burke says, implies delicacy, clear colour, and moderate size: the sublime implies great scale (the ocean, or starry skies), obscurity and mystery, dramatic illumination (lightning), majesty and difficulty of achievement (Stonehenge), and above all great power and the thought of infinity, which fill the mind with 'delightful horror' (II. viii). Burke's sense of these qualities, so alien to the classical code, marks an epoch in the analysis of moods. By such introspection many subtle and unaccountable instincts found their way into the forefront of attention, and both prose and poetry turned to a more sensitive consciousness of them.

The vogue of feeling shows itself in philosophy. With Hume and Adam Smith we enter the realm of expansive good nature: as with Shaftesbury and Hutcheson the tone of their writing is almost as significant as the sense. Virtue, fixed as in a frost by the intellectualists, is to be thawed out: the springs of human nature are to be freed from the clear but icy crust of reason and are to flow and bubble from their inmost source. Since philosophy is linking moral qualities to feeling the consequence seems to be that the deeper one's virtue the stronger one's emotions. There is a novel degree of fervour in Hume and Adam Smith as they write on such subjects: 'the sentiments of humanity', Hume declares, are so agreeable that they

> brighten up the very face of sorrow and operate like the sun, which shining on a dusky cloud or falling rain paints on them the most glorious colours which are to be found in the whole circle of nature.
>
> *Essays Moral, Political and Literary:* 'The Stoic'

Such enthusiasm over sorrow and sympathy is typical. Hutcheson had already imagined a benevolence coextensive with humanity and even with astral space—if, he said, we knew of rational beings 'in the most distant planets' we should wish them well. For Hume, benevolence is no less unbounded; he describes our sensibility as analogous to the sympathetically-vibrating strings of violins, and a glowing sense of public spirit as being almost the summit of human nature:

> No qualities are more readily intituled to the general goodwill and

approbation of mankind than beneficence and humanity, friendship and gratitude, natural affection and public spirit, ... and a generous concern for our kind and species.
Enquiries Concerning the Human Understanding, ed. Selby-Bigge (1902), 299–300

Hume's ideal man, in all the delightful complacency of his rich, harmonious and sentimental feelings, can be portrayed only in the words of his creator's essay 'The Stoic', already cited:

> The softest benevolence, the most undaunted resolution, the tenderest sentiments, the most sublime love of virtue, all these animate successively his transported bosom. What satisfaction when he looks within, to find the most turbulent passions tuned to just harmony and concord, and every jarring sound banished from this enchanting music!

Adam Smith's *Theory of Moral Sentiments* (1759) breathes the same intoxicating air—intoxicating not because good sense has been forgotten but because the feelings are indulged and inhibitions relaxed. His panegyrics on sympathy, 'the amiable virtue of humanity', recall the novels of sensibility in their transports and tears. The unfortunate, we learn (I. i. 2),

> by relating their misfortunes ... in some measure renew their grief. Their tears accordingly flow faster than before. ... They take pleasure, however, in all this, and it is evident are sensibly relieved by it, because the sweetness of the bystander's sympathy more than compensates the bitterness of their sorrow.

Sufferer and sympathiser harmonise with each other, the former moderating his anguish, the latter sharing his situation with all the delicacy of the generous heart. As in Hume, these impulses are the outcome not of reason but of 'immediate sense and feeling'.

As such sympathy spread, Fielding was able to praise the vogue of charity—'this virtue hath shone brighter in our time than at any period which I remember in our annals' (*The Champion*, 16 February, 1740)—and to mention 'a vast number of schemes' for helping the poor (*Covent-Garden Journal*, 5 May, 1752). In 1755 the public contributed £100,000 for the victims of the Lisbon earthquake, and this disinterested generosity for those of another nation and faith was widely approved. Johnson's *Idler* (6 May, 1758) said that whenever the public was asked to help in a good cause,

every hand is open to contribute something, every tongue is busied in solicitation, and every art of pleasure is employed for a time in the interest of virtue.

Smollett observed an 'extraordinary growth' of benevolence; John Brown's *Estimate of the Manners and Principles of the Times* (1757) avowed that 'the spirit of Humanity is natural to our nation', and Goldsmith's Chinese sage in *The Citizen of the World* remarked England's 'exalted virtue' in the cause of charity.

The century's moral evolution was a complicated general trend in which, far from being sacrificed to reason, 'the passions' received abundant honour and even at times an adulation which at last brought sensibility into disrepute. If the literary moods of the late Augustans are in general warmer and more indulgent than those of the early, the credit must go in a marked degree to the philosophers whose thought had given prestige to feeling and the encouragement of psychological theory to the promptings of emotion.

vi. 'THE NEW PHILOSOPHY'

Give me to learn each secret Cause;
Let Number's, Figure's, Motion's Laws
    Reveal'd before me stand;
These to great Nature's scenes apply,
And round the Globe, and through the Sky,
    Disclose her working hand.
                    AKENSIDE
            Hymn to Science

IF one cause more than another imbued Augustan thought with optimism it was the triumphs of science. What Akenside called

The scholiast's learning, sophist's cant,
The visionary bigot's rant,
    The monk's philosophy

was being swept away as an enormous encumbrance. The seventeenth century in England and France saw a movement towards intellectual clarification and collaboration such as Italy had developed since the fifteenth and sixteenth centuries, and one great sign of it was the founding of the Royal Society for the purpose Bacon had promulgated, 'the enlarging of the bounds of human empire, to the effecting of all things possible'.

One of the Society's founders, Dr. John Wallis, wrote an *Account of Some Passages in his own Life*, which was published (of all unlikely places) in Thomas Hearne's 1725 edition of Langtoft's mediaeval *Chronicle*. In 1645, Wallis relates, he met several men interested 'in what hath been called the *New Philosophy*, or *Experimental Philosophy*', who met weekly in London 'to consider of *Philosophical Enquiries*'. Partly dispersed during the Civil War, towards the end of the Commonwealth they were reunited in London at Gresham College, and in 1662 they received Charles II's charter as the Royal Society.

The Society was interested in knowledge, in Boyle's words, 'as it hath a tendency to use'. Its early *History* (1667) by Thomas Sprat is no mere record of 'pure' science; it deals with technological improvements, developments in the American colonies, and a hundred other 'real' things. Yet not all its investigations were as practical as these; indeed, those most influential in enlarging the mind were such as explored the minutiae of living organisms or the magnitudes of astronomy. Their results were not the special province of the expert; early science was largely the hobby of gentlemen amateurs like Cowley, Pepys, Evelyn and Dryden, and most of the Society's *Philosophical Transactions* lay within the compass of the general reader. Public lectures like the Boyle series disseminated the new ideas, and there was as yet little fear either that the amateur and the specialist might come to inhabit different worlds or that science and religion might prove hostile. The world of knowledge was one, and all men were free of it. The early Boyle lecturers, for instance, were chosen by Archbishop Tillotson (with Evelyn's help), and often applied the new thought to the confirmation of faith. Samuel Clarke considered 'the Being and Attributes of God', 'the

Obligations of Natural Religion', and 'the Truth and Certainty of the Christian Religion'. Later the reverend William Derham spoke on astro-theology and physico-theology, 'or a Demonstration of the Being and Attributes of God from his works of Creation'. Such an alliance of science and faith had been one of Bacon's strongest intentions, and it was furthered by the greatest seventeenth-century scientists like Newton and the naturalist John Ray, whose *Wisdom of God Manifested in the Works of the Creation* (1691) was widely influential. Science had its victories no less renowned than faith, but in no spirit of rivalry, and this confidence in united purposes is impressive and moving.

A series of virtual miracles was revealed throughout Nature. The telescope probed the vastness of the sky and the microscope the details of minute organisms. Nature's infinite variety called for systematisation, and in the hour of need there was Newton with his *Principia* (1687) to explain the heavens and Ray with his great *Historia Generalis Plantarum* (1686–1704), fifty years before Linnaeus, to methodise the world of vegetables. In the field of natural history the eighteenth century cast its net widely by sending naturalists on voyages of exploration, a precedent for Darwin's famous *Beagle* expedition (1831–6). When Cook made his first voyage in *Endeavour* (1768–71), he was accompanied by Joseph Banks, a wealthy and brilliant young amateur of botany, and by a pupil of Linnaeus, and Botany Bay owes its name to the wealth of material they found in that part of Australia. Banks was later knighted and became President of the Royal Society; on Linnaeus's death in 1778 he induced an English naturalist, Sir James Edward Smith, to buy his books and collections which thereby became, as they still are, the Linnean Society's property.

Through such men and through the passion they spread for natural observation the later eighteenth and the nineteenth centuries reaped a rich harvest of amateur natural history; the wonders of creation were manifested not only to specialists but to hundreds of patient amateurs, and instilled a reverent naturalism which has ever since remained as a refreshment to the national spirit. Of the early amateurs, Erasmus Darwin the grandfather of Charles has his niche for propounding the evolutionary inheritance of acquired characteristics; Thomas Pennant is still known as a topographer and zoologist; and it is to that fortunate friendship between Pennant, Daines Barrington and Gilbert White that we owe White's *Natural History of Selborne* (1789). The general reader was not forgotten; Erasmus Darwin wrote his extraordinary *Botanic Garden* (1789–91) in the palatable form of heroic couplets 'to inlist the imagination under the banner of science' and achieved a fourth edition by 1799, and *The Botanical Magazine* and the Linnean Society's *Transactions* were started in 1787 and 1791 respectively.

In planning this admirable universe it was natural to think that the Creator had borne particularly in mind his favourite creature, Man. This was one of the many strands of the eighteenth century's mediaeval inheritance: man had always seemed the centre of the universe, to which the forces of nature had an especial reference—the fruits of the earth grew to feed him and the rain fell to nourish them. There were, it is true, some like Shaftesbury whose broad outlook saw that nature exists for itself and not for humanity, and like Pope who satirised the man 'who thinks all made for one, not one for all'. Yet at least in a temperate climate there was some excuse for thinking Man to be the beneficiary of a great benevolent institution. Nehemiah Grew's *Cosmologia Sacra* (1701: typical title) asserts that those birds which are good to eat fly in flocks and so are easily detected, and that animals useful to man multiply faster than others. Grew was secretary to the Royal Society (1677–9), and not negligible as a scientific thinker. William Wollaston's *Religion of Nature Delineated* (1724) notes how the plane of the earth's equator intersects that of its orbit 'and makes a proper angle with it, in order to diversify the year and create a useful variety of seasons', and Joseph Priestley repeats this same example of divine beneficence in his *Institutes of Natural and Revealed Religion* (1772–4). Hartley's *Observations on Man* (1749) praises God for making the vegetable kingdom green, 'which is the middle colour of the seven primary ones, and consequently the most agreeable to the organ of sight'. Why this chromatic benevolence did not extend to the sea and the sky might admit, as Sir Thomas Browne would say, of a wide solution. All this is simultaneously naïve and magnificent. Pleasure at man's special position was natural enough, and on the whole, despite warnings against pride by Swift, Pope and others, the Augustans could hardly be blamed for their self-congratulations.

Three aspects of the universe above all struck their minds—its magnitude, complexity, and order. These again were age-old impressions yet science provided so much new evidence about them that they were felt almost as revelations. Addison's *Spectator*, No. 565, declares that were the solar system annihilated it would 'not be missed more than a grain of sand upon the sea-shore'. Wollaston proves God's infinite power by 'the insupportable glory and lustre' of the sun with its 'vast distance, magnitude and heat'. Thomson prays Nature (*Autumn*, 1353-6) to

> *Snatch me to heaven; thy rolling wonders there,*
> *World beyond world, in infinite extent,*
> *Profusely scatter'd o'er the void immense,*
> *Shew me.*

The shining heavens proclaimed their great Original—'such regions of matter about us', said Wollaston, 'in which there is not the least particle that does not carry with it an argument of God's existence'. Young summed it up with his usual dogmatic italics—'an *undevout* astronomer is *mad*'. The assurance of this belief, expressed often and fervently, is striking: the suspicion that all might not be for the best in the best of possible worlds was shouldered aside as the petulence of conceit, criticising a Creator whose purpose it was too petty to fathom. Pope did so in the *Essay on Man*, and Thomson and others elsewhere, and by the time one arrives at the level of Priestley and Paley the degree of gratification is almost repellent. Not all opinions coincided, it is true; Butler's *Analogy* admits both life and nature to be flawed and Voltaire and Johnson pilloried the optimists in *Candide* and *Rasselas* (both 1759). Not everyone could, like *Rasselas*'s philosopher, 'concur with the great and unchangeable scheme of universal felicity'. Yet it was not unreasonable to view the scheme of things with confidence and see the universe adding the confirmation of natural religion to the tenets of revealed, working through infinite wisdom for the greatest good of the whole.

There is however one important consequence of science with a different bearing. Some men distrusted it, either through distrust of human capacities, or because it encouraged pride, or because natural philosophy seemed inferior to moral, or because it sometimes appeared ridiculous.

The Augustans were not blind to the limitations of the human mind. Locke did not make excessive claims for it, though like Bacon he believed in its great potentialities if rightly used. Swift and his fellows of the Scriblerus Club tried to counter the adulation showered on Newton which (despite Pope's famous epigram of praise) they thought excessive. Man might explore nature, the *Essay on Man* argued, but he could not understand himself. Even Newton, 'whose rules the rapid comet bind', could not 'describe or fix one movement of his mind' (ii. 35–6).

Was it not, then, absurd to be elated at scientific skill? Was science indeed life's true business? For Pope as for all humanists the prime subject of enquiry was the moral nature of man, and the end of *The Dunciad* is a warning against the scientists' materialism and the rationalism of their metaphysics. Years before, in the 408th *Spectator*, Pope had asserted that human nature is 'the most useful Object of humane Reason', and that moral philosophy

as much exceeds all other Learning, as it is of more Consequence to adjust the true Nature and Measures of Right and Wrong, than to settle the Distance of the Planets and compute the Times of their Circumvolutions.

Johnson too, in the *Life of Milton*, asserts the primacy of humane studies:

The truth is, that the knowledge of external nature, and the sciences which that knowledge requires or includes, are not the great or the frequent business of the human mind. Whether we provide for action or conversation, whether we wish to be useful or pleasing, the first requisite is the religious and moral knowledge of right and wrong.

Shebbeare considered the biologists' collecting mania contemptible and 'even the sublimer parts of philosophy' like astronomy to be 'infinitely inferior to that of the studying man'.

The humanists found ammunition in apparent absurdities. The apparently absurd, of course, may lead to the fundamental, but this is not always evident at first sight. A broadcast on the brain included, to quote *The Radio Times* (8 March, 1949), the sound of ' "brain-waves" recorded in the laboratory, and a running commentary on an octopus undergoing memory training'. What, one wonders, would Swift or Johnson have made of an octopus undergoing memory training? The modern mind is accustomed not to find such things odd, whereas Augustan sceptics found many things very odd indeed. Samuel Butler, for instance, did so, and wrote *The Elephant in the Moon: a Satire on the Royal Society* (1676) about an astronomer misled by a fly on his lens. Even the progressive Addison makes free with those who 'amuse themselves with the stifling of cats in an air-pump, cutting up frogs alive or impaling of insects upon the point of a needle' (*Spectator*, No. 21), and Goldsmith's Chinaman cheerfully despises research:

> I am amused, my dear Fum, with the labours of some of the learned here. One shall write you a whole folio on the dissection of a caterpillar; another shall swell his works with a description of the plumage on the wing of a butterfly; a third shall see a little world on a peach leaf, and publish a book to describe what his readers might see more clearly in two minutes, only by being furnished with eyes and a microscope.
> *The Citizen of the World*, letter lxxxix

It is of course true that Sprat's *History of the Royal Society*, or the Society's *Transactions*, or such a miscellany as Derham's *Physico-Theology* contains many curiosities. But nature is so manifold that hardly anything is curious enough to be impossible; certainly nothing in early science is odder than the present-day processes of making fleecy fabrics of spun glass, or warming a room by extracting heat from colder air outside. To the incredulous Augustan, experiments 'to make Fire and Flame ponderable', to try the efficacy of snow in the treatment of pleurisies, and to dissect the optic nerves of moles and swordfish (these examples are from Derham) were by their mere nature ridiculous. Derham indeed thinks it necessary to apologise for a long note on the structure of a mole's ear (*Physico-Theology* (1713), 118 fn.):

> I hope the Reader will excuse me for being so particular in this Organ only of the *Mole*, a despised Creature, but as notable an example of God's Work, as its Life is different from that of other Quadrupeds.

Such details, and such information as that 'Dr. Halley' has found the sun to be 119,032,125 miles from the earth and that light travels 264,516 miles a second were satirists' treasure-trove. Swift was perhaps gibing at Derham in *Gulliver's Travels*: Derham discusses how a wasp-sting works, and Gulliver presents three Brobdingnagian specimens to Gresham College. Most of Swift's shafts at Laputan scientists have been traced to the Royal Society's transactions: the attempt to distinguish colours by touch is based on Boyle's account of a blind man alleged to have done so, and the experiment to store sunbeams in cucumbers is a parody of Stephen Hales's work on plant respiration and the effects of sunlight on soil. Swift's onslaught on science is part of that ruthless commonsense which is a shortcoming in him, though it was prompted also by political dislike of the Royal Society (Newton, as Master of the Mint, for example, had testified in favour of Wood's coinage), and also probably by the belief that scientists (he calls them by the unsavoury name of 'Projectors') were gulling the public of money.

There were, then, those who disliked science and this dislike strengthened (despite Shelley) in the Romantic revival. Blake broke out strongly against Bacon; Wordsworth wrote of the 'fingering slave' who would 'peep and botanize Upon his mother's grave'; Keats protested that the rainbow was now 'giv'n In the dull catalogue of common things' (a drastic reversal of the wonder Newton's *Opticks* aroused in the Augustans). The romantics did not want 'philosophical persons' to account for 'things supernatural and causeless': they were apt to be less interested in physical enquiries than in a crazy woman under a thorn bush or in their communings with a 'spiritual' nature. But in the eighteenth century the fuller impact of materialism was not so strongly felt, and from the pages of the Augustans a double impression arises, on the one hand of a surviving preference for humane studies, and on the other of exhilaration at a new discovery of truth.

vii. PHILOSOPHY AND LITERATURE

> Human Nature is the only science of man; and yet has been hitherto the most neglected. It will be sufficient for me, if I can bring it a little more into fashion.
> HUME
> *Treatise of Human Nature*, bk. I, pt. iv, sec. vii.

PHILOSOPHY and literature have never been closer than they were for the Augustans. Banishing the idea that learning was a matter for scholars alone the age admitted all reverent and not oversceptical men to the fields of science, philosophy and theology. Religious congregations, theatre audiences, readers of poetry and periodicals—all formed the public for moral and scientific enquiries, and shared Addison's desire to naturalise philosophy 'in clubs and assemblies, at tea-tables and in coffee-houses' (*The Spectator*, No. 10).

The first requisite for this purpose, as well as for clear thought, was a plain prose. The best-known sign of the new taste is that found in Sprat's *History of the Royal Society* (1667: pp. 112–13):

> Who can behold, without indignation, how many mists and uncertainties these specious *Tropes* and *Figures* have brought on our Knowledge? ... Of all the Studies of men, nothing may be sooner obtain'd, than this vicious abundance of *Phrase*, this Trick of *Metaphors*, this volubility of *Tongue*, which makes so great a noise in the World.

Rejecting 'amplifications, digressions and swellings of style' the Society encourages

> a close, naked, natural way of speaking; positive expressions; clear senses; a native easiness: bringing all things as near the Mathematical plainness,

as they can: and preferring the language of Artizans, Countrymen, and Merchants, before that of Wits or Scholars.

In that spirit, if not so austerely, Bacon and Hobbes had written, and Locke and Swift were to write. 'Positive expressions, clear senses' are the watchword, rather than the passionate rhetoric of Donne, the recondite curiosity of Burton or Browne, the poetic imagery and eloquence of Jeremy Taylor, the picturesqueness of Earle or Walton and the Biblical and colloquial force of Bunyan, 'for truth', says Dennis, '(like the Innocence of our first Parents) loves to appear naked, and Solid Sense, like perfect Beauty, is but hid by Ornament' (*Critical Works*, ed. Hooker, i. 50).

To say that the Augustans quite renounced the heady pleasures of rhetoric would be wrong; men feel as well as think, and like to sway as well as to convince their fellows. Shaftesbury luxuriates in rhapsody even while Locke is at the height of his fame; Addison and Derham soar above their normal levels in the *Glorias* of scientific enthusiasm, and the influences of Cicero, the Bible, Milton, and (later) sensibility counteracted the vogue of the 'close, naked, natural way of speaking'. Speciously in Bolingbroke, magnificently in Burke, the purple patch retains its place.

Yet the trend remains, a standard from which elaboration is a digression or a holiday. Particularly in the sphere of thought the Augustans aim at clarity, though ironically the greatest and apparently clearest of their prose-writers, Swift, is the one about whose precise intentions there is most discussion. As for Locke, Clarke, Hutcheson, Smith, Price, Priestley, Paley, Hume, and Godwin their concern is to explain themselves: in all of them metaphysics calls for aid on sense and philosophy is brought home to men's business and bosoms. If their work is often vulnerable at that level it is because they are speaking of the highest matters in terms attuned to the ears of daily life. The same is true of Addison: Hume praises his 'easy and obvious philosophy' but he strikes us as too easy. Perhaps Hume overestimated the appeal of mere amenity—few modern readers can find Clarke, Priestley or Paley palatable as stylists, despite their lucidity. Nevertheless it is a merit in the Augustans that when they are shallow they do not conceal the fact. Obscurity gives the writer an unfair advantage, and this advantage they rarely take. Whether their ideas are easy or difficult they have the discipline and good manners to be as clear in expressing them as possible.

How far the new interests helped or hindered literature is hard to decide: they extended the imagination's range but impaired its subtlety. On the credit side there is the stimulus of a 'new' cosmology, and here as so often Addison is his time's best representative. The 420th *Spectator* eloquently describes how 'the authors of the new philosophy' enlarge the mind, 'whether we consider their theories of the earth or heavens, the discoveries they have made by glasses, or any other of their contemplations on nature'. From microbes, through 'metals, minerals, plants and meteors', the mind rises to contemplate the whole celestial scheme until it is 'lost in such a labyrinth of suns and worlds, and confounded with the immensity and magnificence of nature'. Astronomy was the supreme though not the only inspiration: Newton had put on a new and rational basis the mediaeval faith that God's love was the prime force moving the spheres. For Pope he was a divinely-appointed instrument to reveal Nature and Nature's laws, and Mallet in *The Excursion* saw his soul shining 'amid the general quire Of saints and angels' through his mathematical corroboration of heavenly love (ii. 160–4):

> *Simplicity divine: by this sole rule*
> *The Maker's great establishment, these worlds*
> *Revolve harmonious, world attracting world*
> *With mutual love, and to their central sun*
> *All gravitating.*

Faith, science, imagination and poetry forge a quadruple alliance; in Richard Glover's words, borrowed by Professor Marjorie Nicolson as the title of her book on these matters, 'Newton demands the Muse'.

Newton moreover received the Muse. Blackmore, influenced perhaps by Derham's physico-theology lectures of 1711, produced *The Creation* (1712), which Dennis compared favourably with

Lucretius's *De Rerum Natura*, Addison judged to be 'one of the most useful and noble productions in our English verse', and Johnson, through whose recommendation Blackmore was included in the *English Poets*, thought to have set its author among the first favourites of the English Muse. It is a long work with a Lockeian preface arguing that man has no innate idea of God but that even 'Bigots in Atheism' should yield to the 'Wonders of Creating Art' the universe displays. Taste is unlikely to witness a Blackmore revival, yet in verse sometimes animated, sometimes prosaic, sometimes impressive and always clear he gives a real sense of the varied wonder and beauty of creation. John Hughes's *Ecstasy* (1720) hailed both Newton's astronomy and his optics. Mallet and Akenside celebrated the harmony of the stellar system. More importantly, Pope played with prismatic discoveries in those brilliant lines on the sylphs (*The Rape of the Lock*, ii. 63-8):

> *Loose to the wind their airy garments flew,*
> *Thin glittering textures of the filmy dew,*
> *Dipt in the richest tincture of the skies,*
> *Where light disports in ever-mingling dyes,*
> *While every beam new transient colours flings,*
> *Colours that change whene'er they wave their wings.*

The Augustans were strong in praise of colour, especially of the prismatic effects of rainbows, rain-drops, dew and gems, or of the composition of light and its richness and variety of tint. As Newton's gravitational work revealed a new majesty in the heavens so his optical discoveries stirred a new curiosity in colour and, Professor Nicolson suggests, countered the Cartesian argument that 'secondary' qualities like colour and sound are less important than 'primary' like solidity and size which are supposedly 'in' their objects. Science then did not necessarily reduce the world's reality to mere matter and motion; it also heightened the beauty of things, and of this heightening Addison's 420th *Spectator* and Akenside's *Pleasures of the Imagination* (1744) are not unworthy records.

Other aspects of science, however, were less nutritious. Locke's cast of thought did not help imagination; in France Descartes was said by Boileau to have cut poetry's throat, and that champion of science Malebranche 'could never without disgust read a page of the finest verses' (Dugald Stewart, *Works*, 1854, i. 150). The Royal Society's criteria of style were signs of an attempt to put the mind directly in contact with its 'objects' and exclude from its dealings with them the shaping spirit of imagination.

Some kinds of 'truth' are less effective than others in sounding the overtones of poetry; they fail to suggest the tremor of feeling, the 'something far more deeply interfus'd'. To say this is not to accept unqualified the romantic depreciation of neoclassic poetry, yet as soon as one turns from the best Augustan poets (Pope, Johnson, Gray, Goldsmith, Cowper and a few others) to the next best the quality of neoclassic poetic language appears to be deficient, and the intimate pulse of life seems to die. In explanation there are various theories accusing the age's classical affiliations in education and criticism, the influence of Milton, and the social aim of writing, with poets as well as prose-writers confining themselves to things which normal men can recognise from their normal experience. Some loss has already been admitted at the end of the chapter on religion; another, and related, loss may come from too strong a sense of the external world as external, as objective matter whose intricacy or majesty arouse admiration but whose impersonality does not collaborate with man's imagination or moods. Augustan poets find new worlds to explore—astronomy, picturesque landscape, the life of nature—yet something is missing; they hear and see the world around yet it remains a set of external facts. Perhaps, as Lessing's *Laökoön* suggests, poets were trying the wrong things, making their poems deal with a detailed factual record of the world more suitable to painting. Whatever the cause, the fault is there; rarely, for instance, does Thomson's pleasure in natural effects make *The Seasons* more than a notebook turned into Miltonics and much the same is true of other Augustan long poems. The external world is too external and not until Blake, Wordsworth and Coleridge is the inner world of man poetically united to the outer world of nature in real partnership.

Yet if attention (particularly in poetry) often remained on the surface, merely 'painting fair the form of things', in some respects (particularly in prose) it prepared to plunge below. The study of morals and psychology, which Hume complained of as neglected, was explored with method and enthusiasm. Early in the *Treatise of Human Nature* (1739) Hume observes that in ancient Greece a century elapsed between the birth of natural science and 'the application of experimental philosophy to moral subjects'. In England, he points out, the same period has passed 'betwixt my Lord Bacon and some late philosophers' (mentioning Locke, Shaftesbury, Mandeville, Hutcheson and Butler) 'who have begun to put the science of man on a new footing, and have engaged the attention and excited the curiosity of the public' (i. 6–7). The moral philosophers' achievement was to display the inner world; Hume speaks of his project in the *Enquiry Concerning Human Understanding* as 'mental geography, or delineation of the distinct parts and powers of the mind', and this 'mental geography' becomes a leading topic of attention. Pamela educates her children after the principles of Locke's *Thoughts on Education* and Sterne takes from associationism the unprecedented narrative manner of *Tristram Shandy*. The philosopher, like the man of letters, is increasingly interested in the life within, and Hume describes the enquirer as needing no more information about moral qualities than introspection can supply:

> He need only enter into his own breast for a moment, and consider whether or not he would desire to have this or that quality ascribed to him and whether such or such an imputation would proceed from a friend or an enemy.
>
> *Essays and Treatises* (1767), ii. 230

The feelings, impulses private or social, 'ruling passions', sentiment, the relations between emotion and reason—these are more and more a part of literary psychology, cultivated in finer shades and more indulgently abundant in the novel and drama of sensibility, in poetry and criticism. Hume's emphasis on sympathy has been called his most important contribution to moral philosophy, and it is the sort of philosophical introspection which deepened literary sensibility by stressing the fellowship between man and the world around him. As the vogue of analysis grows, criticism concerns itself less with judgment by rules or moral orthodoxy and seeks instead the springs of feeling and the personal autonomy of inspiration. Johnson has been called the last of the great judicial critics; after and indeed contemporaneously with him the newer fashion was growing, of closer psychological understanding and subtler poetic response. Shakespearean criticism in particular evolves thus, into a concern for subtleties: Shakespeare's power, in Maurice Morgann's phrase (*The Dramatic Character of Sir John Falstaff*, 1777),

agrees in general so perfectly with that of Nature that it is not only wonderful in the great but opens another scene of amazement to the discoveries of the microscope.

Morgann's essay, with William Richardson's *Philosophical Analysis* (symptomatic phrase) *of Some of Shakespeare's Remarkable Characters* (1774) and Whateley's *Remarks on Some of the Characters of Shakespeare* (1785), marks the emergence of the 'microscopic' interpretation which leads to Coleridge.

Augustan thought, then, directs and affects literature in many ways, accompanying it in exploring the possibilities of life and of nature. Philosophy's precise influence must always be unascertainable in subjects so large and various as life and literature, yet it was part of current thought and its leading ideas were the frequent concern of literary men. Its whole operation, generally speaking, must be seen within the framework of Christian belief; it was a supplementary and not an alternative study of man and his world, and its conclusions about cosmic purposes or the social virtues were reinforcements for enlightened religion. From religion and philosophy alike literature drew its climate of ideas, and the more it is studied the more fraternal, the more harmonious the linkage proves to be in the unified culture of Augustan England.

VI. THE VISUAL ARTS

i. THE POLITE IMAGINATION

> A man of a polite imagination is let into a great many pleasures that the vulgar are not capable of receiving. He can converse with a picture, and find an agreeable companion in a statue.
>
> ADDISON
> *The Spectator*, No. 411

IN his *History of England in the Eighteenth Century* (1878) Lecky observed that the English classical architects 'had touched the very nadir of taste'. The whirligig of time brings in his revenges, and today those architects are extolled as all but infallible. The Augustan arts have never been more admired than in an age which looks back two centuries to the coherence of what seems a golden era of design. That, rather than other art-forms, is the theme of this chapter. Eighteenth-century music, delightful as it is with Handel, the anthems of Greene and Boyce, the chamber works of Arne, and *The Beggar's Opera* with its melodious ballad-offspring, does not show the pressure of Augustan sensibility as strongly as do the visual arts, and its relations with literature are far less organic. Music expressed the social spirit as an accompaniment to masquerades, glee parties, dances and church worship, but until the nineteenth century felt its romantic intoxications the deeper emotions were stirred rather through the eye. It is what the Augustans saw more than what they heard that reveals their nature. The well-to-do Georgian was not always 'a man of a polite imagination' yet on the whole he was civilised enough to build himself a good house, fill it with seemly furniture, hang it with family portraits and Old Masters, and dispose a quantity of statuary in its niches. This was all part of the Augustan code, and the degree of its success is often superlative.

The polite imagination was more than a social grace; it entered (the Augustans felt) into a man's whole character and affected his moral nature, and this harmony between taste and morals was an article of Shaftesbury's faith. He absorbed from Plato a lofty belief in the transcendent significance of beauty, and from the Stoics an advocacy of self-control. He assimilated aesthetics to morality by holding good taste and good conduct to be twin sides of the complete man: morality and art were both forms of beauty. As he put it in *Advice to an Author* (pt. iii, sec. 3; in *Characteristicks*, 1711),

thus are the Arts and Virtues mutually friends; and thus the science of virtuosi and that of virtue itself become, in a manner, one and the same.

For classical architecture, Mr Christopher Hussey has pointed out in prefacing Margaret Jourdain's *Work of William Kent* (1948), Shaftesbury did what Ruskin was to do for Gothic, by 'giving to architectural style the added prestige of moral rightness', identifying spiritual with stylistic qualities and judging art with the high seriousness of ethical purpose. In the sombre light of the twentieth century Shaftesbury's patrician refinement seems superficial, yet his connoisseurship of art and morals enlightened his time with the glow of a luminous humanism. The Augustan cultivation of the arts was paralleled (at least in intention) by the cultivation of virtue.

The writings of Jonathan Richardson the elder are relevant here. A portrait-painter of some merit, and a friend of Pope, he virtually founded art-criticism in England, forerunning Reynolds as a theorist and indeed, according to Johnson's *Life of Cowley*, being the first source of Reynolds's interest in painting. It was to Reynolds that the Strawberry Hill reprint of his works (1792) was dedicated. His influence was exerted through three essays, on *The Theory of Painting* (1715), *The Art of Criticism* (1719) and *The Science of a Connoisseur* (1719), and he wrote to vindicate painting from the idea that it was a 'pleasing superfluity', merely 'one part of our ornamental furniture'. England, he protested, though rich in musicians, writers, philosophers, soldiers and statesmen, was sadly lacking in connoisseurs, and he set out to establish art-appreciation on the noblest possible grounds. Painting, he held, is a source of moral improvement and of knowledge, by which we learn of 'countries, habits, manners, arms, buildings civil and military, animals, plants, minerals, their natures and properties'. An enthusiast for the great masters will feel 'nobler ideas, more love to his country, more moral virtue, more faith, more piety and devotion' than the Philistine, and classical sculptures or Raphael's paintings confirm the Psalmist in placing man little lower than the angels, crowned with glory and honour. Art is an Aristotelian idealisation of man's estate (*Works*, 1792, 113):

> Nature must be raised; and improved not only from what is commonly seen to what is but rarely, but even yet higher, from a judicious and beautiful idea in the painter's mind.

Taste, apprehending this higher reality, is a philosophical quality and produces not only better connoisseurs but better men.

The idea that art aims at ennoblement is characteristic Renaissance doctrine, a natural outcome of an art serving a Church and an aristocracy. It could, however, as appears in the curious specimens of 'criticism' just quoted, become a pedantry fatal to any critical concern for plastic values; Richardson argues for instance that history painting is better than landscape or still-life because these 'cannot improve the mind, they excite no noble sentiments' (p. 119). Such arguments are misguided but they are symptoms of that marriage the age tried to effect between high art and high morals, and the fact that they were put forward is, in a way, creditable to human nature.

Pope's *Epistle to Burlington*, already quoted in more than one connection, surveys taste as a function of the good life. Good taste for Pope is the artistic aspect of good sense, and good sense is the intellectual aspect of good human nature. Bad taste is a form of mania and moral folly, whether in the collector's jumble of 'drawings and designs . . . statues, dirty Gods and Coins', or in the parvenu's ostentation (13–16):

> *For what has Virro painted, built and planted?*
> *Only to show, how many Tastes he wanted.*
> *What brought Sir Visto's ill got wealth to waste?*
> *Some Dæmon whisper'd, 'Visto! Have a Taste'.*

'Imitating fools' have parodied Burlington's enlightenment, with specious monstrosities like Timon's villa, whose master shivers in his Venetian door as the winds sweep through his misconceived mansion. Pope's watchwords (the resource of his time) were 'Sense' and 'Nature' (65-70):

> *Still follow Sense, of ev'ry Art the Soul,*
> *Parts answ'ring Parts shall slide into a whole,*
> *Spontaneous beauties all around advance,*
> *Start ev'n from Difficulty, strike from Chance;*
> *Nature shall join you, Time shall make it grow*
> *A work to wonder at—perhaps a* STOW.

'Sense' means unity, proportion and the rational spirit of 'rightness' which achieves good qualities of mind, beauty allied with convenience, learning with grace, and so on; 'Nature'—that protean term—seems to mean the landscape which must complete the building. Pope had a disciple in James Cawthorn of Tunbridge Wells, a schoolmaster who left an attractive memorial in his poem *Of Taste* (1756). Like other critic-moralists Cawthorn takes taste to be more than an elegant accomplishment (143-6):

> *true taste, when delicately fine*
> *Is the pure sunshine of a soul divine;*
> *The full perfection of each mental pow'r;*
> *'Tis sense, 'tis nature, and 'tis something more.*

That 'something more' is a quality of genius, though taste is to guide and judge where genius is often erratic; taste is genius's critical aspect (161-4), which

> *corrects, by one ethereal touch*
> *What seems too little, and what seems too much;*
> *Marks the fine point where each consenting part*
> *Slides into beauty with the ease of art.*

Taste thus conceived is an important function of human nature; it derives its strength not from mere 'aesthetic emotion' (if there is such a thing) but from reason and ordered feeling, and from mental discipline through a (largely classical) tradition. True taste then shows human nature at its best; false taste is the earmark of the fool. The Augustans were creditably earnest about a faculty which later generations have too much confounded with dilettantism. It is true that the precise definition of true taste was in dispute. Perhaps Wren was its exemplar? But Burlington and the Palladians objected (as did Shaftesbury) that his style was too exuberant—'that dam'd gusto that's been for this sixty years past', said William Kent. Vanbrugh? Certainly not—'Expence and Vanbrugh, Vanity and Show', wrote Cawthorn. The Palladians? They were criticised by Robert Adam, and Robert Adam by Sir William Chambers, and 'natural' gardeners by the formalists, and addicts of *chinoiserie* and the Gothick by the traditionalists. The battle was more than one of styles—its rallying-cries were Nature and Sense, however those terms were construed. No orthodoxy, of course, reigns for ever; in letters and the arts new fashions pressed on the old. But for a long time the general virtues of well-instructed taste kept them healthy and mature.

This was particularly fortunate at a time when building was a national hobby. Prefacing *A Sermon Preached at the Consecration of a Chapel* (1667) Robert South hailed the Restoration zest for construction; God, he noted, 'has changed men's tempers with the times, and made a spirit of building succeed a spirit of pulling down'. The same spirit animated the Augustans; towns displayed their formal squares and terraces, their municipal buildings and private mansions, the country its farms, parsonages and palaces. Even churches, often thought of as neglected in Hanoverian England, multiplied their local variations of Wren, Hawksmoor or Gibbs. Above all, the century triumphed in its aristocratic houses; the great landowners and their architects realised an abundance of superb design.

The polite imagination, then, required an informed taste in architecture. The intelligent man took this as part of his education, and might indeed even practise as an amateur architect without a qualm. At Oxford Henry Aldrich designed most of the handsome Peckwater quadrangle at Christ Church (where he was Dean), and the admirable All Saints', whose Corinthian-columned elevation surmounted by bold square tower and sturdy spire so firmly overlooks the High. A Cambridge counterpart, Sir James Burrough, put up new buildings at Peterhouse and Trinity Hall. Sanderson Miller, a country gentleman of Warwickshire, not only gained fame for his Gothic ruins but produced the fine Palladianism of Hagley Hall there and the excellent Shire Hall at Warwick. The greatest patron-connoisseur of the century was not content to be an onlooker; as Thomson observed, 'numerous domes a Burlington confess'. The credit for these has been at times distributed between Burlington and his protégés such as William Kent, Colen Campbell and Giacomo Leoni, but there seem good grounds for allowing him not only an intent study of Italian styles as a brilliant youth on the Grand Tour (1714–15) but also the design of actual buildings such as the York Assembly Rooms and his Chiswick villa modelled on one of Palladio's at Vicenza. The most remarkable instance of amateur skill is Vanbrugh, who at thirty-five unexpectedly switched his vast energies from writing to building. As Swift commented in *The History of Vanbrugh's House*, 1707,

> *Van's* genius, *without thought or lecture,*
> *Is hugely turn'd to* architecture.

We shall return to Vanbrugh: here he is noticed briefly as an astonishing example of the architect without formal training, the amateur on the grandest scale.

For every amateur who practised there were hundreds who did not but whose informed interest gave prestige to good design. Encouraged by public enthusiasm Augustan styles developed in rich variety, though within the prescriptions of a general sanity which (except for a scattering of 'follies') did not incur the confusion which bedevilled the Victorians. Interest was fostered by vigorous rivalries which kept architects, furnishers and their clients on the alert, and also by the reinforcement of magnificent publications. It is an experience in civilisation to open such works as Knyff's *Britannia Illustrata* in its two great volumes (1708–20) with its double-page engravings of houses and their settings; or Leoni's edition of

Palladio's *Architecture* (1715) with exact plates and a lavish text; or Colen Campbell's *Vitruvius Britannicus* (1717–25), with Burlingtonian eulogies of Palladio and Inigo Jones, three volumes of extreme magnificence; or Robert Castell's *Villas of the Ancients* (1728) nobly produced and dedicated to Burlington as one with 'a great and universal Knowledge in the *Belles Arts*'; or the two great volumes of Robert Wood's *Ruins of Palmyra* (1753) and *Ruins of Balbec* (1757), reconstructing Syrian temples to look like the prototypes of the most patrician Augustan buildings; or Stuart and Revett's *Antiquities of Athens* (1762–1816), four volumes of superb plates in scrupulous detail; or perhaps finest of all Robert Adam's *Ruins of the Palace of the Emperor Diocletian* (1764), dedicated to the King, and the three volumes of *The Works in Architecture of Robert and James Adam* (1778–9, 1822). By the irresistible impressiveness of such works the influence of Burlington's circle, and later of the Adam brothers and of Roman and Greek antiquities spread through all the commonwealth of the connoisseurs. Good taste was fortunate to find an ally in the great wealth of clients and collectors, which if it led sometimes to megalomania led more often to a justified magnificence which architects were gifted enough to achieve in the great country houses.

ii. ORDER AND HARMONY

There is nothing in Nature that is great and beautiful, without Rule and Order; and the more Rule and Order, and Harmony, we find in the Objects that strike our Senses, the more Worthy and Noble we esteem them.
JOHN DENNIS
Critical Works, ed. E. N. Hooker, i. 202

LIKE writers, architects could admire the classics in the belief that there the human spirit was properly expressed and the problems of form and purpose properly solved, whereas with the Gothic, with what Evelyn had called 'heavy, dark, melancholy, monkish piles, without any just Proportion, Use or Beauty compared with the Ancient', the style was too complex, the detail too bewildering, and the purpose too remote from civilised life. Architecture of the classical tradition balanced its lines and masses in mutual peace and carefully wedded its details to the unity of the whole. As Pope wrote in one of his many passing appreciations of the arts (*Essay on Criticism*, 247-52),

> *Thus when we see some well-proportion'd dome,*
> *(The world's just wonder, and e'en thine, O Rome!)*
> *No single parts unequally surprise;*
> *All comes united to th'admiring eyes;*
> *No monstrous height, or breadth, or length, appear;*
> *The Whole at once is bold, and regular.*

A classical building, it has been said, should have the lucidity and completeness of a mathematical equation—but mathematics, one might add, raised to spiritual contentment. Wren, himself a scientist, put definitively the classical ideals of linear order; in 'Tract I' of *Parentalia* (1750), a series of family documents gathered by his son and published by his grandson, he distinguished the 'customary' sense of beauty (when through habit we accept a thing as beautiful) from the 'natural' (which is 'from *Geometry*'). Geometrical figures, he boldly said, 'are naturally more beautiful than other irregular; in this all consent as to a law of Nature'. Of them, the square and circle are the most beautiful, and next the parallelogram and oval: 'strait lines are more beautiful than curve; next to strait Lines, equal and geometrical flexures'. The scientist liked forms found not so much in the physical world as in the abstracting and intellectual powers of the human mind, and those were the forms classical architecture embodied.

Order, coherence and unity, then are the conditions of the 'new' style. They make art intelligible. One of the best of aesthetic critics, Geoffrey Scott in *The Architecture of Humanism* (1924), puts it that architecture (particularly 'humanist' or classical architecture) realises the order implicit in natural law but obscured by nature's heterogeneity (p. 238):

Order in Nature bears no relation to *our* act of vision. It is not humanized. It exists, but it continually eludes us. This Order, which in Nature is hidden and implicit, architecture makes patent to the eye. It supplies the perfect correspondence between the act of vision and the act of comprehension. . . . Style, through coherence, subordinates beauty to the pattern of the mind and so selects what it presents that all, at one sole act of thought, is found intelligible, and every part re-echoes, explains and reinforces the beauty of the whole.

The order of a Gothic cathedral may be masterly. But it is complex, and the Augustans did not on the whole see that it evinced powers of mind greater than those which evolved the classical style. The Gothic was not always disparaged, but though prepared to be romantic-reverential about it the Augustans seldom saw it as intellectually magnificent too.

The humanised world, then, is the particular sphere of Augustan building. For years, Carlyle relates, he had passed Wren's Chelsea Hospital without consciously noticing it, until one day he realised that it had always given him subconscious pleasure. Then he looked at it 'and saw that it was quiet and dignified and the work of a gentleman'. In other words, it considers its company, is clear without pedantry, and has a self-command which comes not from lack of spirit but from an instinct for social order.

The last chapter of *The Architecture of Humanism* is called 'Humanist Values'. It analyses how we respond to architecture by projecting our feelings into it, and by interpreting its language by our sensations. 'We transcribe ourselves into terms of architecture' by instinctively identifying ourselves with a building's construction; we feel unstable before what looks unbalanced, and oppressed by what looks ponderous. We also 'transcribe architecture into terms of ourselves'; arches 'spring', domes 'swell', vistas 'stretch', Greek temples are 'calm' and baroque façades 'restless', and spires, instead of pressing downwards as dead weights, seem light and aspiring. 'The whole of architecture is in fact unconsciously invested by us with human movement and human moods'. Vertical lines seem to soar, horizontal ones to be stable and settled. Symmetry and continuity cause a satisfied rhythm of feeling; sudden breaks mean aesthetic and emotional shock. Classical design (unless it has the baroque's drama and movement) suggests equipoise, forms so adjusted as to '*cancel all suggested movement*, [whereby] our consciousness is sustained at a point of rest'.

Such equipoise satisfies the mind and stabilises the feelings, for we seek in the outer world fulfilment of our inner needs (p. 235):

> The humanist instinct looks in the world for physical conditions that are related to our own, for movements which are like those we enjoy, for resistances that resemble those that can support us, for a setting where we should be neither lost nor thwarted.

Some proportions, spaces and volumes, therefore, harmonise with our nature; others (a wide room with low ceiling, a narrow room with high ceiling, a vast elevation with small windows) do not. And man's civilised desires, his social qualities as a human being, find their fulfilment best in the classical styles, in the styles of mental order, in 'architecture that is spacious, massive and coherent, and whose rhythm corresponds to our delight'. Form is here coherent and intelligible, the emotions are harmonised, and architecture becomes humane.

The buildings which this analysis so well elucidates preserve the normal dignity of human nature. They are sometimes extravagant and overweening, sometimes sedate and dull, but generally they speak for sanity and for living achieved in a mood of civilised pleasure. Their derivation is naturally from the well-springs of humanism, classical antiquity and the Italian Renaissance. Italy was (as indeed it had been earlier and still remains) a place of pilgrimage, the home of both eras of humanism, and tradition in literature and art was an inheritance from classical precedent though interpreted with native vigour. Amid the dilapidated grandeur of Rome Addison felt 'Immortal glories' revive in his mind (*Letter from Italy*, 1703, 70), and Dyer's *Ruins of Rome* (1740) observes the connoisseurs amid Piranesian splendours (49–52):

> *here advent'rous in the sacred search*
> *Of antient arts, the delicate of mind,*
> *Curious and modest, from all climes resort,*
> *Grateful society!*

Greece and Rome seemed, as Reynolds called them in his seventh *Discourse*, 'the fountains from whence have flowed all kinds of excellence'. Yet while classical antiquity provided the ultimate inspiration it was Renaissance Italy which, with its churches, palaces and private villas, had best solved the problems facing the modern architect. In particular, cultivated taste turned to the Palladian buildings of Vicenza. 'This sweet town', said Evelyn, 'has more well-built palaces than any of its dimensions in Italy,' and Lord Chesterfield advised his son to study the work of Palladio, so well represented there (*Letters*, 7 August and 17 October, 1749). Palladio (1518–80) was a happy influence on English design because of his relative purity of style (more 'correct' than the exuberant baroque) on which English architects could model themselves and by which they were disciplined. The boldest innovation in English architecture was Inigo Jones's importation of Palladianism into a still largely-mediaeval England, a century ahead of the general movement of taste, in the Queen's House at Greenwich (1617–35), the Whitehall Banqueting House (1619–22), St. Paul's in Covent Garden (1635–8), and the great house of Wilton (1649 onwards) with its famous double-cube room nobly suited to its Vandyke portraits. Reacting against Wren's wealth of style, Lord Burlington's circle later reverted to Italy and Palladio who (said Colen Campbell) 'seems to have arrived at the *Ne Plus Ultra* of his Art', and whose statue together with that of the twin-deity Inigo Jones presided over the stairway leading to Burlington's Chiswick villa.

To hundreds of young men and their tutor-companions the Grand Tour revealed a finer world. Many of them returned unreasonably prepossessed by things antique or Italianate—in Congreve's *Way of the World* (1700) Mirabell wishes that Parliament would 'prohibit the exportation of fools'. But many blossomed under cosmopolitan experience which enriched and did not devitalise their native character. As for artists and architects, the spirit in which they studied the ancients and the Italians was that blend of discipleship and independence which Dryden, Pope and Johnson exemplify in literature. Reynolds is the clearest example because he describes his intentions at length, but hardly less notable are the architects who published their great volumes of classical studies and then designed in the full energy of their own instructed tastes. Worship of the masters resulted not in sterility but in rich and novel invention. So Burlington and his circle studied Palladio and then produced Holkham and Houghton, Moor Park and the Horse Guards. So Robert Adam studied Diocletian's palace and the ornaments of Herculaneum and Pompeii, and then produced Osterley Park, Syon and Kedleston. Honouring tradition did not hamper the Augustan architect; his styles might be more suitable for a Mediterranean than a British climate, yet his buildings were generally triumphantly unservile and vigorous.

Within the accepted language there was, as in literary style, great personal variety. Wren's inventive virtuosity showed itself in his dozens of City churches; his manner was admirably modified in different ways by Hawksmoor, Gibbs, Archer, Flitcroft and others, and Vanbrugh, Kent and the Burlingtonians led major divergences from it, to yield later to the new refinement of the Adams or the neo-Grecians, while the strong conservative fashion stood firm in Ware, Vardy and the great Chambers. Within what seems stability and continuity there was continual change, and an expert can recognise personal styles and estimate dates within a narrow range of error. A like combination of the stable general theme with vigorous personal variations, of accepted convention with individual interpretation is found in the other arts—in painting where personal styles blend easily with the general idiom, and in furniture design. The range of variation is smaller than in the centuries before and after, but it is sufficient to allow the arts as well as the letters of the time to reveal more and more human personality the more they are studied. Long experience, far from resulting in satiety, finds an astonishingly freshly-renewed appeal within the accepted tradition.

iii. THE MAIN STREAM

> When the Artist has conceived in his imagination the image of perfect Beauty, or the abstract idea of Forms, he may be said to be admitted into the great Council of Nature.
>
> REYNOLDS
> Du Fresnoy's *Art of Painting* (trans. Wm. Mason), Note III

ADVOCATES on the one or the other side dispute the supremacy in English architecture as between Inigo Jones and Sir Christopher Wren, between the brilliant student of Italian originals and the great inventive scientist with his intuition for volume and outline and his unsurpassed sense of construction. The adjudication of the contest is unimportant; the two men stand as twin sources of the major Augustan styles. Wren's experience was less cosmopolitan; he travelled only to Paris, and that briefly, and his classicism, wonderfully rich through the imaginative and intellectual power of his mind, has perhaps a freer and stronger spirit. Born in 1632 he seems to have started as an architect about 1661, a satisfactory date in view of the general evidence that 1660 marks a new era. He had already been and he continued to be a scientist—Gresham Professor of Astronomy at twenty-five, Savilian Professor at Oxford at twenty-eight. In 1663 he began the Sheldonian Theatre at Oxford and the admirable chapel of Pembroke at Cambridge and in 1665 travelled to France and watched the building of the Louvre—'a School of Architecture', he said, 'the best probably at this Day in Europe'. In 1661 Evelyn, always alert in matters of taste, had him summoned from Oxford as assistant to Sir John Denham the poet, Surveyor-General of His Majesty's Works, whom he succeeded in 1669, so becoming responsible for the rebuilding of London after the Fire. His views on town-planning were perhaps acquired abroad, for his famous scheme for London was something novel in England, too novel indeed for the citizens. The first stone of the new St. Paul's was laid in 1675, the choir was opened in 1697 with a thanksgiving service for the Treaty of Ryswick, the dome was ready in 1708, and in 1710 he watched his son place the top stone on the lantern. Simultaneously he had rebuilt the City churches with astonishing energy and inspiration—no fewer than eighteen were begun in 1670. There was also the Chelsea Hospital which so pleased Carlyle, the magnificent completion of Inigo Jones's work at Greenwich Palace, and the masterly reconstruction of Hampton Court, along with many smaller but hardly less noble buildings like Trinity chapel at Oxford and Emmanuel chapel and the great Trinity Library at Cambridge. Wren lived to see St. Paul's completed—lived indeed to the age of ninety-one, by which time the current of fashion had veered and caused his supersession from his official posts. Yet if refined tastes like Shaftesbury's and Burlington's were disturbed by his magnificence, with much of the great seventeenth-century eloquence still in it, there were many like Berkeley and Defoe who not being faddists for elegance spoke in its praise. These fluctuations have long come to rest; what remains is that superb contribution to London's sky-line, more obscured now than it was then, but still to be recaptured in its pristine splendour in the paintings and drawings Canaletto did from Richmond and Somerset House. In these the cathedral dominates everything, its whole upper order standing clear of the surrounding buildings, and the spires of the City churches rise in vital and picturesque variety. St. Paul's has been called the perfect union of humanistic ideals in art with robust English churchmanship, and indeed Wren's greatness, like Milton's, lies in the achievement of the full grandeur of humanism within a strong confident national idiom.

His younger contemporaries came under his influence and formed a distinguished group. The grandeur that Wren developed in public buildings the lesser but not negligible William Talman (c. 1650–1720) was introducing into private mansions: Dyrham, in Gloucestershire, attains it beautifully on a modest scale, and the more famous Chatsworth monumentally on the largest. Unfortunately for himself he had a gift for irritating prospective clients and was outmanœuvred by his far more brilliant rival Vanbrugh, so that his recorded buildings are few. More striking in accomplishment was Nicholas Hawksmoor (1661–1736), who entered Wren's office, superintended his building work for thirty years and was one of the architects for the 'fifty' new churches planned under Queen Anne (only a dozen or so were built). His London work is bracingly bold and dramatic; St. George-in-the-East at Stepney, bombed but due for restoration, raises a great openwork tower like a stone beacon of gleaming white over dockland in a conception of true grandeur; St. Anne's Limehouse, internally dignified, with a touch of poetry, and externally rising into another admirable open tower, invests that part of the Commercial Road with something finer than grandeur; St. Alfege's Greenwich, with its later fine tower by John James, holds its own with the nearby palace by Inigo Jones and Wren; Christ Church Spitalfields erects a striking obelisk-like steeple on a highly-original tower over a vaulted portico; St. Mary Woolnoth confronts King William Street with another highly-original tower rising above a rusticated base into curious twin-turrets; and St. George's Bloomsbury, in the small degree to which it is not masked by vast office blocks, adds a Roman pomp to that part of Holborn, with its immense Corinthian portico above a flight of steps and its western tower rising above columns to a stepped pyramid surmounted in extreme lordliness by the statue of St. George. All these, together with the quadrangle and library at Queen's College which are high among the masterpieces of Oxford (as the pseudo-Gothic towers of All Souls among the curiosities) stamp Hawksmoor as one of the most daring and inventive of English architects. Next there is James Gibbs (1682–1754), a Scot who came under Wren's eye and was another architect for the 'fifty' churches. His St. Mary-le-Strand, St. Martin's-in-the-Fields, and his spire to Wren's St. Clement Danes are among the most famous classical buildings in London after St. Paul's itself, and outside London there are the Senate House and King's College buildings at Cambridge, the dramatic and monumental Radcliffe Camera at Oxford, and the impressive nave of All Saints' Derby (now the cathedral). There are lesser men too like John James of Greenwich with his spire at St. Alfege's and his massive St. George's in Hanover Square, Henry Flitcroft (known as 'Burlington Harry' from his discipleship of the Earl) who designed St. Giles-in-the-Fields, Holborn, with its trim nave and delightfully Gibbsian spire (on a larger scale he also did the vast Palladian Wentworth Woodhouse in Yorkshire), and Thomas Archer, a follower of Vanbrugh, who put some of his master's happy valiancy into St. Paul's Deptford and St. John's Westminster, besides getting a wealth of curve into his tower of St. Philip's Birmingham, which has the true baroque flavour.

To the work of these men and of the superbly grandiose Vanbrugh the label of 'baroque' is affixed in recognition of the dramatic movement of their lines, the picturesque interrelationships of their masses, and the greater exuberance of their details than in the more poised classic which was to come. There is something appropriate, in an age stirred by the passions of Queen Anne's reign and the earlier Georges, in a style which has the robustness of the seventeenth century rather than the more critical refinement of the eighteenth. In the case of Vanbrugh, Augustan bravura shows itself in spectacular strength. Castle Howard, Blenheim and Seaton Delaval are almost superhuman. They have not often been thought convenient for living in, but that is another matter; the baroque has a flair for the picturesque and Vanbrugh indulged it to the full. One enters Blenheim's vast park, for instance, from Woodstock through a great arched stone gate and sees a serpentine lake like a reach of the Thames (a later embellishment, this, by 'Capability' Brown), spanned by the curve of a monumental bridge. The road turns through trees and at last plunges through the outer court gateway, a massive entrance with converging pilasters not unlike an Egyptian temple, to reveal a cloister of severe arches and a third gate surmounted by an elaborate turret. Through this lies the great forecourt of paved walks, the house embracing it on three sides with grand open colonnades of honey-coloured stone right and left, sweeping back in quadrants to join the central mass of the house, which rises loftily with its Corinthian portico. The design has a scale and boldness that are almost stupefying, yet are if anything outdone by the corresponding south front facing on the great lawn, with strong rusticated corner-blocks, a fine sweep of round-headed windows binding the whole façade together with an irresistible rhythm, and a great portico surmounted by a white bust of Marlborough, serenely superior to mortal men, behind which on a summer's day the clouds float in equal serenity. There is immense grandeur here, grandeur rather than beauty but not the less compelling for that, a sense of size at once magnificent and humane (children playing round the great columns are not at all out of place), a blend of opulence and Roman severity. Robert and James Adam's *Works* (preface, p. 1) define 'movement' in design as

the rise and fall, the advance and recess, with other diversity of form, in the different parts of a building, so as to add greatly to the picturesque of the composition,

and Vanbrugh's façades, his sweeping colonnades and advancing and receding masses are animated and picturesque. He was, said Reynolds in his thirteenth *Discourse*, 'a Poet as well as an Architect', and in his play of light and shadow showed 'a greater display of imagination' than any rival.

So much for the baroque. Already, however, we have heard the Burlingtonians complaining of its 'dam'd gusto' (a word here as apt in its modern as in its original meaning). The Palladian countermovement was not towards simplicity (to apply that word to the style of Kent is to make nonsense of it) but towards rich refinement within and elegant restraint without. In reverting to an earlier style ('Jones and Palladio to themselves restore', Pope counselled) Burlington perhaps saved architecture in England from the exuberance that befell it on the Continent and saved it from excess in a time of abundant wealth. Refinement and 'correctness' were the ideals of his circle as (still more evidently) of the Adam brothers later. A notable series of buildings went up in the approved style—a new front to Burlington House in Piccadilly, his own Palladian villa at Chiswick, the York Assembly Rooms, Holkham House in Norfolk for Thomas Coke, Raynham (altered for Lord Townshend), the fine town house at 44 Berkeley Square, London, with a famous staircase and, best-known, the Horse Guards building. These activities took about twenty-five years, from the late 1720s onwards, and for most of them Burlington and his favourite disciple William Kent were responsible. Among the other Burlingtonian achievements were

Moor Park in Hertfordshire by Giacomo Leoni, a Venetian whom the Earl brought over, and Houghton Hall in Norfolk by Colen Campbell for Sir Robert Walpole. Magnificent outside and in, columned and panelled in marble, with great doorways, ceremonial flights of stairs, richly coffered ceilings and gilded mouldings, handsome fireplaces surmounted by mirrors or paintings, these palatial places are the glories of Hanoverian England, those which today it is at once most necessary and most difficult to preserve. Along with the work of the great traditionalists like Chambers at Somerset House or his pupil Gandon in Dublin, the almost hyper-sensitive elegances of Robert Adam, and the admirable provincial work of men like the elder and younger Wood of Bath or John Carr of York, these Palladian buildings are the great symbols of Augustan humanism, designed for a human scale of living and an ordered if often elaborate sense of beauty.

Less magnificent than the palaces but far more numerous are those dwellings which are today perhaps the most attractive of all possible residences, the houses of the moderately well-to-do. No vast porticoes here, no outlying wings and sweeping quadrants, no princely suites hung with Continental treasures; instead, a simple front of stone or brick, a plain pedimented porch and well-proportioned rooms with tall sash-windows. They may be modest places indeed, homes of middling farmers, of parsons or professional men; they may be a shade finer, like Shenstone's 'elegant' Leasowes; or they may be almost splendid, like the house Sir Charles Grandison prepares for his bride (*Sir Charles Grandison*, letter of 9 December):

> The situation is delightful. The house is very spacious. It is built in the form of an H; both fronts pretty much alike. The hall, the dining-parlour, two drawing-rooms, one adjoining to the study, the other to the dining-parlour . . . are handsome, and furnished in an elegant but not sumptuous taste. . . . The dining-room is noble, and well-proportioned: It goes over the hall and dining-room parlour. It is hung with crimson damask, adorned with valuable pictures. . . . The best bed-chamber adjoining is hung with fine tapestry. The bed is of crimson velvet, lined with white silk; chairs and curtains of the same. . . . The gardens and lawns seem from

the windows of this spacious house to be as boundless as the mind of the owner, and as free and open as his countenance.

Augustan buildings and their contents had the same end in view—harmonious splendour for the aristocracy, harmonious comfort for the gentry.

As for Augustan painting, there is much in it that is individual but little that insists on individualism. Hogarth and Blake struck out lines of their own (though Blake is so little an Augustan in his sense of style that to include him is a distraction). Painters generally kept to the conventions and the most pressing of these was that of portraiture, in which the age did its major work. The next most pressing was that of landscape deriving from the various styles of Claude, Salvator Rosa and the Dutch school. Though in both categories English painters developed qualities of their own—and indeed in landscape were soon to give the rest of Europe a fresh vision—there was almost nothing of the revolutionary individualism which the nineteenth century was increasingly to stamp on the art of painting.

Except for religious art, the main demand had always been for portraiture. 'Portraits always have been and always will be popular in England,' said Hogarth, and Johnson characteristically strengthened the assertion to the effect that he would prefer the picture of a dog he knew to all the allegorical paintings in the world. No-one not a portraitist, Shebbeare complained, not even Canaletto, could make a living; in England, he said pungently, 'self is the most delightful object that self can behold'. From Holbein to Kneller this demand was satisfied largely by foreign artists, though with the addition of an occasional Briton like the Elizabethan miniaturist Nicholas Hilliard. Tudor and Stuart portraiture, though it can be inexpressive, can also be technically and psychologically brilliant, and many of the canvases, for instance, in the National Portrait Gallery seem to lose nothing of their subjects' spectacular personal vitality. Augustan portraiture is as different as Augustan literature; the gleam and brilliance goes and is replaced by a steadier solider manner, just as the varied Elizabethan physiognomy gives place to a general experienced worldliness. Kneller (1646–1723) painted many prominent figures from the days of Charles II onwards, among them Charles himself, Locke, Wren, Evelyn, Pepys, Wycherley and the invaluable Kit-cat series in the National Portrait Gallery which includes Congreve, Steele, Addison, Garth, Vanbrugh, Walsh and Tonson. Dryden praised him as a brother in the arts, and on his death an anonymous poet lamented him as irreplaceable (*A Session of Painters*, 1725):

> Mourn, England, mourn, since Kneller is no more,
>   Who can his place supply?
> What genius can the mighty art restore,
>   Or must it vacant lie?

'Shakespeare in poetry and Kneller in painting, damme!' was the reproof the young Reynolds, just back from Italy with a new style, received from John Ellys the King's Painter. Kneller's women, like those of Pope's epigram, mostly have no character at all. But his men, shrewd, bluff, cynical, alert, honest or dull as the case may be, are well-understood and well-communicated.

The interval between Kneller and Reynolds was vigorously filled by Hogarth, who animates his satirical paintings (in their original oils glowing with colours that engraving has to forego) with the liveliest formulas of type-characterisation—for instance, the *Marriage à la Mode* series in the National Gallery—and who in his serious portraits shows a truer sense of individual personality than anyone else in his century. There were also portraitists in another art, that of sculpture, for this was the age of Scheemakers and Rysbrack from Antwerp and Roubiliac from Lyons. The portrait bust was particularly popular; there was a brisk market for heads of Shakespeare, Bacon, Inigo Jones, Milton, Locke and other Augustan idols, and from St. Paul's and Westminster Abbey downwards churches began rapidly to fill with monumental sculpture of unprecedented abundance.

In the second half of the century, though sculpture maintained its hold, the pendulum of interest swung strongly again to painting, and Reynolds, Gainsborough and Romney, and later Raeburn and

Lawrence, provided the age's triumph. The boast of heraldry, the pomp of power, were interpreted in that rich idealisation to which the humanist spirit liked to rise. Above all it was Reynolds who gave his sitters that supernal distinction of bearing, the aristocratic grace of the society lady, the commanding stance of the warrior, the thoughtful wisdom of the statesman. He was himself a friend of the great, companion of wits and writers, a man of sociable and equable temper. He was not primarily a psychologist, yet it was the person and not the station that interested him, and there are few finer things than the famous portrait of Mrs. Siddons as the Tragic Muse, the vividly animated and roguish Garrick, and the various portraits of Johnson—that heavy pugnacious face, eyes half-closed with concentration, lips half-open with a challenging impromptu, a face almost brutal but also both judicious and swiftly-responsive. Such portraits are either in the grand style, like the Mrs. Siddons, or the portrait of Lord Heathfield with the keys of Gibraltar, or show a kinship with the grand style by choosing their subjects' best rather than their normal qualities. Flattery? Not really —it is the humanist tradition. Reynolds's children are almost ideal children, enchanting and innocent creatures. His warriors like Captain Orme, Lord Heathfield and Admiral Keppel (his first patron) are honourable men with direct eyes and sturdy faces lit by stormy sunlight against a background of symbolic cloud (it was of course the tradition of heroic portraiture). His great ladies have a queenly grace. Hogarth would have put more significance into them: Gainsborough would have managed a lighter touch, more poetry, a more luminous texture—when a Reynolds portrait lacks character there is little interesting detail to compensate, despite the harmonious disposition of form and tone. But there the portraits are, the best that humanity (without losing itself in complacency— these are real people, however favourably interpreted) thought of itself in the age of Johnson.

It is not to the point here to go into different styles. In his fourteenth *Discourse* Reynolds himself touches on Gainsborough's manner, more intuitive than his own, with wonderful sympathy for natural atmosphere, and with a 'lightness of effect' which came from the deft speed of his brush rather than the studied care of Reynolds's own. Gracious and subtle, refined and sensitive at once, both in portraiture and landscape Gainsborough is exquisite; here too the humanist tradition, poetically interpreted and crossed with a delicate new sense of landscape, achieves some of its loveliest results. The other painters of the time are numerous and delightful—Romney, Allan Ramsay, Zoffany, Highmore, Arthur Devis, Benjamin West, Angelica Kauffmann and the rest; in individual portraits or pleasant conversation pieces they give the countenance of the social world, a little stiff sometimes, a little posed, sometimes over-lavish in dress, now and then naïve, but charmingly appropriate to a gentleman's walls, and in the case of Richard Wilson achieving a Claudeian poetry of landscape that can be truly great painting.

As the great houses were not only private residences but show-places to be publicised by admiring tourists and artists (the eighteenth century is the first great age of guide-books and scenic drawings), so paintings were not only private possessions but were popularised by means of prints, the vogue for which grew apace as did the technique of making them. Portraits, caricatures, sporting scenes, views of country seats and local scenery were not an oligarchical monopoly but were widely shared. It is not helpful to bring the word 'democracy' into all this, for codes of rank and taste were far from equalitarian. Still, more extensively than ever before the pleasures of civilisation were spread through books and pictures, and if Johnson could speak of the common reader (that is, the ordinary educated person) as the effective standard of taste, the common sightseer or connoisseur was the effective public for a lot of artistic activity.

This wider interest was reflected in the Royal Academy (1768), founded after some vicissitudes by a number of artists who had previously exhibited their work at the Foundling Hospital. On 2 January, 1769, Reynolds as the first President delivered the first of those fifteen annual *Discourses* which so heightened the prestige of art criticism. Patrons, led by George III, were generous, the earnings and the social repute of the fashionable painters mounted rapidly, facilities for art education were improved, and a code of orthodoxy was established which has irritated the unorthodox ever since. From the beginning the Academy was the centre of interest, and Reynolds's first *Discourse* was an almost jubilant assurance of success:

> There are, at this time, a greater number of excellent artists than were ever known before at one period in this nation; there is a general desire among our Nobility to be distinguished as lovers and judges of the Arts; there is a greater superfluity of wealth among the people to reward the professors; and above all, we are patronised by a Monarch who, knowing the value of science and of elegance, thinks every art worthy of his notice, that tends to soften and humanise the mind.

In the applied arts the position was no less happy. In the designing of furniture the names of Chippendale, Sheraton and Hepplewhite stand in the public mind as signs of supreme excellence. Yet scholarship has begun to distribute the credit more widely by depriving these three of much that was wrongly supposed to be theirs, and by identifying scores of obscure draughtsmen whose due some of it really is. Great skill was widely spread, and good design was a widely-based national art. The general wealth of invention, the harmony of furniture with its setting, the achievement of detailed and of unified beauty—these qualities comprise one of the richest fields of pleasure in the whole English inheritance. Not only furniture but silver- and iron-ware, glass and porcelain, carpets and needlework took their place in a coherent design which seemed as well able to deal with small as with large composition, with intimate interiors as with terraces and crescents, or buildings related to half a town or a whole countryside.

Nothing of this should imply that the eighteenth century was an aesthete's paradise. Though its art stemmed from certain specialised circles it spread rapidly into a broad range of society; it was hardly 'art' in a specialised sense at all. It was art, rather, created in admiration of a worthy tradition and with a bracing desire to do all things well, art as the product of a whole national life, by great good fortune finding the formula not for one kind of distinction only but for many, and existing not for self-expression but to be reflected back upon the whole quality of social living—'applied art', indeed, whether 'fine' or merely useful. Admiring it nowadays we may be excused a touch of idolatry.

iv. DIVERGENT CURRENTS

It is one thing to make an idea clear, and another to make it affecting to the imagination.
BURKE
The Sublime and the Beautiful, pt. ii, sec. iv

INVENTIVE vigour, however, cannot long be controlled within traditional forms, even if these evolve as strongly as did the Augustan. The Augustan achievement is one of great positive energy held in place by commanding conventions of taste and skill. There is nothing negative about it: the positive energy of Wren and Hawksmoor and Vanbrugh is tremendous, as is that of Kent's or Chippendale's furniture, or Pope's or Johnson's verse, or *The Beggar's Opera* or a Fielding novel. We live with these things nourished and unsatiated because of the inward strength embodied in them and harnessed to social life, the fullness of their creative energy united with splendid sociability. This is a display of positive power, not of negative restraint. Critics are misleading; they talk of polish and decorum, but these qualities no more account for the character of a Johnson essay or a Robert Adam building than a set of brakes explains why a motor-car goes.

The Augustan imagination seemed steadily settled in a neoclassic tradition, but its steadiness was that of energy held in check which a novel impulse might release. The impulse from the East, already mentioned in connection with trade, was something which disturbed it with a new life. From the late seventeenth century *chinoiserie* had its slaves and its satirists, and the whole movement is a delightful curiosity. The Victoria and Albert Museum has a great cabinet of 1670 on a thoroughly Italianate stand of cherubs, garlands and acanthus, the cabinet itself, however, illustrating the newer mode by being black-japanned and deliciously panelled in silver, green, gold, pink and purple, with herons, bulrushes, wild ducks, lotus, angular trees, kiosks and gravity-defying rocks that rise from lakes like the humps of some arthritic amphibian. In the same collection there is a famous bed from Badminton, where the Duke of Beaufort went in for such things, with bristling dragons at each corner, and the Chinese furniture made by Chippendale for Garrick, exquisite with green and cream decorations of weeping willows, little figures under pyramidal hats, pagodas, palaces, plantains and elliptical crags. Towards the middle of the century Chinese wallpapers began to arrive as presents from merchants and ambassadors, complexly elegant with gnarled trees sprinkled with fronds, flowers, vases and bird-cages, and inhabited by herons, peacocks and long-tailed pigeons. Mrs. Montagu, Queen of the Bluestockings, had such a room in the exquisite house James Stuart designed for her in Portman Square, 'lined', she said in a letter, 'with painted paper of Pekin, and furnished with the choicest moveables of China'. The inhabitants of Richmond in the 1750s had the honour of observing the Duke of Cumberland afloat in his 'mandarin yacht', an astonishing craft with kiosk amidships, a high mast hung with crescents and ornaments like open umbrellas, topped with a nightmare weathercock like a vast grasshopper, and a hull along which undulated a Chinese dragon. Chambers, commissioned as gardener at Kew to the Dowager Princess of Wales in 1757, ran the whole gamut of exotic taste with a House of Confucius, a mosque, a 'Gothic' cathedral, a Roman arch and the famous Pagoda, which still stands as witness to a potent fashion, though shorn of the glittering iron griffins which used to adorn its every corner. Not only the well-to-do succumbed to the new romanticism: *The World*, on 14 February, 1754, announced that hardly an oyster-stall or chandler's shop between Hyde Park and Shoreditch was without its Chinese or Gothic ornaments, or a combination of both.

It is time to look North instead of East, to the twin-divergence of the Gothic, a vogue which showed that something in the nation's consciousness, some desire for a revival, was awakening. Whereas Reason spoke for order and geometrical figure, for the square and circle, the oblong and oval, as signs of man's intellectual dominance, Instinct spoke for the unpredictable, the intricate and the irregular.

To the rational taste of Queen Anne's day, the Gothic was triply distasteful. Its first fault was barbarism, for were not the Goths the destroyers of Rome? Its second was its confusion, instead of unity and grace. Its third was its provinciality, its quaint and local character instead of the civilised and cosmopolitan. Addison in the 62nd *Spectator* spoke of it as 'the extravagance of an irregular fancy', like the ill-judged wit of metaphysical poetry. The Gothic was uncouth; Tickell's *Oxford* (1707) mentioned 'thick-skull'd Heroes of the *Gothique* line' and Millamant in *The Way of the World* (1700) scorned the boorish Witwoud as 'rustic, ruder than Gothic'. Christopher Wren junior pronounced an anathema in *Parentalia* (1750); let any man of taste, he said, look at Henry VII's deplorable Chapel in Westminster Abbey (p. 308), with its

sharp Angles, Jetties, narrow Lights, lame Statues, Lace and other Cutwork and Crinckle-Cranckle... taking off from that noble Air and Grandeur, bold and graceful Manner, which the Ancients had so well, and so judiciously established.

Such a style could only be the detritus of barbarism.

Yet men cling to old things not only from pedantry but from a deep sentiment of attachment. Local masons still practised the old style, and antiquaries liked its overtones of history. Even classical architects—Wren, Hawksmoor, Kent, Adam—tried it on occasion. The face of England was still largely mediaeval, with open fields and ancient towns; old buildings were everywhere. Indeed unless we feel the classical style coming like a breath of fresh air into the midst of crumble and clutter we underestimate its impact as the sign of a new life: we can sense this impact wherever Georgian houses of bombed towns are rebuilt, their original newness recaptured in primrose-yellow or rose-red brick glowing across the grey streets and showing for the first time since the eighteenth century the astonishing gaiety of their trim façades so long dirt-hidden. But while admiration attached to the new, affection often clung to the old. Antiquaries like Dugdale, Anthony à Wood and Thomas Hearne can surprise us with their romantic emotion, their 'melancholy delight', as Wood calls it, in ivy-grown ruins and historic houses. No wonder that Scott, so rich in these feelings himself, admired his predecessors; indeed it is by reading him, absorbing his sense of the past and his generous affection for old places, that we best appreciate what the recovery of the old-fashioned meant for his generation, and how the sentiment of history warmed the romantic imagination as it did that of the antiquaries who kept open the lines of communication with the past.

Much of this is latent even in the days of Burlington. Defoe, staunchly progressive as he was, praises Gothic buildings in his *Tour*. He is enthusiastic about Canterbury, Winchester, Salisbury, Wells, Hereford, Chester and Lichfield, along with St. George's Windsor and King's Chapel Cambridge. 'Very gay things', he calls them. Even better than a gay thing is York, 'the beautifullest church of the old building that is in England'. A contemporary, Thomas Gent, went further in his *History of the Famous City of York* (1730), showing a quite unclassical pleasure in the cathedral's mediaeval sculpture:

> Here are antick postures, both of Men and Beasts; in one Place and in another, is a Man cut out Half Way as if he was thrusting and striving, with all his Strength, to get out of a Window, or some narrow passage. In another are several Faces, having different Aspects, as one crying, another laughing, a third making wry Mouths, Etc. And what is very ingenious, in another Place is to be seen an old bald-pated Fryer, kissing a young Nun in a Corner; And in the Chapiters of the Pillars near are the faces of several other Nuns as well old as young, peeping and laughing at the old amorous Fryer.

An eye for the odd could lead to the Gothic, though only to the least significant aspect of it. Yet of course there was a goblin-quality in it which the connoisseur would think contemptible. If like Evelyn one found it 'melancholy and monkish', or like Addison were amused, or like Berkeley called it 'fantastical and for the most part founded neither in nature or reason', could it be more than a freak?

Much depended on what one thought 'natural' to man. To one mind the natural is the orderly and intelligible, to another the intricate and mysterious. The struggle to vindicate Gothic was akin to that to vindicate Shakespeare and Spenser as artists and not mere eccentrics of genius, for to like Shakespeare and Spenser with their multifarious detail was to like something analogous to Gothic. John Hughes prefaced his edition of *The Faerie Queene* (1715) thus (p. lx):

> To compare it therefore with the Models of Antiquity, wou'd be like drawing a Parallel between the *Roman* and the *Gothick* Architecture. In the first there is doubtless a more natural Grandeur and Simplicity: in the latter, we find great Mixtures of Beauty and Barbarism, yet assisted by the Invention of a Variety of inferior Ornaments; and tho the former is more majestick in the whole, the latter may be very surprizing and agreeable in its Parts.

In his edition of Shakespeare (1725) Pope compared his author's work to 'an ancient majestick piece of *Gothick* Architecture', 'more strong, and more solemn' than a modern structure, with 'much the greater variety and much the nobler apartments', and he claimed that despite the frequent triviality of details 'the Whole' arouses a greater reverence. At length Pope's own editor Warburton popularised the idea that a Gothic building imitates a grove of trees (Pope himself told Spence that he would like to plant an avenue to imitate a cathedral—Nature imitating Art). The Goths, he said, overran Spain but yearned for their native woods and so invented a new architecture 'upon original principles and ideas much nobler than what had given birth even to classical magnificence', by which their buildings resemble groves as nearly as architecture can (*The Works of Pope*, 1751, iii. 46). This misguided theory recurs in Smollett's *Humphry Clinker*, where also the tetchy Matthew Bramble complains to his friend Dr. Lewis that the 'Saracen' style (Wren had urged the claims of the Saracens rather than the Goths as its inventors) is much too cold for England (Letter of 4 July). The forest-glade notion was fanciful, yet by admitting the Gothic to be unified (like a colonnade of trees), 'natural' and—a remarkable admission

—'nobler' than even the classic it created a favourable prejudice. Gothic buildings, like Shakespeare's plays, were increasingly admitted to show artistry: 'have not many Gothic buildings a great deal of consistent beauty in them?' Hogarth asked in *The Analysis of Beauty* (1753), and he praised Westminster Abbey for its 'established and distinct character in building'.

Gradually, then, the century awoke to a new experience. Unfortunately the cultivation of moods took the place of architectural understanding; Gray's friend Richard Bentley, for example, engraved the ivy-mantled church tower of the *Elegy* within a decorative gothic arch of stucco dropping away from its plain brick substructure—thereby betraying that 'Gothic' was taken not as a method of building but as a superficial trapping to evoke a mood. Ruins were an incentive to the agreeable languor of melancholy, Gothic ruins above all (though the classical too would serve), and sham ruins were better than no ruins at all. In this respect, it must be admitted, Augustan taste was absurdly at fault, as satirists were happy to prove. Mrs. Delany wrote to Swift on 24 October, 1733, that an antiquary had mistaken an old cabin, disguised by Lord Bathurst on his Cirencester estate as a 'venerable castle', for a relic of King Arthur. A visitor, it was said, guessed it to be six hundred years old and was told by the custodian that his lordship planned another six hundred years older still. In Richard Graves's *Spiritual Quixote* (1772) the antiquary Mr. Townsend fears that sham relics will bemuse the future historian. Fortunately for the safety of historical studies these silly affairs, often of lath and plaster, have mostly disappeared, though some survive as mementoes of a sentimental cult.

The most famous of mood-provokers was Walpole's house at Strawberry Hill, which he bought in 1747 and fitted with battlements, vaulting, tracery, painted glass, suits of armour and 'Gothic' bookcases. Its subsequent owners have conscientiously maintained it much in Walpole's style, but his reputation would have stood higher had it long ago crumbled. It is a monument of execrable taste by which his connoisseurship is damned to everlasting fame. It is flimsy, gaudy and dishonest; it is a large curio, just as the bric-à-brac with which he filled it was small curio. Visitors did not know whether to admire it as a museum, worship in it as a chapel, or laugh at it as an oddity. Walpole wrote to George Montagu (17 May, 1763) of 'the air of enchantment and fairyism which is the tone of the place', but the enchantment is morbid and the fairyism sinister. Fortunately the Gothic was not always as drearily and falsely picturesque as in sham ruins and Strawberry Hill: it was often used lightly and gaily as a charming frivolous flavour in decorations outside and in, and in literature it lent a spice to comic as well as serious mediaevalism. Gothic fun did not have to wait for Peacock in the nineteenth century; here, from Mary Leapor, the daughter of a Northamptonshire gardener, who became a cook-maid (which may partly account for the following) and composed some pleasant verses, is part of the agreeably-named *Crumble-Hall* (1748):

> That Crumble-Hall, whose hospitable door
> Has fed the wanderer, and reliev'd the poor;
> Whose Gothic towers, and whose rusty spires,
> Were known of old to knights, and hungry squires;
> There powder'd beef and warden-pies were found,
> And pudding smok'd within her spacious bound . . .
> With humming beer her vats were wont to flow,
> And ruddy nectar in her vaults to glow.
> Here came the wights who battled for renown,
> The sable friar, and the russet clown;
> The loaded tables sent a sav'ry gale,
> And the brown bowls were crown'd with simp'ring ale;
> While the guests revell'd on the smoking store,
> Till their stretched girdles could contain no more.

There is the spirit of Peacock's *Misfortunes of Elphin* anticipated in the year of *Roderick Random*.

But the most famous novelty in Augustan taste is the development of the 'natural', and even more potent the 'picturesque' in landscape. The garden, so formal under William and Mary, cast off its shackles and was allied with the surrounding country; straight avenues and geometrical waterworks gave way to serpentine paths and meandering streams. Here again the satirists found their game:

Mrs. Lennox in *The Female Quixote* (1752) derides an estate where 'the most laborious efforts of art had been used to make it appear like the beautiful product of wild uncultivated nature'. But the laborious efforts of art as exerted by Bridgeman, Kent and 'Capability' Brown produced not only 'wild uncultivated nature' but sweeps of tranquil greensward with apparently casual groupings of trees whose 'natural' charm was more than unaided Nature could achieve. Indeed, the work of Kent and Brown, and of Repton at the end of the century, modelled scores of landscapes with the utmost beauty, with easy generosity of scale, peaceful vistas through trees now grown (as they were not when satirists mocked) to their full maturity, and the varying green slopes and levels of English parkland.

The ingredients of landscape, and of Burke's distinction between beauty and sublimity, were gradually compounded into a new philosophy of scenery. 'The beautiful' was the ideal of humanised landscape, but the sublime was coming into its own as an aesthetic experience. Nature's wildness and grandeur were invoked as signs of her elemental power; the appeal strengthened of such painters as Salvator Rosa and Ruysdael, who convey the 'delightful horror' of wild scenery. Salvator's lights and shadows, broken trees, beggars and banditti gave the Augustans a change from their own stability. Ruysdael's dark masses of rocks and shaggy foliage, his stormy gleams of light and passing glooms, formed the essence of 'the picturesque'—a word then unweakened by the sense of trivial quaintness which now debases it. 'The picturesque' came to be used specifically as a term for whatever had the dramatic variety, the chiaroscuro, the varied texture and colour which would attract a painter. The masters of the picturesque, besides Salvator and Ruysdael, were Claude Lorrain (in a serene way), many of the Dutch painters, and at home George Morland, with his gypsies, crumbling cottages, and rough forest clearings. Whereas the portrait and conversation piece reinforced the conventions of society, the picturesque landscape subverted them.

Its great exponent (though by no means its inventor, for poets, prose-writers, philosophers and artists had long cultivated it) was

William Gilpin, born in 1724 in the suitably romantic Scaleby Castle near Carlisle, graduating from Oxford and eventually receiving the living of Boldre in the New Forest, where he passed his life as a good parish priest from 1777 until his death in 1804. His hobby was the 'picturesque tour', and he published his observations in a series which started with the Wye (written in 1770, published in 1782), and continued with the Lakes, the Highlands of Scotland, the New Forest, and so on. Jane Austen was an admiring reader, though she made fun of the picturesque vogue, and William Combe and Thomas Rowlandson immortalised the practice in the *Tours of Dr. Syntax in Search of the Picturesque* (1812–21)—though Syntax is not Gilpin, who was already dead.

Gilpin's theory is grounded in Burke's *Enquiry*, but he extends the analytical process by distinguishing the picturesque from the beautiful and the sublime, since neither 'beauty' nor 'sublimity' accounts for the appeal of Nature's dramatic irregularity. Ruins, which are Nature's dealings with man's handiwork, are picturesque by their broken masses, and Gilpin thanks Henry VIII and Oliver Cromwell for providing so many—'these two masters', he calls them, as though landscape were a canvas and old buildings a kind of pigment. Furness Abbey, he notes, 'has suffered from the hand of time only such depredations as picturesque beauty requires'. Tintern is less satisfactory; the gables are too regular. 'A mallet judiciously employed', he suggests (and then withdraws the vandalism) 'might be of service'. His connoisseur tone is agreeable; time has adorned Tintern with 'mosses of various hues, with lychens, maiden-hair, penny-leaf and other humble plants', which give 'those full-blown tints which add the richest finishing to a ruin'.

Gilpin's detail is often amusing, but his achievement was serious. His were aesthetic adventures. He admired storms, gloom intensified by shafts of light, and the Dutch painters for their tempests and flying clouds. He knew a romantic scene when he saw one and could describe it so that the reader sees it too. Here is a storm in the Lakes:

> The sky floating with broken clouds—the mountains half-obscured by driving vapours, and mingling with the sky in awful obscurity—the trees

straining in the blast—and the lake stirred from the bottom, and whitening every rocky promontory with its foam. . . . Some broad mountainside, catching a mass of light, produces an astonishing effect amidst the leaden gloom which surrounds it. Perhaps a sunbeam, half-suffused in vapour, darting between two mountains, may stretch along the water in a lengthened gleam, just as the skiff passes to receive the light upon its swelling sail; while the sea-gull, wheeling along the storm, turns its silvery side, strongly illumined, against the bosom of some lurid cloud, and by that single touch of opposition gives double darkness to the rising tempest.
Observations on the Mountains and Lakes of Cumberland and Westmoreland, 2nd ed., (1788), i. 134–5

That is certainly more dramatic than sensitive, too strenuous and intent on exemplifying a formula. It is also ominously the germ of bad Victorian painting. Yet in its own way its melodramatic manner is effective, and it accords with Ruskin's brilliant comments (in *Modern Painters*, part IV, chapter xvi) on the development of romantic taste for storm and transience in landscape.

The Chinese, the Gothic, and the Picturesque, then, meant visual experiences evoking strange ranges of feeling, and broke radically with the Augustans' normal styles. In his essay *The Northanger Novels* (1927) Mr. Michael Sadleir distinguishes two suggestive qualities of the Gothic (present also in the Picturesque, but only partially in the Chinese). The first is that of escape from the stable lines of classical form through an addiction to verticals (Burke makes somewhat the same point). Gothic lines soar into points and pinnacles, and so do crags and trees. The second quality has contrary implications—it is the crumbling of man's work in ruin, symbol of Nature's supremacy. Not only the English romantics felt this, nor did the feeling arise only from Gothic ruins: Piranesi is rich in it, and Rome perhaps its greatest instance. It is by a striking complexity of emotion that the picturesque movement should have run to these opposites—to transcendence which spurns the earth (much neo-Gothic building is exaggeratedly tall, as Fonthill Abbey was), and to submission to Nature's power. Both point to Byron's flamboyance, and in *Childe Harold* (IV. cvii) the second of them is lavishly indulged in the description of Rome:

> *Cypress and ivy, weed and wallflower grown*
>   *Matted and massed together—hillocks heaped*
>   *On what were chambers—arch crushed, column strown*
>   *In fragments—choked-up vaults, and frescos steeped*
>   *In subterranean damps, where the owl peeped*
>   *Deeming it midnight;—Temples—Baths—or Halls?*
>   *Pronounce who can: for all that Learning reaped*
>   *From her research hath been, that these are walls.*
> *Behold the Imperial Mount! 'Tis thus the Mighty falls.*

That almost exultant acceptance of transience is the antithesis of humanism, yet something perhaps as deep in Augustan feeling as humanism itself, less visible but never distant, the sense of mystery.

V. THE ARTS AND LITERATURE

> *Like friendly Colors our kind arts unite*
> *Each from the mixture gathering sweets and light*
> *Their birth, their features with resemblance strike*
> *As Twins they vary and as Twins are like.*
>   POPE: *To Mr. Jervas* (first version), 19–22

AUGUSTAN arts and letters, it is natural to think, are akin in their aims and conventions. But in what does the kinship consist, apart from general traits such as a growing sense of landscape, or the emotional enrichment of picturesque wildness and mystery?

The central stream of taste, in the first place, had a social rather than an individual reference. Artists and writers were not strange creatures haloed with the integrity of a personal 'vision'. Art and letters were parts of a communal culture, not separate and superior worlds of individual aspiration. The system of patronage contributed something to this, since looking to a patron for an income was not much use if one had the temperament of a Blake. The dominant forms contributed something too; the periodical essay, the satirical poem, the social novel, the portrait and conversation piece were hardly the media for a self-devoted individualist, and the client brought up on Wren or Palladio was generally cool towards architectural revolutions. But these are symptoms rather than causes; the basic cause was general consent as to what the arts were for, that they preserved the outlook on life that the Augustans had settled as being good. The arts tend towards the social centre; the century's strong central magnetism holds its vigorous and various parts together.

In the second place this magnetism is the force of humanism, which insists on the dignity and interest of human beings and their capacity for the rational good life. Georgian buildings are on the whole the most pleasing yet devised in this country for social living, the most harmonious in proportion and the most satisfying in their implications about human nature. Georgian painting is sociably inclined and pleasantly civilised. Georgian writing is the most completely devoted to the theme of man not alone but with his fellows.

And in the third place, the canons of critical judgment were similar, whichever art was in question. They derived from the whole neoclassic movement and were not peculiar to the Augustans, but in England it was with the Augustans that they found their fullest expression.

The first of them asserted the prestige of 'the ancients'. 'Know well each ancient's proper character,' Pope advised: 'Look upon what the ancients have done,' Jonathan Richardson commanded. Reynolds traced all excellence ultimately to them. For both literature and art tradition was a vital learning drawn from antiquity; a learned traditionalism is as characteristic of a painter like Reynolds as of a writer like Johnson, and these two men provide almost identical philosophies of their respective arts, a similarity strengthened by their friendship but also inherent in the time. 'The ancients' were supplemented by the critics, artists and architects of the Renaissance, and the resulting tradition was one of rich accumulated human experience to be studied in no slavish sense but with a view to enabling the individual to realise his best powers in original work. As Reynolds puts it in the sixth *Discourse*,

> a mind enriched by an assemblage of all the treasures of ancient and modern art will be more elevated and fruitful in resources, in proportion to the number of ideas which have been carefully collected and thoroughly digested.

Yet devotion to tradition is not servility. The experience of the ages might be epitomised in rules, but, as Reynolds said, these were not to be 'the fetters of genius'—they fettered only those without genius. Pedants might overrate them but good judges were more generous. 'There is always an appeal open from criticism to nature,' Johnson observed in the *Preface to Shakespeare*, and for Reynolds the study of tradition is (like all education) the preliminary learning on which the student then achieves his own powers, disciplined and stimulated to a higher attainment than mere self-expression could reach. The best expression combined the individual perception with the tuition of history. The rules were guides not to the lower but to the higher 'imitation', not mere obedience but the attainment by the example of models of a higher art than the models themselves had reached. The Augustans did not, perhaps, suppose that antiquity would be outshone, but they did suppose that the way to outshine it (if possible) was first to borrow its light. Let the great masters uplift you, Reynolds advises in the sixth *Discourse*, and your mind will become more magnanimous:

> Whoever has so far formed his taste as to be able to relish and feel the beauties of the great masters, has gone a great way in his study; for merely from a consciousness of this relish of the right, the mind swells with an inward pride, and is almost as powerfully affected as if it had itself produced what it admires. Our hearts, frequently warmed in this way by the contact of those whom we wish to resemble, will undoubtedly catch something of their way of thinking, and we shall receive in our own bosoms some radiation at least of their fire and splendour.

Many questions are begged here—whether 'the beauties of the great masters' are the most fruitful models (the Augustans, it must be admitted, knew little other painting, and did not like primitives), whether discipleship does not stultify, and so on. An individualist will throw Reynolds and neoclassicism overboard, as Blake explosively did. Yet in a general sense Reynolds is right, in that an artist's inspiration may often come from another artist's work, and for most of the Augustans this particular tradition was still potent and fruitful.

There was a potent canon, too, of intelligibility. 'Whatever professes to benefit by pleasing', said Johnson in the *Life of Cowley*, 'must please at once'. 'A picture', Reynolds insisted, 'should please at first sight and appear to invite the spectator's attention.' The arts exist for the public's benefit and it is the public's taste which counts. So Johnson at the end of the *Life of Gray* speaks of 'the common sense of readers uncorrupted with literary prejudices' (that is, not the specialist or expert) as the arbiter of fame. Immediate public judgment may err, but 'about things on which the public thinks long it commonly attains to think right' (*Life of Addison*), and Reynolds declares that 'the well-disciplined mind . . . submits its own opinion to the public voice'. This is indeed plain common sense rather than the property of one critical fashion, yet its Augustan emphasis shows how much the public was thought fit to be trusted and its preferences respected. Here again 'the ancients' had an advantage, being upheld by the suffrages of the ages, and here again society exerted its authority over the individual.

Another canon requires coherence and unity. In Pope's words,

> *In wit, as nature, what affects our hearts*
> *Is not th' exactness of peculiar parts;*
> *'Tis not a lip, or eye, we beauty call,*
> *But the joint force and full result of all.*
> Essay on Criticism, 243–6

The poet's business, says Imlac the philosopher in *Rasselas*, 'is to examine not the individual but the species; to remark general properties and large appearances'. Reynolds is in accord: obtrusive detail is 'worse than useless'. The Metaphysical poets, Johnson protests, lost 'the grandeur of generality' by protracting their ideas into minutiae, and Reynolds thinks that concentration on particulars is actually contrary to the habits of human attention:

> to express [generality] in painting is to express what is congenial and natural to the mind of Man, and what gives him by reflection his own mode of conceiving.
>
> *Eleventh Discourse*

Details, then, must conduce to an easily-apprehended whole. They may be beautiful in themselves, or even abundant, as in the applied arts, but they must not thwart the mind seeking intelligible and unified beauty.

The last main canon is that of 'Nature', of the normal course of life and the human mind. It is often merely a cliché, preferred to engage automatic approval. But in fact it could be either the *normal* or the *best* aspect of life. Following Nature might mean simple realism, but it generally meant the attainment of representative 'truth' about life (in this sense Shakespeare followed Nature and the Metaphysicals did not), and also the attainment of the 'higher' rather than the 'lower' truth. Neoclassic critics often stress the supremacy of the epic, because that is the loftiest form in which the 'nature' of life can be expressed; it is ideal and heroic narrative with the extra dignity of verse and is therefore suited to express man's 'proper' quality. The painter likewise should, ideally, aim at the 'higher' truth: Dryden's *Parallel of Poetry and Painting*, much read, sets itself firmly in the Renaissance tradition of artistic idealisation. The portrait-painter, according to Jonathan Richardson, 'is chiefly concerned with the noblest and most beautiful part of human nature' (the face), and may within reason idealise his sitters to show mankind's true beauty and dignity. Study the world attentively, says Reynolds, 'but always with those masters [of antiquity and the Renaissance] in your company': portray the nobler aspects of life, which are as real as the ignoble, and more 'natural' to man as nearer his true quality.

These counsels apply differently to different arts. Literature was the most varied and the least amenable to critical laws. Still, the characteristic admiration of antiquity, the recognition of (if not always obedience to) traditional practice, the aims of clarity, coherence and harmony—these are the background to literature as well as the other arts, and are as prominent in Dryden, Pope, Fielding and Johnson as in Richardson, Reynolds, and the architects.

Certain parallels in style, too, suggest themselves, though it is easy to be fanciful in drawing them. Wren, Hawksmoor and Vanbrugh show a large, dramatic and often surprising sense of form and rhythm which recalls the eloquence of seventeenth-century prose or of Milton's poetry. The similarity is far from exact: the architects are manly, and inventively bold, rather than complex and subtle; they combine the magniloquence of the earlier era with the strong clarity of a Dryden, speaking of an age vivid, confident and varied, not yet settled into a steady rhythm of life. As in all such analogies one cannot say that art is precisely like literature; the connection is that they both show in various ways the dominant character of the time, and in the case of the early Augustans it is a dominant character of almost exuberant power. The next age sees Addison, Berkeley, Pope and the Burlingtonians: it suggests less exuberance and more concern to set in order, to improve and illuminate the accepted conventions, a sense for 'polite' civilisation and for intelligence not higher than in the Restoration but more judiciously refined, and a reverence for classical practice quieter though not less profound. Generalisations are treacherous; the Restoration's hurly-burly did not quickly subside into settled order, unruly brilliance did not entirely accept communal rule, and some of the greatest men (Swift and Hogarth, for instance) are laws to themselves. Yet by the time of Pope and Burlington the Augustan code had two generations behind it; its novelties were familiarised and both literature and the visual arts were expressing their inner strength in styles often (though not always) less robust yet with an admirable assurance and discipline.

In the middle of the century several strands may be distinguished. Subversive movements like *chinoiserie* and the Gothic affect various arts. In the central tradition there is a conservative strength in the paintings of Reynolds, the buildings of Chambers, Vardy, the Dances and Gandon, and in the prose of Fielding, Johnson and

Gibbon, while a sophisticated brilliance enlivens Zoffany, Robert Adam, Sheridan and Horace Walpole. Here again the analogies are loose, yet social life does in fact express itself on the one hand in robustness and on the other in vivacity. One might even trace a third quality, of temperate rational clarity reduced to a somewhat flat good taste, in the cool prose of men like Paley, in the sobriety of Regency stucco, and the devitalised neo-Greek sculpture of Flaxman. But that suggestion, though not misrepresenting those cognate aspects of the different arts, may well be too glib.

Another bond, at least between painting and poetry, lies in certain aims. The idea of a poem as a speaking picture and a picture as a visual poem affected the practice of both arts. In painting it encouraged anecdotage, a practice from which, except in landscape, painting hardly freed itself until the late nineteenth century. It is true that painters were interested in technique as well as subject-matter, in formal qualities and the texture of paint, but a picture was taken as something translatable into literary terms. A portrait rendered character and social circumstances; a social scene reported an incident—fête, masquerade or regatta. History paintings recorded heroism; allegorical paintings were moral lessons; caricatures were satiric commentary. Most of this is always true—artists and writers say many of the same things. Georgian art wanted to say the same things about life as literature did; fortunately it also kept a sound sense of how to use its own language of paint.

If painting had literary aims (Jonathan Richardson and Reynolds are clear about them) poetry was often pictorial by choice. Pope was friendly with both Richardson and Charles Jervas, under whom he studied painting, and he drew to a remarkable degree on his technical knowledge, enriched at least his early work by abundance of colour, showed a direct knowledge of painters and their styles, and proved in *Windsor Forest* to be sensitive to the composition and graduated colour of pictorial landscape. Poets had often taken pleasure in the country, but Pope was among the earliest to look at landscape methodically, though he expresses himself with epigrammatic sharpness rather than with contemplative steadiness. In spite of this his 'painted Scene of Woods and Forests in Verdure and

Beauty, Trees springing, fields flow'ring, Nature laughing', as he describes it to Caryll, is a foretaste of more elaborate landscape in later poets.

Many an Augustan displayed his subject as a succession of prospects, a habit due partly to the notion of poetry as formal composition and partly to the cultivation of topography as one of the visual arts. Thomson in *The Seasons* does so continually: he accompanies Lord Lyttelton through Hagley Park, for instance, with 'excursive eye', noting 'the dale With woods o'erhung and shagg'd with mossy rocks', the 'solemn oaks that tuft the swelling mounts', and finally (*Spring*, 1746, 946–52)

> *the Height, from whose fair Brow*
> *The bursting Prospect spreads immense around;*
> *And snatch'd o'er Hill and Dale, and Wood, and Lawn,*
> *And verdant Field, and dark'ning Heath between,*
> *And Villages embosom'd soft in Trees,*
> *And spiry Towns by surging Columns mark'd*
> *Of household Smoak.*

Abundantly demonstrative, he tries to substitute words for draughtsmanship:

> *Behold yon breathing Prospect bids the Muse*
> *Throw all her Beauty forth . . .*

> *See, where the winding Vale its lavish Stores,*
> *Irriguous, spreads . . .*

> *At length the finish'd Garden to the View*
> *Its Vistas opens, and its Alleys green . . .*

If his success is only moderate it is because his language, strained to include everything, is lacking in suggestive subtlety. Dyer too, amateur painter as well as poet, is confessedly pictorial: *Grongar Hill* invites the 'nymph' of Painting to

> *Come with all thy various hues,*
> *Come and aid thy sister Muse,*

and it proceeds by vignettes, one of the pleasantest topographical poems, descriptive poetry rather than a mere offshoot of painting yet obviously in the pictorial convention.

And finally, personification as the Augustans used it in poetry is akin to painting. Gray's 'rosy-bosom'd Hours, Fair Venus' train' or 'Youth at the prow and Pleasure at the helm' recall such mural decorations as Sir James Thornhill's adorning his ceiling at Greenwich or his dome at St. Paul's or, along with Laguerre's, heightening the splendour of Blenheim. The figures who fleet through Gray's odes—'the fury Passions', 'Disdainful Anger', 'Pallid Fear' and the like—are pictorial shadows, like the spirits who cry to Mrs. Siddons as the Tragic Muse, in Reynolds's portrait. Gray is sometimes indebted to Milton, but he reduces the strong Miltonic life to a generality such as would fill an allegorical canvas. The Johnson who disliked allegorical paintings also, we recall, disliked Gray's 'cumbrous splendour'. One of the more effectively pictorial figures, though not a personification, is that of the Bard;

> *On a rock, whose haughty brow*
> *Frowns o'er old Conway's foaming flood,*
> *Robed in the sable garb of woe*
> *With haggard eyes the Poet stood;*
> *(Loose his beard, and hoary hair*
> *Stream'd, like a meteor, to the troubl'd air)*
> *And with a Master's hand, and Prophet's fire,*
> *Struck the deep sorrows of his lyre.*

The immediate sense is of a figure of art, and then one happens on Gray's note: 'The image', it says, 'was taken from a well-known picture of Raphael.' The corroboration is satisfactory but was hardly needed. Collins's personifications too bring painting to mind:

> *Ah* Fear! *Ah frantic* Fear!
> *I see, I see thee near.*
> *I know thy hurried Step, thy haggard Eye!*
> *Like Thee I start, like Thee disorder'd fly.*
> *For Lo! what* Monsters *in thy Train appear!*
> *Danger, whose limbs of Giant Mold*
> *What mortal Eye can fix'd behold?*

These abstractions are not richly-felt figures; they are the shadows of allegorical murals. Such a derivation cannot be proved absolutely; the Latin poetry on which the Augustans were reared is itself full of personified passions. But the Augustan fashion, with its histrionic gestures and melodramatic figures (and indeed its explicit reference to vision) undoubtedly suggests this particular kinship. The same is true of the heroic poem. Addison's *Campaign* is the usual substance of historical painting (Thornhill and Laguerre at Blenheim are here a precise parallel)—the general riding the whirlwind and directing the storm (the Angel who ostensibly does so is, as Johnson remarked, virtually Marlborough himself), the haughty French Household Guards advancing, the sturdy redcoats, the young officer who 'fill'd with England's glory smiles in death'. The poem does things a painting cannot do; it has movement, variety, a sense of nations rather than mere armies engaged, and a rhetoric which if rather repellent has still resonance and force. But the kind of inspiration it suggests is that of the historical panorama, and its heroic gestures are the common idiom of heroic painting.

The genres of literature, then, are like those of painting—landscape, allegory, conversation piece, portrait and caricature. In this last category the influence of Hogarth is all-important, and Fielding acknowledges more than one debt to him. His incisive satire, his exaggerated forceful outlines and his grotesque comedy prompt many a portrait in Fielding and in Smollett too—perhaps also Richardson's grotesques. Hogarth not only expresses much of the Augustans' fierce comedy and moral conventions but gives literature a graphic mode of portrayal which survives at least into Dickens. In many ways the eye seems to preside over Augustan literary procedure, over its characterisation for instance and also its poetic imagery. Yet the coincidence of this with the vogue of the visual arts may be deceptive; the underlying relationship is probably that (as far as literary sensitivity was concerned) theories of perception laid far more stress on sight than on anything else. The content of the mind, about which philosophers were so exercised, is furnished mostly through the eye. And lastly, a kinship between the arts emerges in the degree to which they all rely on formal pattern—the symmetry of buildings, the careful composition of portraits, the discipline of the couplet, or of prose rhythms. These things are evidence in the different arts (one could cite too the ordered patterns of Georgian music) of the control the Augustan mind sought over its experiences, and they are the hallmark of that confident civilisation which the twentieth century in many ways envies and admires.

F. M. Eden, *The State of the Poor*: A. Young, *Six Weeks Tour through the Southern Counties*, *The Farmer's Letters to the People of England*, *Six Months Tour through the North of England*, and *The Farmer's Tour through the East of England* (4 vols.): T. Pennant, *Journey from Chester to London*, *Tour from London to the Isle of Wight 1787*, and *Account of London*: H. B. Chancellor, *The Eighteenth Century in London* (1920) H. B. Wheatley and P. Cunningham, *London Past and Present* (3 vols., 1910): J. Ashton, *Social Life in the Reign of Queen Anne* (1883): W. and A. E. Wroth, *London Pleasure Gardens* (1896): W. Besant, *London in the XVIIIth Century* (1902); H. B. Wheatley, *Hogarth and his Times* (1909): O. H. K. Spate, 'The Growth of London', in *Historical Geography of England before 1800* (ed. H. C. Darby, 1936): W. E. Mead, *The Grand Tour in the XVIIIth Century* (1914).

THE WORLD OF BUSINESS

A

Among contemporary documents may be recommended: Defoe, *Tour Thro' the Whole Island of Great Britain*, *Plan of the English Commerce*, *The Compleat English Tradesman*, *Essay on Projects*, and the major novels: Adam Smith, *The Wealth of Nations*: *The Spectator* (espec. Nos. 2, 3, 69, 174, 283, 552): Dyer, *The Fleece*: Voltaire, 'Sur le Commerce' in *Lettres Philosophiques*: Burke, *Observations on 'The Present State of the Nation'*, *Letters on a Regicide Peace*, No. iii, and the American speeches. Later authorities are: P. Mantoux, *The Industrial Revolution in the Eighteenth Century* (trans. M. Vernon, 1928): E. Lipson, *Economic History of England* (3 vols., 1931): W. Cunningham, *The Growth of English Industry and Commerce*, vol. ii. (6th ed., 1922): T. S. Ashton, *The Industrial Revolution* (1948): W. G. East, 'England in the Eighteenth Century', in *Historical Geography of England before 1800* (ed. H. C. Darby, 1936).

B

T. Mortimer, *Elements of Commerce, Politics and Finances* (3 vols.): Josiah Tucker, *Elements of Commerce*: Henry Homer, *Means of Preserving the Publick Roads*: R. H. Tawney, *Religion and the Rise of Capitalism* (1926): H. M. Robertson, *Aspects of the Rise of Economic Individualism* (1933): F. C. Dietz, *Economic History of England* (New York, 1942): J. L. and Barbara Hammond, *The Village Labourer 1760–1832* (1911), *The Town Labourer 1760–1832* (1917), *The Skilled Labourer 1760–1832* (1919): H. J. Habakkuk, 'English Landownership 1680–

1740' in *Economic History Review*, vol. x, no. 1: A. S. Collins, *Authorship in the Days of Johnson* (1927) and *The Profession of Letters 1780–1832* (1928): F. A. Mumby, *Publishing and Bookselling* (1930): W. H. R. Curtler, *Enclosure and Redistribution of our Land* (1920): F. D. Klingender *Art and the Industrial Revolution* (1947): A. Raistrick, *Dynasty of Iron Founders: the Darbys and Coalbrookdale* (1953).

PUBLIC AFFAIRS

A

Among contemporary documents may be recommended: J. Locke, *Second Treatise of Civil Government* (ed. by J. W. Gough, 1946): Swift, *Journal to Stella* (ed. H. Williams, 2 vols., 1948), *Examiner* papers, and pamphlets on English and Irish affairs *passim*: Halifax, *Character of a Trimmer*: Bolingbroke, *Letters on the Spirit of Patriotism* and *On the Idea of a Patriot King*: Burke, espec. American and Indian speeches, *Reflections on the Revolution in France, Appeal from the New to the Old Whigs, Letters to the Sheriffs of Bristol, Speech to the Electors of Bristol*, and *Two Letters to Gentlemen in the City of Bristol*. Later authorities are: G. M. Trevelyan, *The English Revolution 1688–1689* (1938): H. J. Laski, *Political Thought from Locke to Bentham* (1925): F. J. C. Hearnshaw (ed.) *Social and Political Ideas of Some English Thinkers of the Augustan Age* (1928): L. B. Namier, *The Structure of Politics at the Accession of George III* (2 vols., 1929): R. Lodge, *Political History of England 1660–1702* (1910): I. S. Leadam, *Political History of England 1702–60* (1909): W. Hunt, *Political History of England 1760–1801* (1905): and Clark, Williams and Lecky as in 'General A' list.

B

Tracts and Pamphlets of Richard Steele (ed. Rae Blanchard, 1944): D. Defoe, *True-Born Englishman*, and numerous prose pamphlets: S. Johnson, *Taxation no Tyranny, The False Alarm, The Falkland Islands*: H. Fielding, *Don Quixote in England, Historical Register for 1736, Pasquin, Jonathan Wild, The Jacobite's Journal, Serious Address to the People of Great Britain*: D. Hume, *Theory of Politics* (ed. F. Watkins, 1951): W. Godwin, *Political Justice*: T. Paine, *The Rights of Man*: Mary Wollstonecraft, *The Rights of Women*: G. Canning, G. Ellis and J. H. Frere, *Poetry of the Anti-Jacobin*: W. Coxe, *Memoirs of Sir Robert Walpole* (3 vols.). Later authorities are: G. M. Trevelyan, *England Under*

Queen Anne (3 vols., 1930–4): C. H. Firth, 'Political Significance of Gulliver's Travels' in *Essays Historical and Literary* (1938): H. N. Brailsford, *Shelley, Godwin and their Circle* (1913): J. W. Gough, *John Locke's Political Philosophy* (1950): T. Wright, *Caricature History of the Georges* (1868): J. R. Sutherland, *Defoe* (1937) and 'The Circulation of Newspapers and Literary Periodicals 1700–1730' (in *The Library*, vol. xv, 1935): P. Magnus, *Edmund Burke* (1939).

RELIGIOUS LIFE

A

Among contemporary documents may be recommended: J. Locke, *The Reasonableness of Christianity*: R. Steele, *The Christian Hero*: Addison, *The Spectator*, passim: W. Law, *Serious Call to a Devout and Holy Life*: J. Butler, *The Analogy of Religion Natural and Revealed*: *The Guardian* (espec. Nos. 3, 18, 19, 20, 26, 39): Swift, *The Examiner* (espec. Nos. 16, 22, 23, 30, 32, 34, 40, 43), *Argument Against Abolishing Christianity*: Berkeley, *Principles of Human Knowledge*, *Alciphron*: Goldsmith, *Vicar of Wakefield*: C. Smart, *Hymn to David*: Cowper, *Olney Hymns*: miscellaneous hymns of Watts, the Wesleys, Addison, Byrom, Doddridge, Perronet, Newton, Olivers, Toplady: Johnson, *Prayers and Meditations*, *Rambler*, *Vanity of Human Wishes*, *Rasselas*: Burke, *Reflections on the Revolution in France*: J. M. Creed and J. S. Boys Smith (edd.), *Religious Thought in the Eighteenth Century as Illustrated from Writers of the Period* (1934). Later authorities are: C. J. Abbey and J. H. Overton, *The English Church in the Eighteenth Century* (1878): C. J. Abbey, *The English Church and its Bishops* (1887): G. M. Trevelyan, *The English Revolution 1688–1689* (1938): W. E. H. Lecky, *History of England in the Eighteenth Century* (8 vols., 1878–90): J. H. Overton and F. Relton, *The English Church from the Accession of George I to the End of the Eighteenth Century* (1906): N. Sykes, *Church and State in England in the Eighteenth Century* (1934), and in *Johnson's England* (ed. Turberville, 1933): T. B. Shepherd, *Methodism and the Literature of the Eighteenth Century* (1940).

B

Contemporary works include: Joseph Butler, *Fifteen Sermons* and *Charge to the Clergy, 1751*: W. Law, *Practical Treatise on Christian Perfection* (ed. L. H. M. Soulsby, 1901), and *Address to the Clergy, 1761*: John Wesley, *Journal* (abridged in 2 vols. 1902 or complete, ed. N.

Curnock, 8 vols., 1909–16), and *Letters* (ed. J. Telford, 8 vols., 1931): James Woodforde, *Diary of a Country Parson 1758–1802* (ed. J. Beresford, 5 vols., 1924–31; or abridged in one vol., 1935): T. Tickell, *On the Death of Mr. Addison*: R. Graves, *The Spiritual Quixote*: W. Cole, *Blecheley Diary 1765–67* (ed. F. G. Stokes, 1931): John Toland, *Christianity Not Mysterious*: M. Tindal, *Christianity as Old as the Creation*: W. Wollaston, *Religion of Nature Delineated*: Hume, 'Superstition and Enthusiasm' in *Philosophical Works*, vol. iii (ed. T. H. Green, 1872): W. Paley, *Evidences of Christianity*. Later authorities are: J. H. Overton, *Life in the English Church 1660–1714* (1885), *The Non-Jurors* (1902), *William Law* (1881): B. L. Manning, *Hymns of Wesley and Watts* (1942): D. Davie, 'The Classicism of Charles Wesley' in *Purity of Diction in English Verse* (1952): G. Sampson, 'The Century of Divine Songs' in *Seven Essays* (1947): H. N. Fairchild, *Religious Trends in English Poetry*, vols. i and ii (1939, 1942): H. O. Wakeman, *Introduction to the History of the Church of England* (rev. S. L. Ollard, 1914): W. J. Amherst, *History of Catholic Emancipation 1771–1820* (2 vols., 1886): J. Wickham Legg, *English Church Life from the Restoration to the Tractarian Movement* (1914): J. Stoughton, *History of Religion in England*, vols. v, vi. (4th ed., 1901): D. Coomer, *English Dissent under the Early Hanoverians* (1946): G. R. Cragg, *From Puritanism to the Age of Reason* (1950): H. W. Clark, *History of English Nonconformity*, vol. ii (1913): G. C. B. Davies, *Early Cornish Evangelicals* (1951): G. R. Balleine, *History of the Evangelical Party in the Church of England* (1908): L. Tyerman, *Life and Times of John Wesley* (3 vols., 1870–1): R. Southey, *Life of Wesley* (2 vols. 1820): D. Cecil, *The Stricken Deer* (1929): A. T. Hart, *Life and Times of John Sharp Archbishop of York* (1949): E. Carpenter, *Thomas Tenison, Archbishop of Canterbury* (1948): G. W. O. Addleshaw and F. Etchells, *The Architectural Setting of Anglican Worship* (1948): M. Whiffen, *Stuart and Georgian Churches outside London* (1949).

PHILOSOPHY MORAL AND NATURAL

A

Among contemporary documents may be recommended: J. Locke, *Essay Concerning Human Understanding*: A. A. Cooper, third Earl of Shaftesbury, *Characteristicks* (2 vols., ed. J. M. Robertson, 1900): F. Hutcheson, *The Original of our Ideas of Beauty and Virtue, Concerning*

Moral Good and Evil, The Nature and Conduct of the Passions, and *System of Moral Philosophy*: D. Hume, *Treatise of Human Nature, Enquiry Concerning Human Understanding, Enquiry Concerning the Principles of Morals,* and *Essays Moral and Political*: D. Hartley, *Observations on Man*: Adam Smith, *Theory of Moral Sentiments*: G. Berkeley, *Principles of Human Knowledge, Three Dialogues between Hylas and Philonous, Alciphron, The Theory of Vision*: J. Bentham, *Principles of Morals and Legislation*: W. Godwin, *Political Justice*: B. de Mandeville, *The Fable of the Bees* (ed. F. B. Kaye, 2 vols., 1924): G. White, *Natural History of Selborne*: L. A. Selby-Bigge (ed.), *British Moralists* (2 vols. 1897). Later authorities are: L. Stephen, *History of English Thought in the Eighteenth Century* (2 vols., 1876): B. Willey, *The Seventeenth-Century Background* (1934), *The Eighteenth-Century Background* (1940): A. N. Whitehead, *Science and the Modern World* (1929): T. Fowler, *Locke* (1880), and *Shaftesbury and Hutcheson* (1882): S. Alexander, *Locke* (1908): R. L. Brett, *The Third Earl of Shaftesbury* (1951): W. R. Scott, *Francis Hutcheson* (1900).

B

Contemporary works include: T. Sprat, *History of the Royal Society*: R. Cumberland, *Treatise of the Laws of Nature* (trans. J. Maxwell, 1727): Rev. John Gay, *Fundamental Principles of Virtue*: John Ray, *Wisdom of God Manifested in the Works of the Creation*: W. Derham, *Physico-Theology, Astro-Theology*: R. Price, *Review of the Principal Questions and Difficulties in Morals*: E. Darwin, *Zoönomia, The Botanic Garden*. Later authorities are: H. R. Fox Bourne, *Life of John Locke* (2 vols., 1876): W. E. H. Lecky, *Rise and Influence of the Spirit of Rationalism in Europe* (2 vols., 1865): E. A. Burtt, *Metaphysical Foundations of Modern Physical Science* (1925): C. Singer, *Short History of Biology* (1931): G. R. Cragg, *From Puritanism to the Age of Reason,* chs. iii 'The Cambridge Platonists' and v 'Impact of the New Science' (1950): Maynard Mack, intro. to *An Essay on Man* (Twickenham edition of Pope, 1950): A. E. Case, *Four Essays on Gulliver's Travels* (1945): A. D. McKillop, *The Background of Thomson's Seasons* (Minneapolis 1942): M. H. Nicolson, *Newton Demands the Muse* (Princeton, 1946): K. Maclean, *John Locke and English Literature of the Eighteenth Century* (New Haven, 1936): Sir Henry Lyons, *The Royal Society* (1944): C. E. Raven, *John Ray, Naturalist* (1942): R. F. Jones and others, *The Seventeenth Century, Studies in the History of English Thought and Literature from Bacon to Pope* (Stanford, 1951):

Joan Bennett, 'An Aspect of Seventeenth-Century Prose', in *Review of English Studies*, vol. 17 (No. 67): R. Blanchard, intro. to Steele's *Christian Hero* (1932): C. A. Moore, 'Shaftesbury and the Ethical Poets in England 1700–1760' in *Publications of the Modern Language Association of America*, xxxi, 1916: John Butt, 'Science and Man in Eighteenth-Century Poetry', in *Durham University Journal*, June 1947.

THE VISUAL ARTS

A

Among contemporary works may be recommended: the periodicals, espec. *The Spectator* and *The World*, for miscellaneous material; Hogarth's cartoons, *The Analysis of Beauty*, and *The Drawings of William Hogarth*, by A. P. Oppé (1948): Pope, especially the *Epistle to Burlington*: E. Burke, *The Sublime and the Beautiful*: Sir J. Reynolds, *Discourses*. Later authorities are: *Johnson's England* (ed. A. S. Turberville, 1933), vol. ii: A. E. Richardson, *Georgian England* (1931): J. Summerson, *Georgian London* (1945), *Architecture in Britain 1530 to 1830* (1953) and *Sir Christopher Wren* (1953): M. Whiffen, *Stuart and Georgian Churches outside London* (1949): R. Edwards and Margaret Jourdain, *Georgian Cabinet-Makers* (1946): Margaret Jourdain and F. Rose, *English Furniture, The Georgian Period 1750–1830* (1953): M. Jourdain, *English Decoration and Furniture* (1922), *The Work of William Kent* (1948), *English Interior Decoration* (1950): Dorothy Stroud, *Capability Brown* (1950): R. Edwards, *Georgian Furniture* (1947): G. Scott, *The Architecture of Humanism* (1914): B. Sprague Allen, *Tides in English Taste* (2 vols., Harvard, 1937): J. Steegman, *The Rule of Taste* (1936): C. Hussey, *The Picturesque* (1927): Sir R. Blomfield, *History of Renaissance Architecture in England 1500–1800* (2 vols., 1897, or a *Short History*, 1 vol., 1900): K. Clark, *The Gothic Revival* (revised 1950): E. K. Waterhouse, *Reynolds* (1941) and *Painting in Britain 1530 to 1790* (1953): J. Lees-Milne, *The Age of Adam* (1947): S. Sitwell, *British Architects and Craftsmen* (1945).

B

Contemporary works include: Jonathan Richardson, *Theory of Painting, The Art of Criticism*, and *The Science of a Connoisseur*: H. Walpole, *Anecdotes of Painting*: W. Gilpin, *Observations on the River Wye, Observations on the Mountains and Lakes of Cumberland and Westmoreland, Observations on . . . the Highlands of Scotland, Remarks on Forest Scenery*,

INDEX

Page-numbers without further specification are for passing or self-evident references.

Abbey, C. J. 138
Adam, James 83, 233
Adam, Robert 221, 228, 234, 240, 242, 256; Adelphi 83; publications 223, 233; his models 228
Addison, Joseph 1, 19, 31, 43, 71, 84, 91, 92, 108, 129, 141, 162, 180, 186, 236, 243, 255; rustic etiquette 37; social order 49; trade 52, 78–9, 95; Bank of England 56–7; politics 103, 106, 127–8; *Campaign*, 127, 259; religious questions 139, 160–1, 165–6; 'enthusiasm' 157; hymns 164, 169–70; sentiment 189; science 206, 208, 212; popularisation of ideas 210–11; on Blackmore 213; on taste 217; classical antiquity 226; on Gothic 242
Addleshaw, G. W. O. 150
Akenside, Mark 90, 111; religious optimism 164; science 189, 202, 213
Aldrich, Henry 221
Amhurst, Nicholas 111, 136
Anderson, Robert 93
Anne, Queen 104–6, 146, 148, 154, 162, 191, 231–2, 242
Anson, George 76–7
Anti-Jacobin, The 118
Arabian Nights, The 96
Arbuthnot, John 111; and John Bull 48
Archer, Thomas 228, 232

Arne, Thomas 19, 217
Arnold, Matthew 121
Atterbury, Francis 106, 153; his trial 140–1
Austen, Jane 248

Bacon, Sir Francis 179, 181, 198, 207, 211, 236; semasiology 181–2, 184; intellectual progress 203–4
Bage, Robert 85; on India 80
Baker, Henry 3
Bakewell, Robert 64
Banks, Sir Joseph 204
Barrington, Daines 205
Barry, James 83
Barry, Spranger 18
Bathurst, Allen, Lord 245
Beaufort, Duke of 241
Beckford, William 96
Bedford, Duke of 120
Behn, Aphra 80
Bentham, Jeremy 188
Bentley, Richard 245
Berkeley, George 138, 141, 162, 173, 255; on St. Paul's 151, 230; 'free-thinking' 158, 161, 166; divine order 165–6, 171; *Theory of Vision* 186; on Gothic 243
Berridge, John 146
Blackmore, Sir Richard 212–13
Blake, William 70, 83, 146, 175, 177, 198, 214, 235, 250, 253; science 209
Boileau-Despréaux, Nicholas 214

271

Bolingbroke, Henry St. John, Viscount 211; rural retreat 40–1; *Idea of a Patriot King* and Locke 103, and unity 104, 108, 120, 130; Secretary for War 105; rivals Harley 105–6; opposes Walpole 111–12, 128; political enthusiasm 126; *Works* published 162
Boscawen, Mrs. Frances 19
Boswell, James 8, 23, 43–4, 152, 162; London 6, 22, 173; titles 84; on Culloden 132
Bougainville, Louis Antoine de 78
Boulter, Archbishop Hugh 109
Boulton, Matthew 87; his enterprise 70, 84
Bourne, George 31, 40
Boyce, William 38, 217
Boyle, Robert 190, 198, 203, 209
Boyle Lectures, The 192, 203–4
Bridgeman, Charles 247
Bridgewater, Francis Egerton, Duke of 76
Brindley, James 76
Brooke, Henry 126
Brown, John ('Estimate') 202
Brown, Lancelot ('Capability') 232, 247
Browne, Sir Thomas 205, 211
Budgell, Eustace 33, 86
Bunyan, John 164, 211
Burgess, Daniel 151
Burke, Edmund 18, 91, 102, 108, 111, 127, 130–1, 211; trade and industry 11, 72; India 80, 116–17; supports 1688 99; Ireland 110–11; American colonies 113–16; France 117, 120–1; political philosophy 119–22, 131, 196; on Parliament 123, 125; religious matters 138, 141–2, 145, 148–9, 157, 161–3; sublimity, mystery and imagination 150, 199–200, 240, 247, 249; on Locke 183
Burke, William 116
Burlington, Richard Boyle, third Earl of, recipient of Pope's *Epistle* 5, 61, 229; as patron 92, 221, 223, 228, 255; his buildings 222; Palladianism 227–8, 233
Burney, Fanny 10, 15; trial of Warren Hastings 117
Burns, Robert 175
Burrough, Sir James 222
Burton, Robert 211
Butler, Joseph 138, 141, 164, 173, 214; *Analogy*'s impact 139, and sombre tone 167, 206; 'free-thinking' 141, 158, 161; 'enthusiasm' 157
Butler, Samuel 157, 208
Byng, John, Viscount Torrington 30, 38
Byrom, John, political nonchalance 129; on Law 158; 'Christians awake!' 169
Byron, Captain John 77
Byron, George Gordon, Lord 94, 96, 249

Cambridge Platonists, the 174, 182, 191, 197–8
Campbell, Colen 222; *Vitruvius Britannicus* 223; Palladio 227; Houghton Hall 234
Canaletto, Antonio 230, 235
Canning, George 118
Carlyle, Thomas 89, 225
Caroline, Queen 44
Carpenter, Edward 143
Carr, John 234

INDEX

Carteret, John, Earl Granville 110
Caryll, John 257
Castell, Robert 223
Cawthorn, James 220–1
Chambers, Sir William 221, 228, 234, 241, 255
Charles II 134, 203, 236
Charlotte, Queen 72
Chaucer, Geoffrey 175
Chesterfield, Philip Stanhope, Earl of, on Parliament 123; on religion 160; on Palladio 227
Chippendale, Thomas 239–41
Chubb, Thomas 161
Churchill, Charles 152; clerical poverty 155
Cibber, Colley 18, 143
Cicero 211
Clark, G. N. 130
Clarke, Samuel 145, 180, 211; his intellectualism 191–2
Clarkson, Thomas 81
Claude Lorrain 235, 247
Clive, Kitty 18
Cobbett, William 7, 65
Coke, Thomas William, Earl of Leicester 64
Cole, William 141, 156
Colepepper, William 148
Coleridge, Samuel Taylor 148, 175, 187, 214; on Defoe 49; and criticism 216
Collection of Parliamentary Debates 55
Collier, Jeremy 143
Collins, William 175; *Persian Eclogues* 96; personifications 258–9
Colman, George, the younger 19, 33
Combe, William 248
Common-Sense; or, the Englishman's Journal 112, 137

Congreve, William 45, 92, 227, 236, 242
Cook, Captain James 77, 80, 204
Cornwallis, Archbishop Frederick 153
Cotman, John Sell 83
Cowley, Abraham 3, 157, 181, 203
Cowper, William 4, 19, 31, 126, 141, 164, 169, 173, 214; rural conditions 28, 30; slavery 81; Calvinism 146, 164, 175, 177; religious gravity 171
Crabbe, George 40, 175; rural conditions 28–9; clerical office 152
Craftsman, The 107, 111–12, 136
Croft, Herbert 161–2
Croft, William 38
Cromwell, Oliver 132, 144, 248
Cumberland, Bishop Richard 188
Cumberland, William Augustus, Duke of 46, 241

Dalton, John 87
Dampier, William 77
Dance, George (elder and younger) 255
Darby, Abraham 69, 86
Darwin, Charles 204
Darwin, Erasmus 84, 204–5
Davies, David 28
Defoe, Daniel 5, 9, 19, 21, 27, 44, 65, 72, 87, 90–1, 95, 126–9, 146; national development 1, 4, 54, 66, 79; London 7, 11–12, its surroundings 14–15, 26; the Thames 10–11; social evils 20, 85; *True-Born Englishman* and drunkenness 20, popularity of 107, on religious disputes 139; social relationships 26, 49; rural development 26–7, 61, 65;

provincial society 36–7; commercial projects 54; South Sea Bubble 57; *Robinson Crusoe* 61, 79, profits on publication 93, and primitive society 95; industrial grime 69; roads 74–5; overseas trade 78–80, 95; his style and imagery 94–5, 133; debt to Locke 102; political activities 104, 108, 148–9; religious controversy 139, 142; on Sacheverell 140–1; religious position 148; St. Paul's 151, 230; on Gothic 243
Delany, Mrs. Mary 245
Denham, Sir John 35, 229
Dennis, John 211–12, 223
Derham, William 204, 211; *Physico-Theology* 208–9, 212
Descartes, René 198, 213
Devis, Arthur 238
Dickens, Charles 43, 259
Doddridge, Philip 169
Dodington, George Bubb, Baron Melcombe 128
Dodsley, Robert 4
Donne, John 211
Dryden, John 11, 19, 157, 203, 227, 236, 254–5
Du Fresnoy, Charles Alphonse 229
Duck, Stephen 28–9
Dugdale, Sir William 242
Dyer, George 28, 118
Dyer, John, *Grongar Hill* 36, 257–8; *The Fleece* and sheep-farming 40, 66–9; on commerce 53, 79, 95; drainage 64; industry 70; *Ruins of Rome* 226

Earle, John 211
East India Company 12, 80, 111; Burke on 116–17

Edgeworth, Richard Lovell 84
Elers, John Philip 72
Eliot, T. S. 175
Elizabeth I, Queen 132
Ellys, John 236
Empson, William 50
Etchells, F. 150
Evelyn, John 203, 223, 227, 236, 243; sponsors Wren 229
Examiner, The, on political parties 107; moderation 108; religious position 147–8; clerical poverty 154

Falconer, William 95
Farquhar, George 23
Fielding, Henry 3, 9, 22, 32, 43–4, 91, 128–9, 134, 162, 240, 255; theatrical taste 18; on poverty 19–21; Hogarth 21, 259; representative characters 49; *Jonathan Wild*'s social import 50; *Author's Farce* and literary profession 92; *Tom Jones*, its profitableness 94, the 1745 112–13, clerical hypocrisy 152, 190, rationalism 190–1; *Amelia*, its profitableness 94, social evils 117; prose style 94, 134; *True Patriot* 104, Walpole attacked in *Historical Register*, *The Champion*, *Pasquin* and *Jonathan Wild* 108, 112, 123, 134; politics 108; anti-Stuart propaganda 112–13, 157; *Joseph Andrews* and Trulliber 152, clerical poverty 154, faith 156, 'enthusiasm' 157; religious stability 174; benevolence 201
Firth, Sir Charles 110
Flaxman, John 256

INDEX

Fleming, Sir Michael le 23
Flitcroft, Henry 228, 230
Foote, Samuel 17–19; *The Nabob* 80
Fox, Charles James 116, 126
Fox, Shadrach 86
Francis, Sir Philip 116
Franklin, Benjamin 86, 90
Froude, James Anthony 111
Free-holder's Journal, The 134

Gage, General Thomas 115
Gainsborough, Thomas 236–8
Galland, Antoine 96
Gandon, James 234, 255
Garrick, David 18, 162, 236, 241
Garth, Sir Samuel 13, 35, 236
Gay, John (poet) 8, 33, 43, 45, 92, 127; *The Mohacks* 6; on London 6, 9, 12–13; country life 30, 33; *The Fan* 45; *Beggar's Opera* and social patterns 49–50, and Walpole 111; South Sea Bubble 58; successful publication of *Polly* 93; religious themes 163, 167
Gay, John (philosophical writer) 164, 188
Gent, Thomas 243
Gentleman's Magazine, The national development 4; practical interests 54; literary popularisation 93
George I 57, 104–7, 153, 162
George II 153, 162
George III 121, 124, 128, 238–9
George IV, 44
Gibbon, Edward 18, 91, 160, 162, 256; *Autobiography* and the South Sea Bubble 58, on Law 174
Gibbs, James 12, 221, 228; architectural career 230
Gibson, Bishop Edmund 191

Gilpin, William 23; rural poverty 28; picturesque scenery 65, 83, 248–9
Glover, Richard 92, 212
Godolphin, Sidney, Earl of 49, 105
Godwin, William 87, 131, 192, 211; social evils 85, 117–18; *Political Justice* 118, and rationalism 193–4; *St. Leon* and feeling 193
Goldsmith, Oliver 18–19, 49, 96, 173, 175, 214; social evils 21; country society 31–2, 37; enclosures 63; concord 108, 126; political zeal 127; Bangorian controversy 140; preaching 151–2; clerical stipends 154; country civility 156; charity 202; science 208
Grafton, Aubrey Henry Fitzroy, Duke of 134
Grainger, James 95
Graves, Richard 32, 145
Gray, Thomas 31, 150, 214, 245; *Elegy* and social unity 50, and religious stability 175, 178; personification 258
Green, Matthew 4, 5, 129
Greene, Maurice 38, 217
Grenville, George 114
Grew, Nehemiah 205
Guardian, The theatrical manners 17; rural virtue 25, 30; scenery 40; country improvement 61; trade as unifier 52; religious problems 139, 154, 158, 166; St. Paul's 151, 178; style of the Bible 160, 168

Hales, Stephen 209
Halifax, George Savile, first Marquis 108, 133
Hamilton, Sir William 72

Handel, Georg Friedrich 38, 217
Hardy, Thomas 31, 38–9, 156
Harley, Robert, Earl of Oxford 49, 92; political and religious questions 105, 148
Hartley, David 180, 205
Hastings, Warren 80, 116–17
Hawkins, Isaac 86
Hawksmoor, Nicholas 12, 221, 228, 240, 242, 255; architectural career 230–1
Hazlitt, William 119
Hearne, Thomas 143, 203, 242
Heathfield, George, Baron 236
Henry VIII 248
Henry, Robert 94
Hepplewhite, George 239
Hertford, Francis Seymour Conway, Earl of 46
Highmore, Joseph 238
Hilliard, Nicholas 235
Hoadly, Bishop Benjamin 153; political views 102; Bangorian controversy 140–1
Hobbes, Thomas 100, 133, 179, 188, 211; *Leviathan* on epistemology 181–2, 184–6, and rationalism 189
Hogarth, William 3, 9, 15, 19, 21, 86, 235, 255; and character-drawing 48–50, 259; elections 123; parsons 152; portraiture 235; his paintings 236–7; *Analysis of Beauty* and Gothic 245
Holbein, Hans 235
Holcroft, Thomas 85; *Hugh Trevor* and country music 38
Homer 194
Homer, Henry on roads 74–5
Hooker, Richard 102, 179; *Ecclesiastical Politie* on social harmony 180, 182, 190

Horace 3
Howard, John 21, 87
Hughes, John 213; edits *Faerie Queene* 244
Hume, David 1, 127, 160, 162, 179–80; profits of *History* 94; political 'science' 131; reason and passions 192, 194–7; human nature 210, 215
Hussey, Christopher 218
Hutcheson, Francis 1, 179, 200, 214; utilitarianism 188; passions 196; moral sentiment 199
Hutton, William *History of Birmingham* and provincial life 38, commerce 77, 87

Jago, Richard 7
James II 56, 143; his abdication 98–9, 103
James, John 231
Jenyns, Soame 167
Jervas, Charles 250, 256
Johnson, Rev. Dr. 123
Johnson, Samuel 3, 8, 10, 19, 22–4, 30, 35, 43–4, 71, 96, 108, 127, 129, 141, 148, 162, 164, 173, 175, 208, 214, 216, 227, 238, 240, 259; London 5–6; pastorals 39, and allegories 235, 258; social unity 49–50; on *The Fleece* 66; social duty 82; Society of Arts 83; merchants 84; *Rasselas* on daily life 90, and religious faith 175, and moral philosophy 179, against optimism 206; on poverty 91; booksellers 93; Burke 114; political views 119, 123, 130–132; religious questions 140, 149, 164, 171–3, 177, preaching styles 152; episcopal politics 153; 'enthusiasm' 157;

'infidels' 162; reviews Soame Jenyns 167; on Law 173; *Idler* on benevolence 202; *Life of Milton* and moral philosophy 207; Blackmore 213; Reynolds's portraits 237; critical tenets 251–5

Jones, Inigo 229–31, 236; St. Paul's Covent Garden 150; the Burlingtonians 223; Palladianism 227, 233

Jonson, Ben 43, 91, 194

Jourdain, Margaret 218

'Junius' 107, 128; controversial style 134–5

Juvenal 6

Kalm, Pehr 27, 30

Kant, Immanuel 193

Kauffmann, Angelica 238

Keats, John 175, 209

Ken, Bishop Thomas 143

Kendal, Duchess of 110

Kent, Nathaniel 28

Kent, William 92, 222, 228, 233, 240, 242, 247; on Wren 221

Keppel, Augustus, Viscount 237

King, Archbishop William 110

King, William 32, 164

Klingender, F. D. 71, 83

Kneller, Sir Godfrey, Kit-cat portraits 19; his reputation 235–6

Knox, John 255

Knyff, Leonard, *Britannia Illustrata* 13, 222

Lackington, James 38

Lacombe, François 21

Laguerre, Louis 150; at Blenheim 258–9

Lamb, Charles 43, 187

Langland, William 91

Langton, Bennet 114

La Roche, Sophie von, London and its surroundings 10, 14–15, 17; Staines 34; Wesley 153

Lauderdale, James Maitland, Earl of 120

Law, William 138, 141, 158, 162, 164; religious duty 2, 168, 173–4; Bangorian controversy 141; influences John Wesley 145; on schisms 157, and irreligion 159; religious joy 169, 171

Lawrence, D. H. 198

Lawrence, Sir Thomas 237

Leapor, Mary, *Crumble Hall* 246

Lecky, W. E. H., the theatre 18; architecture 217

Lennox, Charlotte, *The Female Quixote* 247

Leoni, Giacomo, 222; Moor Park 234

Lessing, Gotthold Ephraim 214

L'Estrange, Sir Roger, controversial style 132, 135

Letters Concerning the Present State of England 38–9

Lillo, George, *The London Merchant* 85

Linnaeus, Carl 204

Locke, John 1, 92, 103, 113, 119, 122, 145, 179, 194, 198, 211, 236; *Treatises of Civil Government* and liberty 99–102; *Letters concerning Toleration* 100, 144; *Reasonableness of Christianity* and Latitudinarianism 144; God and man 164, 197; *Human Understanding* and epistemology 181, 183–8, 207; on poetry 184, and imagination 213; *Thoughts on Education* and Pamela 215

Longinus 199

Louis XIV 105
Loutherberg, Philip James de, at Coalbrookdale 83
Lucretius 213
Lyttelton, George, Lord 111, 257

Machiavelli, Nicolo 130
Mackworth, Sir Humphry, his mines 71–2
Macpherson, James 94, 97
Malebranche, Nicholas 214
Mallet, David 92; *Amyntor and Theodora* and trade 53; *Truth in Rhyme* 130; publishes Bolingbroke's works 162; *Excursion* and astronomy 212–13
Malthus, Thomas Robert 87
Mandeville, Bernard 215; and ridicule 160
Mann, Sir Horace 16, 113, 124, 128
Manning, Bernard 169
Marlborough, John Churchill, Duke of 105, 128; and Blenheim 232; *The Campaign* 259
Mary, Queen 143
Mason, William 229
Massinger, Philip 91
Mathias, T. J. anti-radicalism 38, 98, 118
Miller, Sanderson, his buildings 222
Milton, John 132, 145, 150, 179, 214, 230, 236, 255, 258
Mist's Journal 107
Mogul Tales 96
Molière, Jean Baptiste Poquelin 185
Montagu, Mrs. Elizabeth 19, 241
Montagu, George 15, 37, 161, 246
Montagu, Lady Mary Wortley 45
Montagu, Lord 92
Montesquieu, Charles de Secondat, Baron de 96; and Burke 120

Monthly Review, The 93
Morgann, Maurice 216
Moritz, Carl Philipp 30; London 9–11, 14; Richmond 14; Haymarket theatre 17; countryside 27; Dartford 35; roads 75; Parliament 126; at Nettlebed 156
Morland, George 247
Mortimer, Thomas, social evils 28; commerce 52, 85, 87–8; farming 59
Murdock, Patrick, on Thomson 168, 198
Murphy, Arthur 19

Namier, Sir Lewis 124
Newcastle, Thomas Pelham Holles, Duke of 125
Newcomen, Thomas 86
Newton, Sir Isaac 92, 140, 145, 177, 190, 194, 204, 207; imaginative impact of his *Opticks* 209, 212–13; Wood's halfpence 209
Newton, John 146, 169
Nicolson, Marjorie 212–13
Nixon, John 32
North, Bishop Brownlow 153–4
North, Frederick, Lord 116, 121; ecclesiastical patronage 153–4
Northumberland, Duchess of, her *Diaries* 16
Nourse, Timothy 179

Oates, Titus 132
Oglethorpe, James Edward 126
Oldfield, Mrs. Anne 18
Olivers, Thomas 169
Orme, Captain 237

Paine, Thomas 118; public executions 21

INDEX

Paley, William 211, 256; British constitution 126; religious faith 159, 206
Palladio, Andrea 222–3, 227—8, 233, 251
Parnell, Thomas 127; *Night Piece on Death* 176
Peacock, Thomas Love 246
Pelham, Henry, and Thomas 124, 162
Pennant, Thomas 205
Pepys, Samuel 203, 236
Percy, Thomas, and country clergy 155
Perronet, Edward 169
Peterborough, Charles Mordaunt, Earl of 105
Piranesi, Giovanni Battista 249
Pitt, William (the elder) 114
Plato 218
Pomfret, John 139; *The Choice* 3–4, 5
Pope, Alexander 3, 5, 9, 22, 43–4, 78, 111, 179, 214, 227, 240, 255; *Epistle to Burlington* and proprietorship 5, 61, on church decoration 150, on taste 219–20, 233; rural life 22–4, 31, 40; social imagery 45; social harmony 49; *Essay on Man* and social interdependence 52, 102–3, and slavery 80, political moderation 108, 128, and stability 129–30; on religious happiness 164, the passions 194–5, benevolence 198, man's humility 205–6, God's beneficence 206, Newton 207, 212; *Dunciad* and poverty 92, philosophy 165, 207; translates Homer 93, 97; *Rape of the Lock* and luxury 95, translucence 213; Persian fable 96; Locke 102; Roman Catholicism 142; *Messiah* 170; religious confidence 174; supremacy of moral philosophy 207; *Essay on Criticism* and 'the whole' 224, 253, and the ancients 251; poetry and painting 250, 256–7
Portland, William Henry Cavendish Bentinck, Duke of 116
Price, Richard, radicalism 103, 145, 162; *Principal Questions in Morals* 193
Price, Sir Uvedale, industrial despoliation 70, 83
Priestley, Joseph 84, 87, 103, 145, 162, 205–6, 211
Prior, Matthew 19, 128–9; patriotic zeal 109; religious spirit 139
Pulteney, William 111
Purcell, Henry 38
Pyle, Edmund 153

Queensberry, Duke and Duchess of 92
Quin, James 18

Radcliffe, Mrs. Anne 94
Radio Times, The 208
Raeburn, Sir Henry 236
Raistrick, Arthur 84
Ramsay, Allan 238
Raphael, Sanzio 219, 258
Ray, John 204
Repton, Humphrey 247
Revett, Nicholas 223
Reynolds, Sir Joshua 218, 236, 258; classical models 227; artistic tenets 229, 251–4; and Vanbrugh 233; his portraiture 237–8; P.R.A. 238–9

Richardson, Jonathan, art criticism 218-19, 251, 254-6
Richardson, Samuel 48, 94, 97; *Sir Charles Grandison* 234-5
Richardson, William 216
Robertson, William 94
Rodney, George, Baron 126
Roebuck, John 87
Romney, George 236, 238
Rooke, Sir George 105
Roscommon, Wentworth Dillon, Earl of 139
Roubiliac, Louis François 236
Rowe, Nicholas 127
Rowlandson, Thomas 248
Royal Academy, The, its foundation 18, 238-9
Royal Society, The, its foundation and results 203-5, 208-9, 214
Ruskin, John 218, 249
Ruysdael, Jakob van, and the picturesque 247
Rysbrack, Pieter Andrias 236

Sacheverell, Henry 105; *The Perils of False Brethren* 107; *The Communication of Sin* 133; his trial 140-1
Sadleir, Michael *Northanger Novels* 249
Salvator Rosa and the picturesque 235, 247
Sampson, George 169
Sancroft, Archbishop William 143
Sandwich, John Montagu, Earl of and Wilkes 44
Savage, Richard, the Thames 11; *Epistle to Walpole* 56; slavery 80-1; *Of Public Spirit* 81-2; attacks venality 111
Scheemakers, Peter 236
Scott, Geoffrey, *The Architecture of Humanism* 224-6

Scott, Helenus, *Adventures of a Rupee* 126
Scott, Sir Walter 94; and history 243
Secker, Archbishop Thomas 158
Shadwell, Thomas 23
Shaftesbury, Anthony Ashley Cooper, Earl of 1, 160, 179, 214; and ridicule 160; religious optimism 164; benevolence 197-9, 200; man's humility 205; aesthetic taste 218, 221, 228, 230
Shakespeare, William 18, 132-3, 148, 168, 175, 182, 194, 236, 244-5, 254
Sharp, Granville 81
Shebbeare, John 30; London 5; country life 30-1, 37; the literary profession 92; 'enthusiasm' 157; on science 208; portrait vogue 235
Shelley, Percy Bysshe 118-19, 131, 183
Shenstone, William 4, 7, 19; 1745 113; The Leasowes 234
Sheraton, Thomas 239
Sheridan, Richard Brinsley 18-19, 23, 49, 93, 128, 256
Siddons, Mrs. 18, 237, 258
Simeon, Charles 146
Smart, Christopher, *Song to David* 170, 176; and Blake 177
Smith, Adam 1, 18, 55, 91, 188, 211; rural progress 25; benefits of commerce 53, 88; *The Wealth of Nations* 88-9, 115; *Theory of Moral Sentiments* 88, 180, and the passions 196, 200-1
Smith, Sir James Edward 204
Smollett, Tobias George 9, 30, 32, 91, 127, 259; rural life 27-8;

riots 28; *Critical Review* 93; prose style 94; *Roderick Random* and sea-faring 95; benevolence 202; *Humphry Clinker* and Gothic 244
Society for the Abolition of Slavery 73
Society for the Encouragement of the Arts 83
Somers, John, Baron 92
Somervile, William 32–3; country life 40; on Addison 170
South, Robert 221
South Sea Company 12; the Bubble 57–8; India 80
Southey, Robert 118
Spectator, The rural conditions 31, 37–8, 61; Bank of England 56; Royal Exchange 78–9; commercial virtues 84, 86–7, 90; Locke 102; politics 106; religion 139, 155, 165–6, 170–1; 'enthusiasm' 157; irreligion 159–61; its public 180; the passions 194; science 206–8, 212–13; popularisation of ideas 210; taste 217; Gothic 242
Spence, Joseph 31, 96, 142, 244
Spenser, Edmund 49; John Hughes on 244
Spinoza, Baruch 133
Sprat, Thomas 203, 208, 210
Stafford, Granville Leveson-Gower, Marquis of 76
Steele, Richard 44, 48, 127–9, 162, 236; commercial life 84–5, 91; expelled from Commons 105; *The Crisis* popular 107; religious matters 159, 170
Stephen, Sir Leslie 113, 138–9
Sterne, Laurence 48, 94; as parson 152–3; associationism 215

St. James's Magazine 39
St. John, Henry, see Bolingbroke
Stuart, James ('The Old Pretender') 105–6
Stuart, James (architect) 223, 241
Sutherland, J. R. 50
Swift, Jonathan 19, 22, 40–1, 44–5, 48, 123, 127–8, 153, 162, 171, 206, 208, 211, 245, 255; London 6, 8–9, 18, 43; country 13, 22, 32, 37; social unity 49–50; South Sea Bubble 58; relations to Harley 92; *Gulliver's Travels*, success 93, and Ireland 110, sectarian quarrels 143; his prose style 93, 133–4, 211; on Whigs 104, 147–8; political dissension 105–8; *Conduct of the Allies*, its effect 107; Ireland 109–11; political 'science' 130–1; religious disputes 139, 143, 146; his religious position 146–8, 157–9; preaching styles 151–2; clerical poverty 154; Addison 170; Locke's semasiology 185; on science 207, 209

Talman, William 230
Tatler, The 37; preaching styles 151–2
Tawney, R. H. *Religion and the Rise of Capitalism* 86–7
Taylor, Jeremy 180, 211
Tenison, Archbishop Thomas 143–4
Thackeray, W. M. 43
Thomson, James 92, 128, 186, 189; *The Seasons* and patriotic zeal 4–5, country scenes 40, 59, theism 176, 206, Shaftesbury 198–9, descriptive methods 214, and scenery

257; *Liberty* and the Thames 11, commerce 53, 79-80, British constitution 100, political virtue 111-12, the Enlightenment 164, 183; *Castle of Indolence* and national progress 53-4; success of *Sophonisba* 93; Biblical influence 168; Burlington 222

Thornhill, Sir James 258-9

Tickell, Thomas 40; *Kensington Garden* 13; *On the Prospects of Peace* 78; Addison 170, 177-8; Gothic 242

Tillotson, Archbishop John, Latitudinarianism 144; the Bible's style 160, 168; Boyle lectures 203

Tindal, Matthew, *Christianity as Old as the Creation* 161, 192; Johnson on 162

Toland, John 161, 176

Tone, Wolfe 110

Tonson, Jacob 236

Toplady, Augustus Montagu 169

Torrington, Viscount, see Byng, John

Townshend, Charles, Viscount 64

Trapp, Joseph 151

Trevelyan, G. M., on country life 24; 1688 94

Tull, Jethro 64

Utilitarianism 188-9

Vanbrugh, Sir John 221-2, 228, 230, 236; his architecture 232-3, 240, 255

Vardy, John 228, 255

Verrio, Antonio 150

Vertue, George 92

Vesey, Mrs. Elizabeth 19

Virgil 194

Voltaire 84, 191-2, 206

Walker, Aaron 86

Walker, Jonathan 86

Waller, Edmund 98, 139

Wallis, John 203

Wallis, Captain Samuel 77-8

Walpole, Horace 10, 17, 32, 38, 91, 127, 256; London scenes 15-16; provincial life 37, 76; 'Jemmy Twitcher' 44; social round 46; industry 70; Gothick 94, and Strawberry 245-6; 1745 113; Burke 123; bribery 124; pessimism 128; Methodists 142; 'freethinking' 161

Walpole, Sir Robert 49, 56, 84, 104, 107, 128; and commerce 55, 114; as patron 92; Wood's halfpence 110; corruption 111, 124, 134; the bishops 153; Houghton 234

Walsh, William 236

Walton, Izaac 211

Warburton, William 162; Locke 103; Sterne 153; *Divine Legation* 179; and Gothic 244-5

Ward, Edward 12, 45; London 8; Dissent 136, 146, 148

Ward, James 30

Ware, Isaac 228

Watt, James 84, 86

Watts, Isaac 169-70, 176

Wedgwood, Josiah 4, 81, 84, 87, 145; pottery industry 72-4

Wendeborn, F. A., *View of England*, on justice 2, London scenes 6, 9, 12, 15-16, 19; social evils 21, 80

Wesley, Charles 145; hymns 169, 177

INDEX

Wesley, John 157; social progress 4; poverty 20, 159; farming 29; Unitarians 145; Methodism 145–6; church apathy 151; on Sterne 153

West, Benjamin 238

Wharton, Thomas, Marquis of 109, 111

Whateley, Richard 216

Whichcote, Benjamin, religious dissension 182–3; moral law 191

Whiston, William 140, 145

White, Gilbert 4; *Natural History of Selborne* 41, 205

Whitefield, George 146

Whitehead, Paul 33, 92

Wilberforce, William 126; on Hull 37; slavery 81; Evangelicalism 146

Wilkes, John, his prosecution 107, 126; Johnson on 130

William III 56, 98, 104, 143, 147

Wilson, Richard 238

Wollaston, William 161; scientific optimism 205–6

Wollstonecraft, Mary 118, 193

Wood, Anthony à 242–3

Wood, John (elder and younger) 234

Wood, Robert 223

Wood, William, his halfpence 109–11

Woolf, Virginia 43

Wordsworth, William 187, 198, 209, 214; Godwin 118–19, 194

Wren, Sir Christopher 12, 227, 231, 236, 240, 251, 255; church design 150, 228, 230; 'gusto' 221; canons of design 224; Carlyle on Chelsea Hospital 225, 230; his architectural career 229–30; Gothic 242, 244

Wren, Christopher, junior, on Gothic 242

Wright, Joseph 84

Wyatt, James 16

Wycherley, William 236

Yalden, Thomas 80; mining 71–2

Yeats, W. B. 175

Young, Arthur 65; roads 30, 38, 74–5; enclosures 62; picturesque industry 84

Young, Edward, *Night Thoughts* and religious dispute 139, its popularity 139, irreligion 159, 162, pessimism 167, science 206; his *Last Day* 172

Zoffany, Johann 238, 256

Revised August, 1964

harper ✦ torchbooks

HUMANITIES AND SOCIAL SCIENCES

American Studies

JOHN R. ALDEN: The American Revolution, 1775-1783.† *Illus.* TB/3011

RAY STANNARD BAKER: Following the Color Line: *American Negro Citizenship in the Progressive Era.‡ Illus. Edited by Dewey W. Grantham, Jr.* TB/3053

RAY A. BILLINGTON: The Far Western Frontier, 1830-1860.† *Illus.* TB/3012

JOSEPH L. BLAU, Ed.: Cornerstones of Religious Freedom in America. *Selected Basic Documents, Court Decisions and Public Statements. Enlarged and revised edition with new Intro. by Editor* TB/118

RANDOLPH S. BOURNE: War and the Intellectuals: *Collected Essays, 1915-1919.‡ Edited by Carl Resek* TB/3043

A. RUSSELL BUCHANAN: The United States and World War II. † *Illus.* Volume I TB/3044
Volume II TB/3045

ABRAHAM CAHAN: The Rise of David Levinsky: *a novel. Introduction by John Higham* TB/1028

JOSEPH CHARLES: The Origins of the American Party System TB/1049

THOMAS C. COCHRAN: The Inner Revolution: *Essays on the Social Sciences in History* TB/1140

T. C. COCHRAN & WILLIAM MILLER: The Age of Enterprise: *A Social History of Industrial America* TB/1054

EDWARD S. CORWIN: American Constitutional History: *Essays edited by Alpheus T. Mason and Gerald Garvey* TB/1136

FOSTER RHEA DULLES: America's Rise to World Power, 1898-1954.† *Illus.* TB/3021

W. A. DUNNING: Reconstruction, Political and Economic, 1865-1877 TB/1073

A. HUNTER DUPREE: Science in the Federal Government: *A History of Policies and Activities to 1940* TB/573

CLEMENT EATON: The Growth of Southern Civilization, 1790-1860.† *Illus.* TB/3040

HAROLD U. FAULKNER: Politics, Reform and Expansion, 1890-1900.† *Illus.* TB/3020

LOUIS FILLER: The Crusade against Slavery, 1830-1860.† *Illus.* TB/3029

EDITORS OF FORTUNE: America in the Sixties: *the Economy and the Society. Two-color charts* TB/1015

LAWRENCE HENRY GIPSON: The Coming of the Revolution, 1763-1775.† *Illus.* TB/3007

FRANCIS J. GRUND: Aristocracy in America: *Jacksonian Democracy* TB/1001

ALEXANDER HAMILTON: The Reports of Alexander Hamilton.‡ *Edited by Jacob E. Cooke* TB/3060

OSCAR HANDLIN, Editor: This Was America: *As Recorded by European Travelers to the Western Shore in the Eighteenth, Nineteenth, and Twentieth Centuries. Illus.* TB/1119

MARCUS LEE HANSEN: The Atlantic Migration: 1607-1860. *Edited by Arthur M. Schlesinger; Introduction by Oscar Handlin* TB/1052

MARCUS LEE HANSEN: The Immigrant in American History. *Edited with a Foreword by Arthur Schlesinger, Sr.* TB/1120

JOHN D. HICKS: Republican Ascendancy, 1921-1933.† *Illus.* TB/3041

JOHN HIGHAM, Ed.: The Reconstruction of American History TB/1068

DANIEL R. HUNDLEY: Social Relations in our Southern States.‡ *Edited by William R. Taylor* TB/3058

ROBERT H. JACKSON: The Supreme Court in the American System of Government TB/1106

THOMAS JEFFERSON: Notes on the State of Virginia.‡ *Edited by Thomas Perkins Abernethy* TB/3052

WILLIAM L. LANGER & S. EVERETT GLEASON: The Challenge to Isolation: *The World Crisis of 1937-1940 and American Foreign Policy* Volume I TB/3054
Volume II TB/3055

WILLIAM E. LEUCHTENBURG: Franklin D. Roosevelt and the New Deal, 1932-1940.† *Illus.* TB/3025

LEONARD W. LEVY: Freedom of Speech and Press in Early American History: *Legacy of Suppression* TB/1109

ARTHUR S. LINK: Woodrow Wilson and the Progressive Era, 1910-1917.† *Illus.* TB/3023

ROBERT GREEN McCLOSKEY: American Conservatism in the Age of Enterprise, 1865-1910 TB/1137

BERNARD MAYO: Myths and Men: *Patrick Henry, George Washington, Thomas Jefferson* TB/1108

JOHN C. MILLER: Alexander Hamilton and the Growth of the New Nation TB/3057

JOHN C. MILLER: The Federalist Era, 1789-1801.† *Illus.* TB/3027

---

† The New American Nation Series, edited by Henry Steele Commager and Richard B. Morris.
‡ American Perspectives series, edited by Bernard Wishy and William E. Leuchtenburg.
* The Rise of Modern Europe series, edited by William L. Langer.
❙ Researches in the Social, Cultural, and Behavioral Sciences, edited by Benjamin Nelson.
§ The Library of Religion and Culture, edited by Benjamin Nelson.
Σ Harper Modern Science Series, edited by James R. Newman.
º Not for sale in Canada.

PERRY MILLER: Errand into the Wilderness TB/1139
PERRY MILLER & T. H. JOHNSON, Editors: The Puritans: A Sourcebook of Their Writings
Volume I TB/1093
Volume II TB/1094
GEORGE E. MOWRY: The Era of Theodore Roosevelt and the Birth of Modern America, 1900-1912.† Illus. TB/3022
WALLACE NOTESTEIN: The English People on the Eve of Colonization, 1603-1630.† Illus. TB/3006
RUSSEL BLAINE NYE: The Cultural Life of the New Nation, 1776-1801.† Illus. TB/3026
RALPH BARTON PERRY: Puritanism and Democracy TB/1138
GEORGE E. PROBST, Ed.: The Happy Republic: A Reader in Tocqueville's America TB/1060
WALTER RAUSCHENBUSCH: Christianity and the Social Crisis.‡ Edited by Robert D. Cross TB/3059
FRANK THISTLETHWAITE: America and the Atlantic Community: Anglo-American Aspects, 1790-1850 TB/1107
TWELVE SOUTHERNERS: I'll Take My Stand: The South and the Agrarian Tradition. Introduction by Louis D. Rubin, Jr.; Biographical Essays by Virginia Rock TB/1072
A. F. TYLER: Freedom's Ferment: Phases of American Social History from the Revolution to the Outbreak of the Civil War. Illus. TB/1074
GLYNDON G. VAN DEUSEN: The Jacksonian Era, 1828-1848.† Illus. TB/3028
WALTER E. WEYL: The New Democracy: An Essay on Certain Political and Economic Tendencies in the United States.‡ Edited by Charles Forcey TB/3042
LOUIS B. WRIGHT: The Cultural Life of the American Colonies, 1607-1763.† Illus. TB/3005
LOUIS B. WRIGHT: Culture on the Moving Frontier TB/1053

Anthropology & Sociology

BERNARD BERELSON, Ed.: The Behavioral Sciences Today TB/1127
JOSEPH B. CASAGRANDE, Ed.: In the Company of Man: 20 Portraits of Anthropological Informants. Illus. TB/3047
W. E. LE GROS CLARK: The Antecedents of Man: An Introduction to the Evolution of the Primates.° Illus. TB/559
THOMAS C. COCHRAN: The Inner Revolution: Essays on the Social Sciences in History TB/1140
ALLISON DAVIS & JOHN DOLLARD: Children of Bondage: The Personality Development of Negro Youth in the Urban South∥ TB/3049
ST. CLAIR DRAKE & HORACE R. CAYTON: Black Metropolis: A Study of Negro Life in a Northern City. Introduction by Everett C. Hughes. Tables, maps, charts and graphs
Volume I TB/1086
Volume II TB/1087
CORA DU BOIS: The People of Alor. New Preface by the author. Illus.
Volume I TB/1042
Volume II TB/1043
LEON FESTINGER, HENRY W. RIECKEN & STANLEY SCHACHTER: When Prophecy Fails: A Social and Psychological Account of a Modern Group that Predicted the Destruction of the World∥ TB/1132
RAYMOND FIRTH, Ed.: Man and Culture: An Evaluation of the Work of Bronislaw Malinowski∥° TB/1133

L. S. B. LEAKEY: Adam's Ancestors: The Evolution of Man and his Culture. Illus. TB/1019
KURT LEWIN: Field Theory in Social Science: Selected Theoretical Papers.∥ Edited with a Foreword by Dorwin Cartwright TB/1135
ROBERT H. LOWIE: Primitive Society. Introduction by Fred Eggan TB/1056
BENJAMIN NELSON: Religious Traditions and the Spirit of Capitalism: From the Church Fathers to Jeremy Bentham TB/1130
TALCOTT PARSONS & EDWARD A. SHILS, Editors: Toward a General Theory of Action: Theoretical Foundations for the Social Sciences TB/1083
JOHN H. ROHRER & MUNRO S. EDMONSON, Eds.: The Eighth Generation Grows Up: Cultures and Personalities of New Orleans Negroes∥ TB/3050
ARNOLD ROSE: The Negro in America: The Condensed Version of Gunnar Myrdal's An American Dilemma. New Introduction by the Author; Foreword by Gunnar Myrdal TB/3048
KURT SAMUELSSON: Religion and Economic Action: A Critique of Max Weber's The Protestant Ethic and the Spirit of Capitalism.∥° Trans. by E. G. French; Ed. with Intro. by D. C. Coleman TB/1131
PITIRIM SOROKIN: Contemporary Sociological Theories: Through the First Quarter of the Twentieth Century TB/3046
MAURICE R. STEIN: The Eclipse of Community: An Interpretation of American Studies. New Introduction by the Author TB/1128
SIR EDWARD TYLOR: The Origins of Culture. Part I of "Primitive Culture."§ Introduction by Paul Radin TB/33
SIR EDWARD TYLOR: Religion in Primitive Culture. Part II of "Primitive Culture."§ Introduction by Paul Radin TB/34
W. LLOYD WARNER & Associates: Democracy in Jonesville: A Study in Quality and Inequality** TB/1129
W. LLOYD WARNER: A Black Civilization: A Study of an Australian Tribe.∥ Illus. TB/3056
W. LLOYD WARNER: Social Class in America: The Evaluation of Status TB/1013

Art and Art History

EMILE MÂLE: The Gothic Image: Religious Art in France of the Thirteenth Century.§ 190 illus. TB/44
MILLARD MEISS: Painting in Florence and Siena after the Black Death. 169 illus. TB/1148
ERWIN PANOFSKY: Studies in Iconology: Humanistic Themes in the Art of the Renaissance. 180 illustrations TB/1077
ALEXANDRE PIANKOFF: The Shrines of Tut-Ankh-Amon. Edited by N. Rambova. 117 illus. TB/2011
JEAN SEZNEC: The Survival of the Pagan Gods: The Mythological Tradition and Its Place in Renaissance Humanism and Art. 108 illustrations TB/2004
OTTO VON SIMSON: The Gothic Cathedral: Origins of Gothic Architecture and the Medieval Concept of Order. 58 illus. TB/2018
HEINRICH ZIMMER: Myths and Symbols in Indian Art and Civilization. 70 illustrations TB/2005

Business, Economics & Economic History

REINHARD BENDIX: Work and Authority in Industry: Ideologies of Management in the Course of Industrialization TB/3035

THOMAS C. COCHRAN: The American Business System: *A Historical Perspective, 1900-1955*　TB/1080
ROBERT DAHL & CHARLES E. LINDBLOM: Politics, Economics, and Welfare: *Planning and Politico-Economic Systems Resolved into Basic Social Processes*　TB/3037
PETER F. DRUCKER: The New Society: *The Anatomy of Industrial Order*　TB/1082
ROBERT L. HEILBRONER: The Great Ascent: *The Struggle for Economic Development in Our Time*　TB/3030
ABBA P. LERNER: Everybody's Business: *A Re-examination of Current Assumptions in Economics and Public Policy*　TB/3051
ROBERT GREEN McCLOSKEY: American Conservatism in the Age of Enterprise, 1865-1910　TB/1137
PAUL MANTOUX: The Industrial Revolution in the Eighteenth Century: *The Beginnings of the Modern Factory System in England*°　TB/1079
WILLIAM MILLER, Ed.: Men in Business: *Essays on the Historical Role of the Entrepreneur*　TB/1081
PERRIN STRYKER: The Character of the Executive: *Eleven Studies in Managerial Qualities*　TB/1041
PIERRE URI: Partnership for Progress: *A Program for Transatlantic Action*　TB/3036

Contemporary Culture

JACQUES BARZUN: The House of Intellect　TB/1051
JOHN U. NEF: Cultural Foundations of Industrial Civilization　TB/1024
PAUL VALÉRY: The Outlook for Intelligence　TB/2016

History: General

L. CARRINGTON GOODRICH: A Short History of the Chinese People. *Illus.*　TB/3015
BERNARD LEWIS: The Arabs in History　TB/1029
SIR PERCY SYKES: A History of Exploration.° *Introduction by John K. Wright*　TB/1046

History: Ancient and Medieval

A. ANDREWES: The Greek Tyrants　TB/1103
P. BOISSONNADE: Life and Work in Medieval Europe.° *Preface by Lynn White, Jr.*　TB/1141
HELEN CAM: England before Elizabeth　TB/1026
NORMAN COHN: The Pursuit of the Millennium: *Revolutionary Messianism in medieval and Reformation Europe and its bearing on modern Leftist and Rightist totalitarian movements*　TB/1037
G. G. COULTON: Medieval Village, Manor, and Monastery　TB/1022
HEINRICH FICHTENAU: The Carolingian Empire: *The Age of Charlemagne*　TB/1142
F. L. GANSHOF: Feudalism　TB/1058
J. M. HUSSEY: The Byzantine World　TB/1057
SAMUEL NOAH KRAMER: Sumerian Mythology　TB/1055
FERDINAND LOT: The End of the Ancient World and the Beginnings of the Middle Ages. *Introduction by Glanville Downey*　TB/1044
STEVEN RUNCIMAN: A History of the Crusades. Volume I: *The First Crusade and the Foundation of the Kingdom of Jerusalem. Illus.*　TB/1143

HENRY OSBORN TAYLOR: The Classical Heritage of the Middle Ages. *Foreword and Biblio. by Kenneth M. Setton* [Formerly listed as TB/48 under the title *The Emergence of Christian Culture in the West*]　TB/1117
J. M. WALLACE-HADRILL: The Barbarian West: *The Early Middle Ages, A.D. 400-1000*　TB/1061

History: Renaissance & Reformation

R. R. BOLGAR: The Classical Heritage and Its Beneficiaries: *From the Carolingian Age to the End of the Renaissance*　TB/1125
JACOB BURCKHARDT: The Civilization of the Renaissance in Italy. *Introduction by Benjamin Nelson and Charles Trinkaus. Illus.*　Volume I　TB/40
　Volume II　TB/41
ERNST CASSIRER: The Individual and the Cosmos in Renaissance Philosophy. *Translated with an Introduction by Mario Domandi*　TB/1097
EDWARD P. CHEYNEY: The Dawn of a New Era, 1250-1453.* *Illus.*　TB/3002
WALLACE K. FERGUSON, et al.: Facets of the Renaissance　TB/1098
WALLACE K. FERGUSON, et al.: The Renaissance: *Six Essays. Illus.*　TB/1084
MYRON P. GILMORE: The World of Humanism, 1453-1517.* *Illus.*　TB/3003
JOHAN HUIZINGA: Erasmus and the Age of Reformation. *Illus.*　TB/19
ULRICH VON HUTTEN, et al.: On the Eve of the Reformation: *"Letters of Obscure Men." Introduction by Hajo Holborn*　TB/1124
PAUL O. KRISTELLER: Renaissance Thought: *The Classic, Scholastic, and Humanist Strains*　TB/1048
NICCOLÒ MACHIAVELLI: History of Florence and of the Affairs of Italy: *from the earliest times to the death of Lorenzo the Magnificent. Introduction by Felix Gilbert*　TB/1027
ALFRED VON MARTIN: Sociology of the Renaissance. *Introduction by Wallace K. Ferguson*　TB/1099
MILLARD MEISS: Painting in Florence and Siena after the Black Death. *169 illus.*　TB/1148
J. E. NEALE: The Age of Catherine de Medici°　TB/1085
ERWIN PANOFSKY: Studies in Iconology: *Humanistic Themes in the Art of the Renaissance. 180 illustrations*　TB/1077
J. H. PARRY: The Establishment of the European Hegemony: 1415-1715: *Trade and Exploration in the Age of the Renaissance*　TB/1045
HENRI PIRENNE: Early Democracies in the Low Countries: *Urban Society and Political Conflict in the Middle Ages and the Renaissance. Introduction by John Mundy*　TB/1110
FERDINAND SCHEVILL: The Medici. *Illus.*　TB/1010
FERDINAND SCHEVILL: Medieval and Renaissance Florence. *Illus.* Volume I: *Medieval Florence*　TB/1090
　Volume II: *The Coming of Humanism and the Age of the Medici*　TB/1091
G. M. TREVELYAN: England in the Age of Wycliffe, 1368-1520°　TB/1112
VESPASIANO: Renaissance Princes, Popes, and Prelates: *The Vespasiano Memoirs: Lives of Illustrious Men of the XVth Century. Introduction by Myron P. Gilmore*　TB/1111

3

History: Modern European

FREDERICK B. ARTZ: Reaction and Revolution, 1815-1852.* *Illus.* TB/3034
MAX BELOFF: The Age of Absolutism, 1660-1815 TB/1062
ROBERT C. BINKLEY: Realism and Nationalism, 1852-1871.* *Illus.* TB/3038
CRANE BRINTON: A Decade of Revolution, 1789-1799.* *Illus.* TB/3018
J. BRONOWSKI & BRUCE MAZLISH: The Western Intellectual Tradition: *From Leonardo to Hegel* TB/3001
GEOFFREY BRUUN: Europe and the French Imperium, 1799-1814.* *Illus.* TB/3033
ALAN BULLOCK: Hitler, A Study in Tyranny.º *Illus.* TB/1123
E. H. CARR: The Twenty Years' Crisis, 1919-1939: *An Introduction to the Study of International Relations*º TB/1122
WALTER L. DORN: Competition for Empire, 1740-1763.* *Illus.* TB/3032
CARL J. FRIEDRICH: The Age of the Baroque, 1610-1660.* *Illus.* TB/3004
LEO GERSHOY: From Despotism to Revolution, 1763-1789.* *Illus.* TB/3017
ALBERT GOODWIN: The French Revolution TB/1064
CARLTON J. H. HAYES: A Generation of Materialism, 1871-1900.* *Illus.* TB/3039
J. H. HEXTER: Reappraisals in History: *New Views on History and Society in Early Modern Europe* TB/1100
A. R. HUMPHREYS: The Augustan World: *Society, Thought, and Letters in Eighteenth Century England* TB/1105
HANS KOHN, Ed.: The Mind of Modern Russia: *Historical and Political Thought of Russia's Great Age* TB/1065
SIR LEWIS NAMIER: Vanished Supremacies: *Essays on European History, 1812-1918*º TB/1088
JOHN U. NEF: Western Civilization Since the Renaissance: *Peace, War, Industry, and the Arts* TB/1113
FREDERICK L. NUSSBAUM: The Triumph of Science and Reason, 1660-1685.* *Illus.* TB/3009
RAYMOND W. POSTGATE, Ed.: Revolution from 1789 to 1906: *Selected Documents* TB/1063
PENFIELD ROBERTS: The Quest for Security, 1715-1740.* *Illus.* TB/3016
PRISCILLA ROBERTSON: Revolutions of 1848: *A Social History* TB/1025
ALBERT SOREL: Europe Under the Old Regime. *Translated by Francis H. Herrick* TB/1121
N. N. SUKHANOV: The Russian Revolution, 1917: *Eyewitness Account. Edited by Joel Carmichael*
Volume I TB/1066
Volume II TB/1067
JOHN B. WOLF: The Emergence of the Great Powers, 1685-1715.* *Illus.* TB/3010
JOHN B. WOLF: France: 1814-1919: *The Rise of a Liberal-Democratic Society* TB/3019

Intellectual History

HERSCHEL BAKER: The Image of Man: *A Study of the Idea of Human Dignity in Classical Antiquity, the Middle Ages, and the Renaissance* TB/1047
J. BRONOWSKI & BRUCE MAZLISH: The Western Intellectual Tradition: *From Leonardo to Hegel* TB/3001
ERNST CASSIRER: The Individual and the Cosmos in Renaissance Philosophy. *Translated with an Introduction by Mario Domandi* TB/1097
NORMAN COHN: The Pursuit of the Millennium: *Revolutionary Messianism in medieval and Reformation Europe and its bearing on modern Leftist and Rightist totalitarian movements* TB/1037
ARTHUR O. LOVEJOY: The Great Chain of Being: *A Study of the History of an Idea* TB/1009
ROBERT PAYNE: Hubris: *A Study of Pride. Foreword by Sir Herbert Read* TB/1031
BRUNO SNELL: The Discovery of the Mind: *The Greek Origins of European Thought* TB/1018
ERNEST LEE TUVESON: Millennium and Utopia: *A Study in the Background of the Idea of Progress.* ▮ *New Preface by Author* TB/1134

Literature, Poetry, The Novel & Criticism

JAMES BAIRD: Ishmael: *The Art of Melville in the Contexts of International Primitivism* TB/1023
JACQUES BARZUN: The House of Intellect TB/1051
W. J. BATE: From Classic to Romantic: *Premises of Taste in Eighteenth Century England* TB/1036
RACHEL BESPALOFF: On the Iliad TB/2006
R. P. BLACKMUR, et al.: Lectures in Criticism. *Introduction by Huntington Cairns* TB/2003
ABRAHAM CAHAN: The Rise of David Levinsky: *a novel. Introduction by John Higham* TB/1028
ERNST R. CURTIUS: European Literature and the Latin Middle Ages TB/2015
GEORGE ELIOT: Daniel Deronda: *a novel. Introduction by F. R. Leavis* TB/1039
ETIENNE GILSON: Dante and Philosophy TB/1089
ALFRED HARBAGE: As They Liked It: *A Study of Shakespeare's Moral Artistry* TB/1035
STANLEY R. HOPPER, Ed.: Spiritual Problems in Contemporary Literature§ TB/21
A. R. HUMPHREYS: The Augustan World: *Society, Thought, and Letters in Eighteenth Century England*º TB/1105
ALDOUS HUXLEY: Antic Hay & The Gioconda Smile.º *Introduction by Martin Green* TB/3503
ALDOUS HUXLEY: Brave New World & Brave New World Revisited.º *Introduction by C. P. Snow* TB/3501
ALDOUS HUXLEY: Point Counter Point.º *Introduction by C. P. Snow* TB/3502
HENRY JAMES: The Princess Casamassima: *a novel. Introduction by Clinton F. Oliver* TB/1005
HENRY JAMES: Roderick Hudson: *a novel. Introduction by Leon Edel* TB/1016
HENRY JAMES: The Tragic Muse: *a novel. Introduction by Leon Edel* TB/1017
ARNOLD KETTLE: An Introduction to the English Novel. Volume I: *Defoe to George Eliot* TB/1011
Volume II: *Henry James to the Present* TB/1012
JOHN STUART MILL: On Bentham and Coleridge. *Introduction by F. R. Leavis* TB/1070
PERRY MILLER & T. H. JOHNSON, Editors: The Puritans: *A Sourcebook of Their Writings*
Volume I TB/1093
Volume II TB/1094
KENNETH B. MURDOCK: Literature and Theology in Colonial New England TB/99
SAMUEL PEPYS: The Diary of Samuel Pepys.º *Edited by O. F. Morshead. Illustrations by Ernest Shepard* TB/1007

ST.-JOHN PERSE: Seamarks TB/2002
O. E. RÖLVAAG: Giants in the Earth. *Introduction by Einar Haugen* TB/3504
GEORGE SANTAYANA: Interpretations of Poetry and Religion§ TB/9
C. P. SNOW: Time of Hope: *a novel* TB/1040
DOROTHY VAN GHENT: The English Novel: *Form and Function* TB/1050
E. B. WHITE: One Man's Meat. *Introduction by Walter Blair* TB/3505
MORTON DAUWEN ZABEL, Editor: Literary Opinion in America Volume I TB/3013
 Volume II TB/3014

Myth, Symbol & Folklore

JOSEPH CAMPBELL, Editor: Pagan and Christian Mysteries. *Illus.* TB/2013
MIRCEA ELIADE: Cosmos and History: *The Myth of the Eternal Return*§ TB/2050
C. G. JUNG & C. KERÉNYI: Essays on a Science of Mythology: *The Myths of the Divine Child and the Divine Maiden* TB/2014
ERWIN PANOFSKY: Studies in Iconology: *Humanistic Themes in the Art of the Renaissance. 180 illustrations* TB/1077
JEAN SEZNEC: The Survival of the Pagan Gods: *The Mythological Tradition and its Place in Renaissance Humanism and Art. 108 illustrations* TB/2004
HELLMUT WILHELM: Change: *Eight Lectures on the I Ching* TB/2019
HEINRICH ZIMMER: Myths and Symbols in Indian Art and Civilization. *70 illustrations* TB/2005

Philosophy

HENRI BERGSON: Time and Free Will: *An Essay on the Immediate Data of Consciousness*[o] TB/1021
H. J. BLACKHAM: Six Existentialist Thinkers: *Kierkegaard, Nietzsche, Jaspers, Marcel, Heidegger, Sartre*[o] TB/1002
ERNST CASSIRER: Rousseau, Kant and Goethe. *Introduction by Peter Gay* TB/1092
FREDERICK COPLESTON: Medieval Philosophy[o] TB/76
F. M. CORNFORD: From Religion to Philosophy: *A Study in the Origins of Western Speculation*§ TB/20
WILFRID DESAN: The Tragic Finale: *An Essay on the Philosophy of Jean-Paul Sartre* TB/1030
PAUL FRIEDLÄNDER: Plato: *An Introduction* TB/2017
ETIENNE GILSON: Dante and Philosophy TB/1089
WILLIAM CHASE GREENE: Moira: *Fate, Good, and Evil in Greek Thought* TB/1104
W. K. C. GUTHRIE: The Greek Philosophers: *From Thales to Aristotle*[o] TB/1008
F. H. HEINEMANN: Existentialism and the Modern Predicament TB/28
IMMANUEL KANT: The Doctrine of Virtue, *being Part II of The Metaphysic of Morals. Translated with Notes and Introduction by Mary J. Gregor. Foreword by H. J. Paton* TB/110
IMMANUEL KANT: Lectures on Ethics.§ *Introduction by Lewis W. Beck* TB/105
WILLARD VAN ORMAN QUINE: From a Logical Point of View: *Logico-Philosophical Essays* TB/566

BERTRAND RUSSELL et al.: The Philosophy of Bertrand Russell. *Edited by Paul Arthur Schilpp*
 Volume I TB/1095
 Volume II TB/1096
L. S. STEBBING: A Modern Introduction to Logic TB/538
ALFRED NORTH WHITEHEAD: Process and Reality: *An Essay in Cosmology* TB/1033
WILHELM WINDELBAND: A History of Philosophy I: *Greek, Roman, Medieval* TB/38
WILHELM WINDELBAND: A History of Philosophy II: *Renaissance, Enlightenment, Modern* TB/39

Philosophy of History

NICOLAS BERDYAEV: The Beginning and the End§ TB/14
NICOLAS BERDYAEV: The Destiny of Man TB/61
WILHELM DILTHEY: Pattern and Meaning in History: *Thoughts on History and Society.*[o] *Edited with an Introduction by H. P. Rickman* TB/1075
RAYMOND KLIBANSKY & H. J. PATON, Eds.: Philosophy and History: *The Ernst Cassirer Festschrift. Illus.* TB/1115
JOSE ORTEGA Y GASSET: The Modern Theme. *Introduction by Jose Ferrater Mora* TB/1038
KARL R. POPPER: The Poverty of Historicism[o] TB/1126
W. H. WALSH: Philosophy of History: *An Introduction* TB/1020

Political Science & Government

JEREMY BENTHAM: The Handbook of Political Fallacies: *Introduction by Crane Brinton* TB/1069
KENNETH E. BOULDING: Conflict and Defense: *A General Theory* TB/3024
CRANE BRINTON: English Political Thought in the Nineteenth Century TB/1071
EDWARD S. CORWIN: American Constitutional History: *Essays edited by Alpheus T. Mason and Gerald Garvey* TB/1136
ROBERT DAHL & CHARLES E. LINDBLOM: Politics, Economics, and Welfare: *Planning and Politico-Economic Systems Resolved into Basic Social Processes* TB/3037
JOHN NEVILLE FIGGIS: Political Thought from Gerson to Grotius: *1414-1625: Seven Studies. Introduction by Garrett Mattingly* TB/1032
F. L. GANSHOF: Feudalism TB/1058
G. P. GOOCH: English Democratic Ideas in the Seventeenth Century TB/1006
ROBERT H. JACKSON: The Supreme Court in the American System of Government TB/1106
DAN N. JACOBS, Ed.: The New Communist Manifesto and Related Documents TB/1078
DAN N. JACOBS & HANS BAERWALD, Eds.: Chinese Communism: *Selected Documents* TB/3031
ROBERT GREEN McCLOSKEY: American Conservatism in the Age of Enterprise, 1865-1910 TB/1137
KINGSLEY MARTIN: French Liberal Thought in the Eighteenth Century: *A Study of Political Ideas from Bayle to Condorcet* TB/1114
JOHN STUART MILL: On Bentham and Coleridge. *Introduction by F. R. Leavis* TB/1070
JOHN B. MORRALL: Political Thought in Medieval Times TB/1076

KARL R. POPPER: The Open Society and Its Enemies
Volume I: *The Spell of Plato* TB/1101
Volume II: *The High Tide of Prophecy: Hegel, Marx, and the Aftermath* TB/1102
JOSEPH A. SCHUMPETER: Capitalism, Socialism and Democracy TB/3008

Psychology

ALFRED ADLER: Problems of Neurosis. Introduction by Heinz L. Ansbacher TB/1145
ANTON T. BOISEN: The Exploration of the Inner World: *A Study of Mental Disorder and Religious Experience* TB/87
LEON FESTINGER, HENRY W. RIECKEN, STANLEY SCHACHTER: When Prophecy Fails: *A Social and Psychological Study of a Modern Group that Predicted the Destruction of the World* ‖ TB/1132
SIGMUND FREUD: On Creativity and the Unconscious: *Papers on the Psychology of Art, Literature, Love, Religion.*§ *Intro. by Benjamin Nelson* TB/45
C. JUDSON HERRICK: The Evolution of Human Nature TB/545
ALDOUS HUXLEY: The Devils of Loudun: *A Study in the Psychology of Power Politics and Mystical Religion in the France of Cardinal Richelieu*§° TB/60
WILLIAM JAMES: Psychology: *The Briefer Course.* Edited with an Intro. by Gordon Allport TB/1034
C. G. JUNG: Psychological Reflections. Edited by Jolande Jacobi TB/2001
C. G. JUNG: Symbols of Transformation: *An Analysis of the Prelude to a Case of Schizophrenia. Illus.*
Volume I TB/2009
Volume II TB/2010
C. G. JUNG & C. KERÉNYI: Essays on a Science of Mythology: *The Myths of the Divine Child and the Divine Maiden* TB/2014
SOREN KIERKEGAARD: Repetition: *An Essay in Experimental Psychology. Translated with Introduction & Notes by Walter Lowrie* TB/117
KARL MENNINGER: Theory of Psychoanalytic Technique TB/1144
ERICH NEUMANN: Amor and Psyche: *The Psychic Development of the Feminine* TB/2012
ERICH NEUMANN: The Origins and History of Consciousness Volume I *Illus.* TB/2007
Volume II TB/2008
C. P. OBERNDORF: A History of Psychoanalysis in America TB/1147
JEAN PIAGET, BÄRBEL INHELDER, & ALINA SZEMINSKA: The Child's Conception of Geometry TB/1146

RELIGION

Ancient & Classical

J. H. BREASTED: Development of Religion and Thought in Ancient Egypt. Introduction by John A. Wilson TB/57
HENRI FRANKFORT: Ancient Egyptian Religion: *An Interpretation* TB/77
WILLIAM CHASE GREENE: Moira: *Fate, Good and Evil in Greek Thought* TB/1104

G. RACHEL LEVY: Religious Conceptions of the Stone Age *and their Influence upon European Thought. Illus. Introduction by Henri Frankfort* TB/106
MARTIN P. NILSSON: Greek Folk Religion. *Foreword by Arthur Darby Nock* TB/78
ALEXANDRE PIANKOFF: The Shrines of Tut-Ankh-Amon. *Edited by N. Rambova. 117 illus.* TB/2011
H. J. ROSE: Religion in Greece and Rome TB/55

Biblical Thought & Literature

W. F. ALBRIGHT: The Biblical Period from Abraham to Ezra TB/102
C. K. BARRETT, Ed.: The New Testament Background: *Selected Documents* TB/86
C. H. DODD: The Authority of the Bible TB/43
M. S. ENSLIN: Christian Beginnings TB/5
M. S. ENSLIN: The Literature of the Christian Movement TB/6
H. E. FOSDICK: A Guide to Understanding the Bible TB/2
H. H. ROWLEY: The Growth of the Old Testament TB/107
D. WINTON THOMAS, Ed.: Documents from Old Testament Times TB/85

Christianity: Origins & Early Development

ADOLF DEISSMANN: Paul: *A Study in Social and Religious History* TB/15
EDWARD GIBBON: The Triumph of Christendom in the Roman Empire *(Chaps. XV-XX of "Decline and Fall," J. B. Bury edition).*§ *Illus.* TB/46
MAURICE GOGUEL: Jesus and the Origins of Christianity.° *Introduction by C. Leslie Mitton*
Volume I: *Prolegomena to the Life of Jesus* TB/65
Volume II: *The Life of Jesus* TB/66
EDGAR J. GOODSPEED: A Life of Jesus TB/1
ADOLF HARNACK: The Mission and Expansion of Christianity *in the First Three Centuries. Introduction by Jaroslav Pelikan* TB/92
R. K. HARRISON: The Dead Sea Scrolls: *An Introduction*° TB/84
EDWIN HATCH: The Influence of Greek Ideas on Christianity.§ *Introduction and Bibliography by Frederick C. Grant* TB/18
ARTHUR DARBY NOCK: Early Gentile Christianity and Its Hellenistic Background TB/111
ARTHUR DARBY NOCK: St. Paul° TB/104
JOHANNES WEISS: Earliest Christianity: *A History of the Period A.D. 30-150. Introduction and Bibilography by Frederick C. Grant* Volume I TB/53
Volume II TB/54

Christianity: The Middle Ages, The Reformation, and After

G. P. FEDOTOV: The Russian Religious Mind: *Kievan Christianity, the tenth to the thirteenth centuries* TB/70
ÉTIENNE GILSON: Dante and Philosophy TB/1089
WILLIAM HALLER: The Rise of Puritanism TB/22
JOHAN HUIZINGA: Erasmus and the Age of Reformation. *Illus.* TB/19

JOHN T. McNEILL: Makers of Christianity: *From Alfred the Great to Schleiermacher* TB/121

A. C. McGIFFERT: Protestant Thought Before Kant. Preface by Jaroslav Pelikan TB/93

KENNETH B. MURDOCK: Literature and Theology in Colonial New England TB/99

GORDON RUPP: Luther's Progress to the Diet of Worms° TB/120

Judaic Thought & Literature

MARTIN BUBER: Eclipse of God: *Studies in the Relation Between Religion and Philosophy* TB/12

MARTIN BUBER: Moses: *The Revelation and the Covenant* TB/27

MARTIN BUBER: Pointing the Way. Introduction by Maurice S. Friedman TB/103

MARTIN BUBER: The Prophetic Faith TB/73

MARTIN BUBER: Two Types of Faith: *the interpenetration of Judaism and Christianity*° TB/75

MAURICE S. FRIEDMAN: Martin Buber: *The Life of Dialogue* TB/64

FLAVIUS JOSEPHUS: The Great Roman-Jewish War, with The Life of Josephus. Introduction by William R. Farmer TB/74

T. J. MEEK: Hebrew Origins TB/69

Oriental Religions: Far Eastern, Near Eastern

TOR ANDRAE: Mohammed: *The Man and His Faith* TB/62

EDWARD CONZE: Buddhism: *Its Essence and Development.*° Foreword by Arthur Waley TB/58

EDWARD CONZE, et al., Editors: Buddhist Texts Through the Ages TB/113

ANANDA COOMARASWAMY: Buddha and the Gospel of Buddhism TB/119

H. G. CREEL: Confucius and the Chinese Way TB/63

FRANKLIN EDGERTON, Trans. & Ed.: The Bhagavad Gita TB/115

SWAMI NIKHILANANDA, Trans. & Ed.: The Upanishads: *A One-Volume Abridgment* TB/114

HELLMUT WILHELM: Change: *Eight Lectures on the I Ching* TB/2019

Philosophy of Religion

RUDOLF BULTMANN: History and Eschatology: *The Presence of Eternity* TB/91

RUDOLF BULTMANN AND FIVE CRITICS: Kerygma and Myth: *A Theological Debate* TB/80

RUDOLF BULTMANN and KARL KUNDSIN: Form Criticism: *Two Essays on New Testament Research.* Translated by Frederick C. Grant TB/96

MIRCEA ELIADE: The Sacred and the Profane TB/81

LUDWIG FEUERBACH: The Essence of Christianity.§ Introduction by Karl Barth. Foreword by H. Richard Niebuhr TB/11

ADOLF HARNACK: What is Christianity?§ Introduction by Rudolf Bultmann TB/17

FRIEDRICH HEGEL: On Christianity: *Early Theological Writings.* Edited by Richard Kroner and T. M. Knox TB/79

KARL HEIM: Christian Faith and Natural Science TB/16

IMMANUEL KANT: Religion Within the Limits of Reason Alone.§ Introduction by Theodore M. Greene and John Silber TB/67

PIERRE TEILHARD DE CHARDIN: The Phenomenon of Man° TB/83

Religion, Culture & Society

JOSEPH L. BLAU, Ed.: Cornerstones of Religious Freedom in America: *Selected Basic Documents, Court Decisions and Public Statements. Enlarged and revised edition, with new Introduction by the Editor* TB/118

C. C. GILLISPIE: Genesis and Geology: *The Decades before Darwin*§ TB/51

BENJAMIN NELSON: Religious Traditions and the Spirit of Capitalism: *From the Church Fathers to Jeremy Bentham* TB/1130

H. RICHARD NIEBUHR: Christ and Culture TB/3

H. RICHARD NIEBUHR: The Kingdom of God In America TB/49

RALPH BARTON PERRY: Puritanism and Democracy TB/1138

WALTER RAUSCHENBUSCH: Christianity and the Social Crisis.‡ Edited by Robert D. Cross TB/3059

KURT SAMUELSSON: Religion and Economic Action: *A Critique of Max Weber's* The Protestant Ethic and the Spirit of Capitalism.‖° Trans. by E. G. French; Ed. with Intro. by D. C. Coleman TB/1131

ERNST TROELTSCH: The Social Teaching of the Christian Churches.° Introduction by H. Richard Niebuhr
Volume I TB/71
Volume II TB/72

Religious Thinkers & Traditions

AUGUSTINE: An Augustine Synthesis. Edited by Erich Przywara TB/35

KARL BARTH: Church Dogmatics: *A Selection.* Introduction by H. Gollwitzer; Edited by G. W. Bromiley TB/95

KARL BARTH: Dogmatics in Outline TB/56

KARL BARTH: The Word of God and the Word of Man TB/13

THOMAS CORBISHLEY, S. J.: Roman Catholicism TB/112

ADOLF DEISSMANN: Paul: *A Study in Social and Religious History* TB/15

JOHANNES ECKHART: Meister Eckhart: *A Modern Translation* by R. B. Blakney TB/8

WINTHROP HUDSON: The Great Tradition of the American Churches TB/98

SOREN KIERKEGAARD: Edifying Discourses. Edited with an Introduction by Paul Holmer TB/32

SOREN KIERKEGAARD: The Journals of Kierkegaard.° Edited with an Introduction by Alexander Dru TB/52

SOREN KIERKEGAARD: The Point of View for My Work as an Author: *A Report to History.§ Preface by Benjamin Nelson* TB/88

SOREN KIERKEGAARD: The Present Age.§ Translated and edited by Alexander Dru. Introduction by Walter Kaufmann TB/94

SOREN KIERKEGAARD: Purity of Heart. Translated by Douglas Steere TB/4

SOREN KIERKEGAARD: Repetition: *An Essay in Experimental Psychology.* Translated with Introduction & Notes by Walter Lowrie TB/117

SOREN KIERKEGAARD: Works of Love: *Some Christian Reflections in the Form of Discourses* TB/122

7

WALTER LOWRIE: Kierkegaard: *A Life*
Volume I TB/89
Volume II TB/90
GABRIEL MARCEL: Homo Viator: *Introduction to a Metaphysic of Hope* TB/97
PERRY MILLER: Errand into the Wilderness TB/1139
PERRY MILLER & T. H. JOHNSON, Editors: The Puritans: *A Sourcebook of Their Writings*
Volume I TB/1093
Volume II TB/1094
PAUL PFUETZE: Self, Society, Existence: *Human Nature and Dialogue in the Thought of George Herbert Mead and Martin Buber* TB/1059
F. SCHLEIERMACHER: The Christian Faith. *Introduction by Richard R. Niebuhr* Volume I TB/108
Volume II TB/109
F. SCHLEIERMACHER: On Religion: *Speeches to Its Cultured Despisers. Intro. by Rudolf Otto* TB/36
PAUL TILLICH: Dynamics of Faith TB/42
EVELYN UNDERHILL: Worship TB/10
G. VAN DER LEEUW: Religion in Essence and Manifestation: *A Study in Phenomenology. Appendices by Hans H. Penner* Volume I TB/100
Volume II TB/101

NATURAL SCIENCES AND MATHEMATICS

Biological Sciences

CHARLOTTE AUERBACH: The Science of Genetics∑ TB/568
A. BELLAIRS: Reptiles: *Life History, Evolution, and Structure. Illus.* TB/520
LUDWIG VON BERTALANFFY: Modern Theories of Development: *An Introduction to Theoretical Biology* TB/554
LUDWIG VON BERTALANFFY: Problems of Life: *An Evaluation of Modern Biological and Scientific Thought* TB/521
JOHN TYLER BONNER: The Ideas of Biology.∑ *Illus.* TB/570
HAROLD F. BLUM: Time's Arrow and Evolution TB/555
A. J. CAIN: Animal Species and their Evolution. *Illus.* TB/519
WALTER B. CANNON: Bodily Changes in Pain, Hunger, Fear and Rage. *Illus.* TB/562
W. E. LE GROS CLARK: The Antecedents of Man: *An Introduction to the Evolution of the Primates.*[o] *Illus.* TB/559
W. H. DOWDESWELL: Animal Ecology. *Illus.* TB/543
W. H. DOWDESWELL: The Mechanism of Evolution. *Illus.* TB/527
R. W. GERARD: Unresting Cells. *Illus.* TB/541
DAVID LACK: Darwin's Finches. *Illus.* TB/544
J. E. MORTON: Molluscs: *An Introduction to their Form and Functions. Illus.* TB/529
ADOLF PORTMANN: Animals as Social Beings.[o] *Illus.* TB/572
O. W. RICHARDS: The Social Insects. *Illus.* TB/542
P. M. SHEPPARD: Natural Selection and Heredity. *Illus.* TB/528
EDMUND W. SINNOTT: Cell and Psyche: *The Biology of Purpose* TB/546
C. H. WADDINGTON: How Animals Develop. *Illus.* TB/553

Chemistry

J. R. PARTINGTON: A Short History of Chemistry. *Illus.* TB/522
J. READ: A Direct Entry to Organic Chemistry. *Illus.* TB/523
J. READ: Through Alchemy to Chemistry. *Illus.* TB/561

Geography

R. E. COKER: This Great and Wide Sea: *An Introduction to Oceanography and Marine Biology. Illus.* TB/551
F. K. HARE: The Restless Atmosphere TB/560

History of Science

W. DAMPIER, Ed.: Readings in the Literature of Science. *Illus.* TB/512
A. HUNTER DUPREE: Science in the Federal Government: *A History of Policies and Activities to 1940* TB/573
ALEXANDRE KOYRÉ: From the Closed World to the Infinite Universe: *Copernicus, Kepler, Galileo, Newton, etc.* TB/31
A. G. VAN MELSEN: From Atomos to Atom: *A History of the Concept Atom* TB/517
O. NEUGEBAUER: The Exact Sciences in Antiquity TB/552
H. T. PLEDGE: Science Since 1500: *A Short History of Mathematics, Physics, Chemistry and Biology. Illus.* TB/506
GEORGE SARTON: Ancient Science and Modern Civilization TB/501
HANS THIRRING: Energy for Man: *From Windmills to Nuclear Power* TB/556
WILLIAM LAW WHYTE: Essay on Atomism: *From Democritus to 1960* TB/565
A. WOLF: A History of Science, Technology and Philosophy in the 16th and 17th Centuries.[o] *Illus.*
Volume I TB/508
Volume II TB/509
A. WOLF: A History of Science, Technology, and Philosophy in the Eighteenth Century.[o] *Illus.*
Volume I TB/539
Volume II TB/540

Mathematics

H. DAVENPORT: The Higher Arithmetic: *An Introduction to the Theory of Numbers* TB/526
H. G. FORDER: Geometry: *An Introduction* TB/548
GOTTLOB FREGE: The Foundations of Arithmetic: *A Logico-Mathematical Enquiry into the Concept of Number* TB/534
S. KÖRNER: The Philosophy of Mathematics: *An Introduction* TB/547
D. E. LITTLEWOOD: Skeleton Key of Mathematics: *A Simple Account of Complex Algebraic Problems* TB/525
GEORGE E. OWEN: Fundamentals of Scientific Mathematics TB/569
WILLARD VAN ORMAN QUINE: Mathematical Logic TB/558
O. G. SUTTON: Mathematics in Action.[o] *Foreword by James R. Newman. Illus.* TB/518
FREDERICK WAISMANN: Introduction to Mathematical Thinking. *Foreword by Karl Menger* TB/511

Philosophy of Science

R. B. BRAITHWAITE: Scientific Explanation TB/515

J. BRONOWSKI: Science and Human Values. *Illus.* TB/505

ALBERT EINSTEIN: Philosopher-Scientist. *Edited by Paul A. Schilpp*
Volume I TB/502
Volume II TB/503

WERNER HEISENBERG: Physics and Philosophy: *The Revolution in Modern Science. Introduction by F. S. C. Northrop* TB/549

JOHN MAYNARD KEYNES: A Treatise on Probability.º *Introduction by N. R. Hanson* TB/557

STEPHEN TOULMIN: Foresight and Understanding: *An Enquiry into the Aims of Science. Foreword by Jacques Barzun* TB/564

STEPHEN TOULMIN: The Philosophy of Science: *An Introduction* TB/513

G. J. WHITROW: The Natural Philosophy of Timeº TB/563

Physics and Cosmology

DAVID BOHM: Causality and Chance in Modern Physics. *Foreword by Louis de Broglie* TB/536

P. W. BRIDGMAN: The Nature of Thermodynamics TB/537

A. C. CROMBIE, Ed.: Turning Point in Physics TB/535

C. V. DURELL: Readable Relativity. *Foreword by Freeman J. Dyson* TB/530

ARTHUR EDDINGTON: Space, Time and Gravitation: *An outline of the General Relativity Theory* TB/510

GEORGE GAMOW: Biography of Physics∑ TB/567

MAX JAMMER: Concepts of Force: *A Study in the Foundation of Dynamics* TB/550

MAX JAMMER: Concepts of Mass *in Classical and Modern Physics* TB/571

MAX JAMMER: Concepts of Space: *The History of Theories of Space in Physics. Foreword by Albert Einstein* TB/533

EDMUND WHITTAKER: History of the Theories of Aether and Electricity
Volume I: *The Classical Theories* TB/531
Volume II: *The Modern Theories* TB/532

G. J. WHITROW: The Structure and Evolution of the Universe: *An Introduction to Cosmology. Illus.* TB/504